THE COMPLETE GU.___
EXERCISE REFERRAL

Working with clients referred to exercise

Debbie Lawrence

BLOOMSBURY

LONDON • NEW DELHI • NEW YORK • SYDNEY

Note
Whilst every effort has been made to ensure that the content of this book is as technically accurate and as sound as possible, neither the author nor the publishers can accept responsibility for any injury or loss sustained as a result of the use of this material.

Published by Bloomsbury Publishing Plc
50 Bedford Square
London WC1B 3DP
www.bloomsbury.com

First edition 2013
Formerly published as *GP Referral Schemes; working with GP referred clients*, 2006
Copyright © 2013 Debbie Lawrence
Copyright © 2006 Debbie Lawrence and Louise Barnett

ISBN (print) 978 1 408 1 7493 7
ISBN (Epub): 978 1 408 1 8741 8
ISBN (EPDF): 978 1 408 1 8740 1

A CIP catalogue record for this book is available from the British Library.

Acknowledgements
Cover photograph © Getty Images
Inside photographs © Shutterstock
Illustrations by David Gardner
Designed by James Watson
Typesetting and page layout by Susan McIntyre
Commissioned by Charlotte Croft
Edited by Sarah Cole

This book is produced using paper that is made from wood grown in managed, sustainable forests. It is natural, renewable and recyclable. The logging and manufacturing processes conform to the environmental regulations of the country of origin.

Typeset in 10.75 on 14pt Adobe Caslon

Printed and bound in India by Replika Press Pvt Ltd

10 9 8 7 6 5 4 3 2 1

CONTENTS

ACKNOWLEDGEMENTS

Updating this edition has proved to be challenging and interesting; there have been a number of developments in the area of exercise referral since the publication of the first edition in 2006.

I would like to acknowledge Louise Barnett who co-authored the first edition of this book, for sharing her wealth of experience working with specialist and referred populations. I would also like to thank the people who contributed feedback to the first edition: Sheena Land, Dr Bill Pomeroy (The Oaks Surgery, Swanley, Kent), Keith Smith and Patrick Ogbonna (Patch).

For this new edition I would like to give thanks to the following people for reviewing and providing feedback and information for specific sections. Thank you to: Victoria Smith, Carlos Mendonca, Fiona Winter, Sandie Keane, Tracy Bell, Lisa Young, Leandra Rizza, Rachel Hubbard, Elaine McNish, Keith Smith.

As always, thank you to my partner Joe for his love and support. Thanks also to all my counselling and personal training clients for sharing experiences and feedback.

Wishing you all a happy and healthy life!

Debbie Lawrence
July 2012

INTRODUCTION

The aim of this book is to provide an introductory practical resource for exercise professionals who work or would like to work with clients referred to exercise by their GP or other health professional. It can be used as a resource by approved training providers and colleges, who are delivering the Level 3 Diploma in Exercise Referral (Qualification & Credit Framework – QCF). The book raises awareness of some of the guidelines and considerations that should inform exercise professionals working with clients with specific medical conditions.

It does *not* replace the need for specialist training for those who work with the specific groups and special populations addressed in this book, *nor* does it replace the need to consult with a healthcare professional to support client work.

It is not the ultimate textbook or education reference for all medical conditions. A compendium of other resources has been researched and referenced to inform the contents. The book aims to introduce some medical conditions and discuss these at a level deemed by the writers to be a sufficient starting point for an exercise professional to develop his or her knowledge and experience. The book is a guide and a starting point for continued research and learning.

The strength of the book is that it makes recommendations and offers suggestions based on research and experience of working with these groups; it offers information on how to adapt exercise to enable participation by referred groups. The intention is to provide basic guidance, but in all instances the specific needs and requirements of the individual, together with any other relevant factors, should be considered and accounted for before making any exercise recommendation. In many instances, referred clients present with multiple rather than isolated conditions, and this may influence whether they are suitable for the scheme (risk stratification) and whether the Level 3 instructor is technically qualified and competent to work with them.

With this in mind, any exercise recommendation *must* be tailored to the individual with reference to all of his or her specific conditions and existing abilities and needs. Consultation with the client's GP regarding the frequency, intensity, time and type of exercise to be administered is also an essential factor in planning an individual schedule.

The book is planned in four parts:

- **Part 1:** Explores the benefits of physical activity, barriers, risks and evidence base to support activity with current recommendations for minimum activity levels. It also provides an overview of the components of fitness and health.

- **Part 2:** Explores the referral process and related information, which includes: risk stratification, roles and responsibilities, initial screening, assessments, and health and safety considerations.

- **Part 3:** Focuses on medical conditions: signs and symptoms, prevalence, exercise limitations and guidelines and other interventions and lifestyle advice (medication and nutrition etc.). NB: Please always check the currency of medications with NICE and BNF guidelines. These often change and may vary both nationally and locally.

- **Part 4:** Looks at how to create a helping relationship and how to help people make changes. There is a new chapter which offers some lesson plans to provide ideas for working with clients. These are not blueprints and will need to be adapted and revised to suit specific needs, but they do offer a starting point for planning. Some alternative activity approaches which may have benefits when working with referred clients are also introduced.

Happy reading!

EXERCISE REFERRAL DEVELOPMENTS

The original guidance for the delivery of exercise referral was outlined in the *National Quality Assurance Framework* report (DoH, 2001), which defined the scope of practice for all persons involved in exercise referral. The report proposed a preliminary risk stratification tool (the risk stratification pyramid) and offered initial guidance for professional competence and medico-legal considerations. The report clearly stated as a boundary that it was not designed to provide a prescribed plan for how schemes should operate or be managed.

In 2006, the National Institute of Health and Clinical Excellence (NICE) commissioned a report to review the effectiveness of exercise referral as a mechanism for increasing activity. The report identified many inconsistencies of practice and procedures throughout the UK and a lack of evidence to support the effectiveness of referral schemes for increasing activity (NICE, 2006a). However, a lack of evidence did not mean that exercise or exercise referral was not effective as a means of preventing or managing disease.

In 2010, the British Heart Foundation National Centre for Physical Activity and Health developed the *Exercise Referral Toolkit* (BHF, 2010) which set out to evaluate the provision of exercise referral across the UK and from this, establish clearer guidance and standards for how schemes should operate, specifically with regard to:

- protocols for operation
- inclusion and exclusion criteria
- risk stratification tools
- team roles, responsibilities and boundaries (including specific guidance on referring to Registered Exercise Professionals)
- monitoring and evaluation

In 2011, the Exercise Referral Advisory Group was established to review all previous guidance and the Joint Consultative Forum was formed. This saw, for the first time, the fitness sector and the royal medical colleges coming together to work toward facilitating the provision for advice to the medical and health professions, the fitness sector, healthcare commissioners and other relevant institutions and agencies on:

a) exercise in the promotion of health
b) exercise in the prevention of ill health
c) the use of exercise in the management of disease

The group's first project was to establish the 'Professional and Operational Standards in Exercise Referral Schemes'. The updated guidance will acknowledge the many developments within exercise referral over the last decade and sets out to establish the way forward for the successful operation and management in the future.

Jean-Ann Marnoch, Registrar
Register of Exercise Professionals
2012

OCCUPATIONAL DESCRIPTION AND QUALIFICATION STRUCTURE

Exercise Referral Occupational Description

'An exercise referral instructor's role includes assessing pre-exercise readiness and designing, delivering, monitoring, adapting and tailoring exercise programmes for individual patients with one or more specific controlled medical condition. They collect and interpret relevant patient information aiming to ensure the safety and effectiveness of exercise programmes and actively encourage patients to adopt regular physical activity and an active lifestyle, employing appropriate motivational strategies to achieve this.'
(Full description available from REPs website)

The National Occupational Standards (NOS) for Exercise Referral (available from the SkillsActive website: www.skillsactive.com) underpin the structure and content of the new QCF Level 3

Diploma in Exercise Referral (2012) which comprises of six units:

1. Anatomy & physiology
2. Understanding the principles of nutrition
3. Professional practice for exercise referral instructors
4. Understanding medical conditions for exercise referral
5. Planning exercise programmes with patients
6. Instructing exercise referral with patients

The pre-requisite requirement for this qualification is a Level 2 Certificate in Fitness Instructing (ETM, Gym or Water Based Exercise).

The Level 3 qualification covers a range of medical conditions and will enable the individual to work with patients who are referred to exercise and within a low to moderate risk stratification.

Level 3	Exercise referral conditions		
Cardio and respiratory	**Metabolic/ Immunological**	**Musculoskeletal**	**Mental health**
• Hypertension • Hypercholesterolaemia • Chronic obstructive pulmonary disease • Asthma	• Obesity • Diabetes type 1 • Diabetes type 2	• Osteoarthritis • Rheumatoid arthritis • Osteoporosis • Simple mechanical back pain • Joint replacement	• Depression • Stress • General anxiety disorder

The REPs recognised Level 4 Specialist Exercise Instructor Qualifications are for instructors who wish to specialise in clients with specific medical conditions and develop their knowledge and skills to support clients with a higher risk stratification.

Level 4	Specialist			
Cardio and respiratory	Metabolic, Immunological, Cancer	Muscular skeletal	Mental health	Neurological
• Cardiac rehabilitation • Chronic respiratory	• Obesity & diabetes • Cancer	• Back pain • Falls prevention	• Eating disorders • Substance misuse • Psychotic disorders • Depressive disorders • Anxiety related disorders (OCD etc)	• Multiple sclerosis • Parkinson's disease • Cerebral palsy • Motor neurone disease • Neuromuscular conditions • Acquired brain injury • Spinal cord injury • Stroke

LIST OF ABBREVIATIONS

1RM	1 repetition maximum
6MWT	6-minute walk test
ABPM	Ambulatory blood pressure
ADL	Activity of daily living
AED	Automated external defibrillator
BDZ	Benzodiazepine
BMI	Body mass index
BP	Blood pressure
bpm	Beats per minute
CABG	Coronary artery bypass graft
CVA	Cerebrovascular accident
CHD	Coronary heart disease
CNS	Central nervous system
COPD	Chronic obstructive pulmonary disease
CVD	Cardiovascular disease
DBP	Diastolic blood pressure
DMARD	Disease-modifying anti-rheumatic drug
ECG	Electrocardiogram
ECT	Electroconvulsive therapy
EELV	End-expiratory lung volume
EIA	Exercise-induced asthma
FEV	Forced expiratory volume
FITT	Frequency, intensity, time and type
FVC	Forced vital capacity
GAD	General anxiety disorder
GTN	Glyceryl trinitate
HbA1c	Haemoglobin A1c
HDL	High-density lipoproteins
HR	Heart rate
HRmax	Maximal heart rate
HRR	Heart rate reserve
HRT	Hormone replacement therapy
IFG	Impaired fasting glycaemia
IGT	Impaired glucose tolerance
ISWT	Incremental shuttle walk test
LDL	Low-density lipoproteins
LTOT	Long-term oxygen therapy
MET	Metabolic equivalent
MHR	Maximum heart rate
MI	Myocardial infarction
mmol/l	Millimoles per litre
MAOI	Monoamine oxidase inhibitor
MRI	Magnetic resonance imaging
NIDDM	Non-insulin-dependent diabetes mellitus
NQAF	National Quality Assurance Framework
NRT	Nicotine replacement therapy
OGTT	Oral glucose tolerance test
PaO_2	Partial pressure of oxygen (in arterial blood)
PCI	Percutaneous coronary intervention
PEF	Peak expiratory flow
PNF	Proprioceptive neuromuscular facilitation
PTSD	Post-traumatic stress disorder
rep	Repetition
REPs	Register of Exercise Professionals
ROM	Range of motion/movement
RPE	Rating of perceived exertion
rpm	Revolutions per minute
SD	Standard deviation
SBP	Systolic blood pressure
spm	Strokes per minute
THR	Training heart rate
TIA	Transient ischaemic attack
TFCO	Transfer factor for carbon dioxide
TPR	Total peripheral resistance
VO_2max	Maximum volume of oxygen
VO_2R	Volume of oxygen reserve

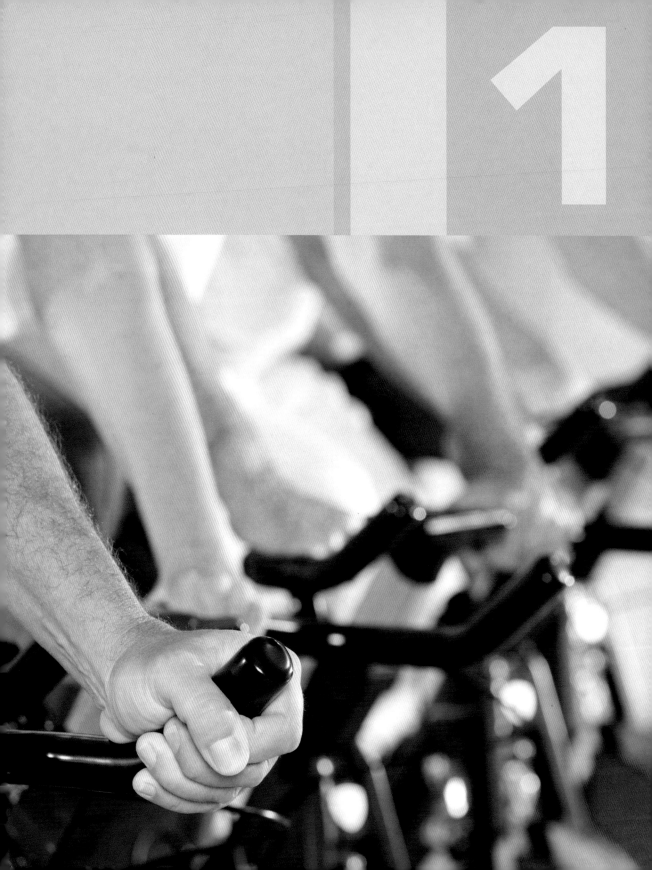

PART **ONE**

PHYSICAL ACTIVITY, EXERCISE AND HEALTH

This section of the book introduces and explains the value of physical activity as a method for improving health and refers to publications defining specific government strategies for further reading. It also discusses the concept of exercise and the components of physical fitness, and provides generalised ideas on how to adapt exercise intensity for persons of a lower fitness level. (Condition-specific considerations are discussed in part 3.) It also introduces the components of total fitness as a model of health and discusses the impact of other lifestyle factors on health.

Leading a physically active lifestyle can improve physical and mental health, reduce the risk of chronic disease and improve life expectancy. It also offers the potential to reduce the financial burden of ill health for the health care services, as well as offering numerous other complementary and indirect benefits (*Joint CMO Report*, DoH, 2011). Yet despite the evidence base to support physical activity and exercise, the activity levels of the British population continue to remain a priority issue for health promotion specialists.

In 2005, the Chief Medical Officer (DOH, 2005a) revealed that levels of physical activity in the British population had declined to a level that had significantly impacted health and well-being and these issues are as relevant today as they were almost a decade ago.

As a nation we continue to suffer in numerous ways and at many levels:

- **Physically** Compared to previous generations, we walk less, cycle less, drive more, drive or use public transport unnecessarily (short journeys and school runs), spend more time watching television and DVDS, spend more time playing with computer games and home technology, and our lifestyles (work, home and leisure) are more sedentary.

- **Nutritionally** We eat more fast, processed and convenience food, eat insufficient fruit and vegetables, eat too many foods high in sugar and fat, consume too much coffee and tea, and drink too little water.

- **Socially** We drink alcohol more regularly (and there are increasing concerns of alcohol misuse, abuse and binge drinking for women, men and teenagers), continue to smoke, and increasingly use illegal drugs for recreational purposes. There are more fast-food restaurants. There are less safe places to be active (parks and fields). Levels of obesity continue to increase, especially among children and young people.

- **Mentally and emotionally** Lifestyles are fast-paced. Self-esteem is lower. Stress, depression, anxiety and other mental health conditions are more prevalent, to the extent that that World Health Organization has indicated that depression may be second only to CHD as the largest contributor to the burden of disease by 2020.

- **Medically** The levels of chronic diseases, such as diabetes, high blood pressure, high cholesterol, stroke, coronary heart disease, depression and obesity, are increasing, and the demands on the NHS continue to be stretched.

- **Spiritually** There are wars and riots, prejudice, intolerance to diversity and difference, power struggles in relationships and a general lack of community.

The whole picture creates a sorry story indeed, especially for a nation of people that can be considered one of the most privileged in the world!

THE ROLE OF PHYSICAL ACTIVITY

1

Physical activity is the umbrella term used for any human movement that results in an increase in energy expenditure above resting level (see table 1.1). This includes activities of everyday living such as:

- getting dressed
- active hobbies and leisure pursuits
- housework
- gardening
- walking or cycling instead of other forms of transport (active travel)
- climbing stairs instead of using escalators and lifts
- manual labour and work (including DIY)
- exercising
- sporting activities.

Table 1.1   Types of physical activity

Physical activity

Everyday activities	Active leisure and recreation	Sport
• Vigorous housework • Gardening • Cleaning the car • DIY • Active travel (walking to the station or walking to school) • Active work • Active play • Using stairs more often	• Exercise and fitness training (e.g. gym, studio and pool) • Health walks • Cycling • Swimming • Dance and movement	• Swimming • Structured competitive activity • Games • Athletics • Outdoor pursuits • Informal sport

Adapted from DoH (2011:9)

RECOMMENDED LEVELS OF PHYSICAL ACTIVITY FOR ADULTS

The current recommendations for physical activity to maintain general health across all age groups were set out in the *Joint CMO Report* (DoH, 2011). These targets are outlined in table 1.2. with examples of activities in table 1.3.

Table 1.2 Recommended activity levels (DoH 2011:7)			
Early years (under 5s)	**Children & Young People (5-18)**	**Adults (19-64)**	**Older Adults (65+)**
• Physically active for at least 3 hours (180 minutes) throughout the day • Floor based play and water based activities	• Moderate to vigorous activity for at least 1 hour (60 minutes) a day • Vigorous activities to strengthen muscles and bones at least 3 days a week	• Accumulate 2.5 hours (150 minutes) of moderate intensity activity over a week. (e.g. 5 days a week 30 minutes per day, in bouts of 10 minutes or more) • OR 75 minutes of vigorous intensity activity • With activities to improve muscle strength on 2 days a week	• Accumulate 2.5 hours (150 minutes) of moderate intensity activity over a week. (e.g. 5 days a week 30 minutes per day, in bouts of 10 minutes or more) • OR for the already active older adults – 75 minutes of vigorous intensity activity • With activities to improve muscle strength on 2 days a week • Some physical activity is better than none • Older adults at risk of falls should include activities to improve co-ordination and balance on at least 2 days a week
For all groups minimise sedentary time			

Table 1.3 Activity examples	
Moderate intensity	Brisk walking, bike riding, swimming, dancing
Vigorous intensity	Gym-based training, sport, aerobic classes, running
Muscle strengthening	Resistance training, carrying heavy loads, body weight exercises (press-ups, sit-ups), heavy gardening
Reduce sedentary behaviour	**Adults and older adults:** Active travel, take regular desk breaks to move, reduce screen time (desk and TV), move more often, climb stairs, walk etc. **Infants:** Reduce time spent in buggies and care seats **Children:** Active travel, play more physical games, visit parks and play outside, limit computer game time

Adapted from DoH (2011:36)

CURRENT LEVELS OF PHYSICAL ACTIVITY

There are numerous opportunities for being more physically active at home and at work, during leisure time and in the way in which we travel. However, the reality is that the majority of people continue to be insufficiently active to improve their health. The Joint Health Surveys Unit, in its reports *The Health Survey for England* (2003) and *The Health of Minority Ethnic Groups* (1999) estimated that:

- 6 out of 10 men were not active enough to benefit their health;
- 7 out of 10 women were not active enough to benefit their health;
- people became less active as they got older;
- South Asian and Chinese women and men were less likely to participate in physical activities;
- Bangladeshi men and women were the least physically active.

The Health Survey for England (2006) found that only 40 per cent of men and 28 per cent of women met the recommended activity levels and this decreased with age, with only 22 per cent of older men and 16 per cent of older women meeting the recommended guidance. Habits maintained in adulthood tend to be formed in childhood and the survey also found that among children, just 61 per cent of boys and 42 per cent of girls met the recommended activity levels for their age category.

More recently, the *Start Active, Stay Active* report from the Chief Medical Officers of the four home countries (DoH, 2011:10) highlighted that:

'Physical inactivity is the fourth leading risk factor for global mortality and accounts for 6 per cent of deaths globally, following hypertension (13 per cent), smoking (9 per cent) and high blood glucose (6 per cent)' (DoH, 2011:10).

The direct cost of inactivity to the NHS across the UK amounts to a conservative estimate of £1.06 billion. This estimate excludes the cost of lost productivity in the workplace from sickness absence (estimated at £5.5 billion per year) and also excludes the costs for some of the conditions that affect older people, such as osteoporosis and falls (DoH, 2011:14).

BENEFITS OF PHYSICAL ACTIVITY

Physical activity as a medium for improving health has featured in many government reports and responsive initiatives over the last two decades. These include:

- *Allied Dunbar National Fitness Survey* (1992)
- *Health Education Authority Survey of Activity and Health* (1999)
- *The National Quality Assurance Framework for Exercise Referral* (DoH, 2001a)
- *Saving Lives: Our Healthier Nation* (DoH, 1999a)
- *NHS Plan* (DoH, 2000b)
- *National Service Frameworks* (NSFs) which include: *Mental Health* (DoH, 1999b), *CHD* (DoH, 2000a), *Cancer* (DoH, 2000c), *Older People* (DoH, 2001d), *Diabetes* (DoH, 2001c), *Children* (DoH, 2004c)
- *The Health Survey for England* (2003, 2006)
- *The Healthy Schools Programme* (www.wired forhealth.gov.uk)

- *Tackling Health Inequalities: A Programme for Action* (DoH, 2003b)
- *Choosing Health* (DoH, 2004b)
- *At Least Five a Week* (DoH, 2004a)
- *A Rapid Review of Exercise Referral Schemes to Promote Activity in Adults* (NICE, 2006)
- *Be Active, Be Healthy* (DoH, 2009)
- *Exercise Referral Toolkit* (BHF, 2010)
- *Start Active, Stay Active* (Joint CMO/DoH, 2011)
- *Professional and Operational Standards for Exercise Referral* (ERAG, 2011)

There is substantial evidence to support the role of physical activity in promoting and managing health (DoH, 2004, 2011:12). Physically active adults have:

- approximately 30 per cent reduced risk of premature death;
- 20–35 per cent reduced chance of developing diseases such as coronary heart disease (CHD) and stroke;
- 30–40 per cent risk reduction for diabetes;
- improved functional capacity;
- reduced risk of back pain;
- increased independence (older people);
- increased bone density and reduced risk of osteoporosis;
- improved psychological well-being;
- 36–68 per cent risk reduction of hip fracture;
- 30 per cent lower risk of colon cancer and 20 per cent lower risk of breast cancer;
- reduced risk of osteoarthritis;
- reduced risk of stress and anxiety;
- reduced risk of clinical depression and dementia in older adults;
- reduced risk of falls (older adults);
- improved functional health;

- improved psychological well-being, self-esteem, mood and sleep;
- improved weight loss and weight management.

The message is clear – we all need to sit down less and move more often! And the more we do, the greater will be the health gains obtained (dose-response relationship) (DoH, 2011).

'Spending large amounts of time being sedentary may increase the risk of some health outcomes, even among people who are active at the recommended levels.' (DoH, 2011:13)

BARRIERS TO PHYSICAL ACTIVITY

There are potentially many real and/or perceived barriers or blocks to being more active. These can be classified as either intrinsic or extrinsic. Intrinsic barriers relate to how the individual feels about physical activity, which can influence both their interest in physical activity and confidence and motivation to take part. This will be influenced by their past experiences (in school, with family etc.) and their beliefs concerning physical activity (instilled by education, family, socialisation and culture) and will also be affected by some mental health conditions (anxiety and depression).

Extrinsic barriers relate to broader issues such as access to and availability of appropriate and affordable physical activity (i.e. in leisure centres, community centres, activity groups), safety in the environment (safety of roads, parks, concerns for personal security, etc.), opportunities for physical activity (at work, school, home) and the attitude and skills of other people (exercise professionals, family, teachers, health professionals, etc.), which will be influenced by culture. These factors can have a disproportionate impact on an individual's ability to respond to the recommended guidance (DoH, 2011).

Whether we realise it or not, health inequalities (barriers) continue to exist for many people and these inequalities will influence participation in sport and exercise.

Lower levels of physical activity are reported among people from the following populations:

- women and girls (men and boys are generally reported to be more active)
- some minority ethnic groups
- people in low-income households
- lower social classes
- people with lower levels of educational attainment
- people performing non-professional and non-managerial status work
- older people
- people with disabilities.
  (DoH, 2005b; Health Development Agency, 2005b; DoH, 2011:8).

People of any age, ethnicity and gender etc. will experience certain barriers to activity and exercise, which may include a lack of:

- **money** (inability to afford the cost to travel to and take part in the activity and/or purchase the clothing and equipment required);
- **interest** (the available and accessible activities may not appeal to them, e.g. they may not want to take part in gym or studio classes);
- **confidence** (they may be fearful of the exercise environment and consider themselves to be too old, too unfit, too fat, too de-conditioned etc. to take part);
- **time** (they may be juggling many other life priorities/responsibilities, such as children, family, work etc. that prevent them from taking time for themselves to be more active);
- **motivation** (they may feel too tired or even just 'can't be bothered' etc.).

Older people may face additional barriers (BHF, 2003a). These may include:

- fear of overdoing it, injuring themselves or aggravating a medical condition;
- embarrassment and feeling they don't fit in or wouldn't be able to keep up;
- safety concerns, such as a fear of falling in some environments (e.g. swimming pools);
- lack of culturally appropriate facilities.

REASONS FOR THE DECLINE IN ACTIVITY

Apart from the barriers to activity cited previously, the decline in physical activity levels in developed countries has been attributed to a number of other lifestyle factors, which include:

- increased use of cars for short journeys such as driving to a local train station and taking children to school;
- perception of the environment as being unsafe for children to play outside the home (parks and fields);
- increase in sedentary leisure and play activities including television, listening to music, reading books and magazines, doing homework and playing computer games;
- decreased participation in sport;
- education (individuals may not be aware of

the health risks of inactivity or the benefits of being active);

• reduced opportunities for physical activity and sporting activities within the school curriculum.

The lifestyle and behaviour of most people will be affected in some way by these trends; these factors are often cited as reasons for some people finding it increasingly difficult to maintain optimal levels of physical activity.

RISKS ASSOCIATED WITH HEALTH-RELATED PHYSICAL ACTIVITY

The benefits of physical activity are substantial and far outweigh any potential risks associated with participation. There is arguably a greater risk posed from being inactive than from being active at an appropriate level! Possible risks associated with exercise and physical activity may include accidents (strains, sprains, fractures, dizziness, fainting, collisions, slips and trips, falls, cramps) and more rarely medical emergencies (hyperglycaemia or hypoglycaemia, exercise-induced asthma, heart attack, hyperthermia etc.) Many of the risks associated with physical activity can be avoided and the greatest risk is among people who:

• do too much exercise (rare);
• take part in more vigorous activity (mainly if previously inactive and deconditioned);
• take part in competitive/contact sport;
• do too much too soon;
• have an existing condition or disease that may require an adapted programme.

People who do too much exercise are rare; however, there are individuals who become obsessive about exercise. They will experience withdrawal symptoms if they have an injury or social engagement that prevents them from exercising. This obsessive behaviour is not caused by exercise, but is more likely to be connected to an underlying psychological disorder and/or maybe an addictive tendency within the personality. For example, people with eating disorders such as anorexia nervosa or bulimia nervosa may use exercise as a way to control weight.

There are also some people with medical conditions, for whom participation in activity would not be recommended. The absolute contraindications for exercise are listed in chapter 4.

PROMOTING PHYSICAL ACTIVITY

All the government initiatives have been set out to promote physical activity at a national and local level. Evidence shows that the people who are most likely to benefit from an increase in physical activity are the least active.

When working with individuals to promote physical activity, it is important that any increase in activity levels starts at a low and steady level and progresses very gradually in relation to frequency, intensity and time. There are various factors to consider prior to making recommendations to promote participation in physical activity. Some of these are listed in table 1.4. (The issues related to specific medical conditions will be explored further through subsequent chapters.)

Table 1.4	Factors to be considered to enable participation
Factors relating to the individual	**Factors relating to the type of environment and type of activity**
• Individual factors e.g. age, gender, disabilities (visual, auditory, physical), culture • Medical history and previous injuries • Muscular-skeletal conditions/diseases e.g. arthritis, low back pain • Existing risk of CHD (high blood pressure, smoking etc.) • Medication (and side effects) • Psychological issues e.g. confidence, self-esteem, motivation or conditions such as depression • Lifestyle factors/behaviours (e.g. smoking, diet, use of alcohol, type of work, perceived time availability etc.)	• Appropriate environment, including the availability of appropriate and safe spaces indoors (pool, studio, home, office, GP surgery, community centre etc.) and outdoors (parks and roads); and the floor surface, temperature, traffic and weather • Clothing and footwear (safety helmet for cycling and appropriate clothing for outdoor exercising) • Level of supervision needed (clinical, personal training, group exercise or unsupervised exercise) • Type of activity (walking, dance or movement-based, pool, gym-based etc.) and components of fitness trained (muscular fitness, cardiovascular, flexibility, motor skills – balance, coordination etc.) • Volume of activity (frequency, intensity, time and type) • Session structure. The inclusion of an appropriate and prolonged warm-up and cool-down is essential for older people and people with CHD

HOW PERSONAL TRAINERS AND EXERCISE PROFESSIONALS CAN HELP

Personal trainers and exercise professionals can contribute to improving activity levels by promoting activity at every available opportunity. They can help to spread the activity message by:

- writing for local papers;
- using social media to share information from other professional organisations and health charities that support activity and health;
- working with local GP surgeries;
- speaking on local radio;
- working with local hospitals;
- visiting and giving talks at schools;
- promoting active travel;
- organising sponsored activity events to support local charities;
- taking exercise back into the community (e.g. in church halls and community centres);
- organising activity sessions in the workplace (lunchtime walks, etc.);
- working with local primary care and commissioning bodies and other local health groups.

They can also make appropriate recommendations as to the frequency, time and type of activity for individuals to make a start towards building their activity levels and promoting healthier living.

Exercise professionals who would like to work specifically with specialist populations and persons referred to exercise should ensure that they are qualified at an appropriate level (see qualifications and standards explained in the introduction). The minimum qualification to work with clients referred to exercise by their GP is the Level 3 Diploma (previously a Certificate) in Exercise Referral.

EXERCISE AND PHYSICAL FITNESS

2

EXERCISE

Exercise can be described as any activity that is planned, structured and performed regularly with a specific goal or purpose in mind, for example: to improve fitness and/or health; to assist management of a medical condition; to feel better; to lose weight. Exercise may involve going to the gym, going for a run, walk, cycle or a swim, or attending a group exercise session.

The amount of exercise people do can be described in terms of frequency, intensity, time and type or mode. The combination of frequency, intensity and time over a fixed period is referred to as the volume of exercise.

PHYSICAL FITNESS

Physical fitness is achieved by performing specific types of exercise in a structured format, at a recommended frequency, intensity and duration/time. There are five components of physical fitness:

1. Cardiovascular fitness
2. Flexibility
3. Muscular strength and muscular endurance (collectively known as muscular fitness)
4. Motor fitness

1. CARDIOVASCULAR FITNESS

Cardiovascular fitness is the ability of the heart, lungs and circulatory system to transport and utilise oxygen and remove waste products efficiently. It is sometimes referred to as cardio-respiratory fitness, stamina, or aerobic fitness.

BENEFITS OF CARDIOVASCULAR TRAINING

To maintain quality of life and the ability to take part in recreational activities it is essential to have an efficient cardiovascular system. Low cardiovascular fitness is associated with an increased risk of chronic diseases such as diabetes, high blood pressure, high cholesterol and coronary heart disease, all of which ultimately cause premature death. Increased physical activity, exercise and improved cardiovascular fitness can assist with the prevention of these diseases, promote better quality of life and reduce some of the unnecessary burden on the National Health Service that these conditions create.

Regular cardiovascular exercise enables the heart to become stronger, which allows it to pump a greater volume of blood in each contraction (stroke volume). The capillary network in the muscles and around the lungs will increase, which allows the transportation of more oxygen to the body cells and the swifter removal of waste products. The size and number of mitochondria, the cells in which aerobic energy is produced, will increase, enabling increased utilisation of oxygen. Cardiovascular training has a positive effect on overall health and specific benefits include:

- achievement and maintenance of weight loss;
- reduced risk of high blood pressure, heart disease and stroke;
- improvement in cholesterol levels;
- prevention of or delaying the development of type 2 diabetes;
- management of type 1 and type 2 diabetes;
- reduced risks of certain cancers.

Recommended training guidelines for developing and maintaining cardiovascular fitness are listed in table 2.1.

ADAPTING CARDIOVASCULAR TRAINING FOR REFERRED POPULATIONS

The frequency, intensity, time and type of the cardiovascular programme recommended should take into account a range of factors including:

- fitness level of the individual;
- the condition(s) with which they have been referred;
- the effects of any medication on the exercise response;
- other lifestyle factors (smoking, alcohol etc.);
- goal, e.g. weight loss;
- client preference (likes and dislikes).

Table 2.1	Recommended guidelines for training cardiovascular for general populations		
Frequency	5 days a week minimum OR	3 days a week minimum OR	3-5 days a week
Intensity Lower intensities may be appropriate for de-conditioned adults to achieve benefits	Moderate intensity 40-<60% VO$_2$R (or 5-6 on the 0-10 physical exertion scale for older adults) OR	Vigorous intensity >60% VO$_2$R (or 7-8 on the 0-10 physical exertion scale for older adults) OR	Combination of moderate and vigorous intensity
Time	30 minutes (can be accumulated – 10 minute bouts) OR	20 minutes OR	As previous, depending on intensity
Type	Cardiovascular endurance, weight bearing exercises For older adults and adults with physical limitations, activities that do not impose excessive orthopaedic stress are recommended (e.g. walking, exercise in water, stationary bike) (ACSM. 2010:193) Increasing the intensity and reducing the frequency increases the risk of muscular skeletal injuries and is not recommended for general populations (ACSM 2010:155)		

Adapted from ACSM. 2010

Previously inactive people will generally have to work at a lower intensity and for a shorter duration initially, and to achieve their goals they may have to gradually increase the frequency and duration of the activity. They may also have lower levels of body awareness and muscular fitness, and their exercise technique may demand more careful attention (observation, correction, teaching) to enable safe participation. The mode of activity will need careful consideration, taking account of physical impairments or limitations such as postural instability or hemiplegia (muscle weakness on one side of the body). For example, a recumbent bike or an upper extremity ergometer may be more appropriate than treadmill walking for an individual with postural instability. A client with hemiplegia may benefit from a combined upper and lower body ergometer, using the unaffected leg and arm to assist with the movement (ACSM, 2005b).

There are specific variants that can be altered to change and adapt the intensity of specific cardiovascular exercise types/modes. These are:

- rate
- resistance
- range of motion
- repetitions
- rest.

Rate/speed

Varying the speed at which cycling, rowing, stepping, walking and running are performed will vary the intensity of the exercise. Working at a slower pace will generally be easier than working at a faster pace. However, it is essential that the exercises remain rhythmical in nature (not too slow or too quick) in order for them to be comfortable and sustainable for an appropriate

Table 2.2	Adapting speed using cardiovascular machines
Cardiovascular machines	**Variant: Rate/speed measure**
Rowing machine	Strokes per minute (SPM)
Cycling machine	Revolutions per minute (RPM)
Treadmill	Miles per hour (MPH) or kilometres per hour (KPH)
Step machine	Number of steps or floors climbed
Cross trainer	Number of stride revolutions

duration. As a general guideline start slower and progressively build the pace to a comfortable, sustainable level. Table 2.2 lists how speed/rate can be varied on different cardiovascular machines.

Resistance/weight

An individual's body weight will automatically add resistance to exercise. It will require more effort from the muscles to lift and move a heavier body weight than a lighter one against the force of gravity. This should be considered when working with people who are overweight or obese or with persons with joint or bone conditions (osteoporosis/osteoarthritis) as even low-impact weight-bearing exercises will already be placing additional stress on their joints. In these instances, prescribed activities should ideally be of a lower impact, such as walking and, for some groups, non-weight-bearing, such as swimming or cycling. Adding propulsion or impact such as jogging on a trampette or running on a treadmill is a way of increasing intensity, but may not be appropriate for all individuals due to increased stress on the lower extremities (joints and muscles).

Swimming and water-based exercise programmes offer greater support to the body and are comparatively less stressful on the joints. Water-based programmes demand the body to move against and through the resistance of water and require the muscles of the upper body to have a much greater involvement to create that movement. Increasing the surface area of the body or moving limbs or using buoyancy equipment (a tube/woggle, water bells, water mitts etc.) will all increase the resistance created and increase the intensity of exercises performed in water. As a general guideline, start the programme without using equipment and progress by building in the use of equipment that increases the surface area/resistance being moved.

Most gym-based cardiovascular machines (rower, cross trainer, cycle, stepper, etc.) offer a variable workload. The intensity or workload can be altered by changing the level of resistance, which can vary (usually between levels of 1 (easiest) to 20 (hardest) depending on specific machines and manufacturers. Lower levels of resistance are generally easier and higher levels are generally harder; however, it is essential to refer to specific manufacturers' guidelines to check the level of resistance. A general guideline is to start at a lower level of resistance and progressively increase to a comfortable working level.

Repetitions/rest

Different methods of training (continuous and interval) can be used to improve cardiovascular fitness. Continuous activity aims to maintain a specific intensity throughout a specified duration. This may not be appropriate for deconditioned individuals starting cardiovascular training, or those with specific conditions such as chronic obstructive pulmonary disease (COPD). These individuals will benefit from a gentle interval training approach with prescribed work and rest times. For example, walking at a faster pace for an established period of time (work ratio) and then lowering the intensity to an easier and more comfortable level for an established period of time (rest ratio) to allow the person to recover. As a general guideline, starting with shorter work times, a lower number of work intervals and longer (and more frequent) rest time intervals is appropriate. Progressively increasing the duration of the work ratios and the number (frequency) of work intervals, and decreasing the time of rest intervals, will provide progression.

Range of motion

To increase or decrease the range of motion (intensity) of cardiovascular activities demands modifications to the size of the movement, for example, by stepping higher, increasing the depth of a knee bend during a squat or increasing the length of a stride during travelling moves. Range of movement can also apply to the upper body during cardiovascular activity (e.g. lifting arms to waist height or above the shoulders while stepping sideways). As a general guideline, start with a smaller range of movement and gradually increase to ensure an appropriate progression of intensity and to reduce the risk of increased stress on the joints. It is also important to consider the speed of movement when increasing the range to avoid a compromise in technique and an increased risk of injury.

EMPATHY TRAINING FOR INSTRUCTORS

It can be useful for trainers and instructors to experience specific workouts with simulations of the restrictions imposed on some referred populations. (This is not always easy – as many conditions cannot be simulated.) Some examples are: extra padding and weights can be worn to demonstrate the restrictions an overweight or obese person may experience when getting onto machines and working at specific intensities/impacts; restrictions could also be made to some ranges of movement of specific joints to help instructors understand limitations of movement.

2. FLEXIBILITY

Flexibility is the ability of the joints and muscles to move through their full potential range of movement. It is sometimes referred to as suppleness or mobility.

BENEFITS OF FLEXIBILITY

Being able to move the joints and muscles through their full potential range of motion is essential for easing the performance of all everyday tasks. Shoulder joint flexibility is needed to reach to change a light bulb, button shirts or cardigans and reach for objects on a high shelf. Hip joint flexibility is needed to lift the knees to climb stairs and take long strides when walking. Spine mobility enables when twisting and turning. Being flexible enables movement to be more efficient and contributes to the maintenance of correct posture and joint alignment. Shortened muscles around the chest and shoulders (pectorals and anterior deltoids) and weak muscles in the upper back (trapezius and rhomboids) can lead to rounding

of the upper back and the postural condition of kyphosis. Shortened and/or tight hamstrings and hip flexors and weak abdominals can lead to the postural condition of lordosis. Improved posture can potentially enhance physical appearance, reduce the incidence of low back pain and assist with the management of joint mobility conditions such as osteoarthritis and rheumatoid arthritis. Being sufficiently flexible contributes to an enhanced quality of life and reduces the risk of injury, especially for older populations. The recommended training guidelines for improving and maintaining flexibility are listed in table 2.3.

Stretching should always be performed when the muscles are warm to avoid injury. To improve flexibility, static stretching should be included in the programme. Static stretching involves the muscle being slowly lengthened to the end of the range of movement, to a point of tightness, but not discomfort. This position is then held for 15–30 seconds. To improve flexibility the stretches should be repeated 2–4 times.

Proprioceptive neuromuscular facilitation (PNF) is a different type of stretching technique that is not recommended for the general population; however, it may be appropriate for specific populations. It involves a 6-second contraction followed by an assisted stretch. This technique requires a partner who is trained in PNF stretching, takes more time and is associated with increased muscle soreness. Activities such as yoga and Pilates can also be used to increase flexibility and may be appropriate for some clients (ACSM, 2005). For further information about stretching, refer to the *Complete Guide to Stretching* (Norris, 2004).

Table 2.3	Recommended guidelines for training flexibility for general populations
Frequency	3–5 days a week (at least 2–3 days a week)
Intensity	Stretch all major muscles > 4 repetitions per muscle group To position of mild discomfort
Time	At least 10 minutes Static stretches held for 10–30 seconds PNF (6-second contraction followed by 10–30 seconds assisted stretch)
Type	Static, dynamic or PNF stretching Older adults static stretches Dynamic stretching (performed safely) for persons whose sport involves these movements (ACSM, 2010:175)

Adapted from ACSM (2010)

ADAPTING FLEXIBILITY TRAINING FOR REFERRED POPULATIONS

The intensity of stretch positions will need to correspond to the:

- range of motion of the individual (variable at each joint);
- condition(s) with which the person has been referred;
- effects of any medication on the exercise response;
- other lifestyle factors.

Previously inactive people and people with specific joint and muscular problems may lack flexibility and will therefore need more supportive and comfortable positions. They may also have less body awareness and their exercise technique may demand more careful attention (observation, correction, teaching) to enable safe participation.

There are specific variants that can be altered to change and adapt the intensity of specific stretches. These are:

- range of motion
- balance
- isolation.

Range of motion

Less flexible participants will generally need to work through a smaller range of motion. Static and passive stretches in supported positions will offer them greater control for performing the stretch and achieving an appropriate range of motion.

Using gravity to assist the stretch, using towels to support levers (quadriceps and hamstring stretch), and trainer-assisted stretches (if appropriate) can be used to help the range of motion and support the stretch position (see figure 2.1.)

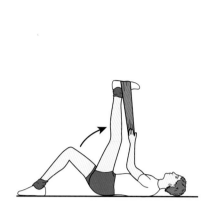 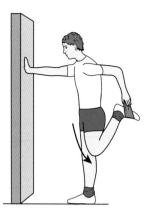

Figure 2.1 Adapting stretch positions

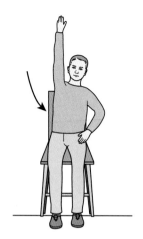

Figure 2.2 Using seated stretch positions

Balance

It may also be necessary to adapt some stretch positions for less flexible people and people with low muscular fitness who may be unable to hold some positions.

Using a wall to provide balance, using floor-based positions (if the person has sufficient functional mobility) (see figure 2.1), and using chair-based stretch positions are all appropriate ways to adapt stretch positions and assist performance (see figure 2.2).

Isolation

Isolating stretches and using easier positions are more appropriate techniques than using stretch positions where multiple muscles are stretched. It is hard to find stretches that totally isolate one muscle; however, some traditional stretch positions are much harder and demand greater flexibility of other muscles and greater work to hold the position than other stretch positions. When working with persons with low levels of flexibility, it is essential to find the most comfortable and supportive position for them.

3. MUSCULAR FITNESS (STRENGTH AND ENDURANCE)

Muscular fitness is a combination of and a balance between muscular strength and muscular endurance and represents the functional fitness needed to maintain correct posture and perform daily activities. Muscular strength is the ability of our muscles to exert a near maximal force to lift a resistance. Muscular endurance requires a less maximal force to be exerted, but for the muscle contraction to be maintained for a longer duration.

BENEFITS OF MUSCULAR FITNESS TRAINING

Muscles need to be strong enough and have sufficient endurance to carry out daily tasks, which require us to lift, carry, pull or push a resistance. These may include carrying shopping, gardening, moving furniture, climbing stairs and lifting our body to/from a chair or into/out of a bath.

Strong muscles will help to maintain the correct alignment of the skeleton. Weakened muscles may cause an uneven pull to be placed on the skeleton. Muscles work in pairs (as one contracts and works, the opposite muscle relaxes). Therefore, any imbalance in workload (if one of the pair is contracted or worked too frequently and becomes too strong and the other is not worked sufficiently or is allowed to become weaker) will cause the joints to be pulled out of the correct alignment. This may potentially cause injury or create postural defects such as rounded shoulders or excessive curvatures of the spine. These are illustrated in figure 2.3.

An imbalance of strength between the abdominal and opposing muscles of the back (the erector spinae) can cause an exaggerated curve or hollowing of the lumbar vertebrae (lordosis). An imbalance of strength between the muscles of the chest (the pectorals) and the muscles between the shoulder blades (the rhomboids and trapezii) can cause rounded shoulders and a humping of the thoracic spine (kyphosis). An imbalance in strength between the muscles on each side of the back can cause a sideways curvature of the thoracic spine (scoliosis). All muscles should therefore be kept sufficiently strong to maintain a correct posture.

Lifestyle may demand that we specifically target certain muscles more than others to compensate for imbalances caused by our work and daily activities. For the majority of persons with a sedentary lifestyle, it is well worthwhile strengthening the abdominal muscles, the muscles in between the shoulder blades (trapezius and rhomboids), and possibly the muscles of the back (erector spinae) and stretching the opposing muscles to these groups (pectorals, erector spinae, hip flexors and hamstrings).

Training for muscular fitness will improve

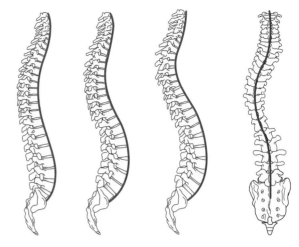

Figure 2.3 Curvatures of the spine

the tone of the muscles and provide a firmer and more shapely appearance. This can contribute to a positive self-image and can enhance psychological well-being and self-confidence.

Muscular fitness improves the strength and health of the bones and joints. The muscles have to contract and pull against the bones to create movement and lift the resistance. In response, the tendons, which attach the muscles to the bone across the joint, and the ligaments, which attach bone to bone across the joint, will become stronger. Therefore, in the long term the joints will become stronger, more stable and at less risk from injury. In addition, increased calcium can be deposited and stored by the bones. This can prevent them from becoming brittle and reduce the risk of osteoporosis.

Muscular fitness training can therefore provide many long lasting benefits that can extend the quality of life for a number of years. The recommended training guidelines for developing and improving muscular fitness are listed in table 2.4.

Table 2.4	Recommended guidelines for training muscular fitness for general populations
Frequency	2–3 days a week same muscle groups on non-consecutive days
	48 hours rest between sessions for the same muscle groups
Intensity and time	I set of 8–12 repetitions for beginners and progressing to 2–4 sets
	60–80% of individual's IRM (to point of fatigue, not failure) Rest of 2–3 minutes between sets
	Older adults and de-conditioned: • I or more sets • 10–15 repetitions per set • 60–70% of IRM
Type	Promote muscle balance (agonist and antagonist work)
	Multi-joint (compound) and single joint (isolation) exercises (ACSM, 2010:169)
	Promote correct technique

Adapted from ACSM (2010)

ADAPTING MUSCULAR FITNESS EXERCISES FOR REFERRED POPULATIONS

As with other components of fitness, the intensity of activities selected should correspond to the following:

- the fitness level of the individual;
- the medical condition(s) with which they have been referred;
- the effects of any medication on the exercise response;
- any other specific lifestyle considerations (work etc.).

Previously inactive people will generally have to work at a lower intensity. They may also have lower levels of body awareness and muscular fitness and their exercise technique may demand more careful attention from the trainer (observation, correction, teaching) to enable safe participation. Fixed resistance machines provide more stability

and support and may be more appropriate than free weights for referred clients beginning resistance training.

There are specific variants that can be altered to change and adapt the intensity of specific muscular fitness exercises. These are:

- resistance
- rate
- range of motion
- repetitions
- rest (between sets or exercises).

Resistance

There are numerous methods for altering the resistance. Muscular fitness activities can be progressed and adapted by:

- increasing (or decreasing) the length of the lever being moved (rear leg raise with bent leg or straight leg);
- adding body weight to (or removing body weight from) the end of the lever (curl-ups

with hands on thighs or hands at side of head);
- working against gravity or working across gravity (push-ups against a wall or floor-based);
- adding an external resistance such as a fixed weight, free weight or exercise band (and altering the resistance);
- using water: water adds resistance to body movements and will alter the type of muscle contraction.

Rate and range of motion

Exercise should always be performed at a controlled speed to promote full range of motion of concentric and eccentric muscle work.

Varying the speed of an exercise will alter the intensity and may also change the focus on the muscle contraction. For example, varying the speed to work faster on the lifting phase and more slowly on the lowering phase will focus on the eccentric contraction range (and vice versa). Caution is advised when lengthening (slowing down) the eccentric phase, as this may cause delayed onset muscle soreness (ACSM, 2005a). It is generally recommended that muscle work be carried out through the full range of motion. However, there are some instances where isometric and static muscle work are more beneficial (and safer) as a starting point, for example in training core stability and posture and for some joint mobility problems (e.g. osteoarthritis).

Repetitions, rest and sets

One set of 8–12 repetitions for all major muscle groups is the traditional guide for muscular fitness improvements for general populations; however, the ACSM (2005) recommends a broader range of repetitions, i.e. 3–20. It is obvious that the number of repetitions and sets can be increased or decreased to meet different fitness goals (strength or endurance). The repetitions will also need to take account of any specific medical conditions the individual presents. For some individuals, as low as one repetition would be an appropriate starting point.

4. MOTOR FITNESS

Motor fitness is primarily a skill-related component of fitness and refers to a number of inter-relatable factors, which include:
- agility
- balance
- speed
- coordination
- reaction time
- power.

BENEFITS OF MOTOR FITNESS

Motor fitness requires the effective transmission and management of messages and responses between the central nervous system (the brain and spinal cord) and the peripheral nervous system (sensory and motor). The peripheral system collects information via the sensory system; the CNS receives and processes this information and sends an appropriate response via the motor system, which initiates the appropriate response.

Motor fitness can have an indirect effect on improving our ability to function in the other components of fitness. Development of specific skills can improve the performance of certain activities and enable more skilful movement and safer exercise techniques. This can help to reduce the risk of injury and will maximise both the safety and effectiveness of performance.

Managing body weight, manoeuvring centre of gravity, coordinating body movements, moving at different speeds, in different directions, and at different intensities, will all in the long term contribute to improving motor fitness.

GUIDELINES FOR TRAINING MOTOR FITNESS

Like all components of fitness, the principles of 'use it or lose it' and 'specificity' apply. What you train for is what improves (Specific Adaptation to Imposed Demand – the SAID principle), so running improves running and stretching the hamstrings makes more flexible hamstrings.

Older populations can sometimes lose the skilfulness of their movement, and therefore motor fitness will need to be retrained. Learning to balance and coordinate movement patterns takes time and it is essential to break the movement down into its simplest parts and progressively build on these. Relearning movement patterns also takes time. As a general guideline, starting more slowly, with isolated movements and simpler movement patterns, and focusing on correct performance help to provide the foundation for developing motor fitness. Patience, encouragement and raising awareness to small changes and progression are essential to maintain motivation.

TOTAL FITNESS AND LIFESTYLE

3

TOTAL FITNESS

Total fitness provides a model for determining and balancing overall health and well-being. It requires balanced 'fitness' or well-being in all the following areas (see figure 3.1).

- **Physically** Achieving recommended levels of physical activity in daily lifestyle and taking part in exercise to maintain physical fitness: cardiovascular, muscular, flexibility and motor fitness as discussed in chapters 1 and 2.
- **Socially** Being able to create and maintain healthy relationships with others and society. Being included and engaged rather than excluded and isolated (referred to as harder to reach groups).
- **Mentally** Having positive mental health, which includes an awareness of personal thinking patterns and being able to manage thinking to assist positive decision making and life choices.
- **Emotionally** Having an awareness of and the ability to manage and express emotions (happy, sad, scared, angry) assertively with respect for self and others.
- **Nutritionally** Eating a balanced diet containing a variety of foods from all major food groups (carbohydrates, fats, protein, vitamins, minerals, water, fibre), eaten within recommended guidelines (see DoH, *The Eatwell Plate*), and maintaining a balanced calorific intake to meet energy demands.
- **Spiritually** Having an awareness of belief systems, which may evolve from family, society, culture and religion, and managing these to make positive decisions for self, others and society. Embracing, accepting and respecting the notion of difference and similarity among people.
- **Medically** Being free from illness and disease and making positive life choices to maintain medical health.

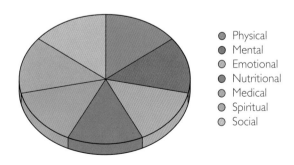

- Physical
- Mental
- Emotional
- Nutritional
- Medical
- Spiritual
- Social

Figure 3.1 Components of total fitness

Total fitness requires a little bit more than just taking part in regular physical activity. It demands that attention is paid to lifestyle, diet, habits, stress levels, emotions and ability to communicate, and asks you recognise that sometimes it is important to quite simply relax, rest and recuperate.

Physical activity, exercise and physical fitness contribute to maintaining health, well-being and total fitness.

SOCIAL FITNESS

Social fitness relates to interaction and communication with other people and the ability to form and maintain healthy, functional relationships within society. Exercise and activity provide opportunities for social interaction and enable individuals to improve their social fitness.

Depressed clients in particular can feel very isolated and alone with the problems that contribute to their depression. In addition, the stigma attached to mental health conditions will influence how they feel about themselves and also how they perceive that others will think of them. It can be hard for them to motivate themselves to seek out a social network; however, the benefits are numerous.

Apart from the physical benefits of exercise and activity, group exercise in particular is an excellent medium for promoting social interaction and benefits. It naturally encourages networking and friendships to blossom among participants, and many additional social opportunities evolve from the relationships developed within the session. Since depression and other health conditions (osteoporosis, high blood pressure, arthritis etc.) are common to many people, support can be found in sharing experiences of how to manage the condition. It will also reduce feelings of being alone or the only person having to deal with the condition(s), which normalises the experience and can increase confidence towards participation in activity and self-management.

MENTAL AND EMOTIONAL FITNESS

Mental and emotional fitness refers to psychological well-being. The pressures of daily life can have a negative effect on mental and emotional fitness, causing people to feel tired, anxious and stressed. The diagnosis of medical conditions (high blood pressure, osteoporosis, cancer etc.) will raise some degree of fear in most people regarding future mobility, independence, suffering and life expectancy.

When people feel stressed, it stimulates the release of hormones that prepare them for fight or flight. As a consequence sugars are released into the bloodstream to provide energy for the necessary physical action. However, all too often action (fight or flight) is not taken and instead people stew on their problems (worry and fear). This has a negative effect on health because the sugars that are released can potentially contribute to atherosclerosis. Stress is therefore a contributory factor to a number of minor and major diseases, including high blood pressure, coronary heart disease, irritable bowel syndrome and anxiety. Long-term stress is also believed to be a contributory factor to depression. It is wise to take some precautionary measures to reduce our stress levels.

As a method of managing stress, some people choose unhealthy habits such as the use of tobacco, alcohol (discussed later in this part), drugs, coffee or unsuitable food to help them manage emotions and provide a short-term fix for feeling better and coping. In the long term all these substances produce a negative effect and involve a further health risk. Information regarding support programmes to assist smoking cessation, management of drug or alcohol misuse and weight management support are available from most local health trusts, hospitals and GP surgeries.

Regular exercise and activity are excellent ways of managing the stress response. Physical exertion offers an excellent release for physical stress and the pressure and tension that build up in the muscles as a consequence of the stress response. It can also distract one from daily hassles or worries and help to clear the mind and assist thinking. Exercise promotes the circulation of endorphins, a compound of hormones that induce a feeling of well-being that can last for much longer than the duration of the activity. In addition, the longer-term benefits of exercise can all contribute to improved self-esteem, self-image and self-confidence.

Some group exercise sessions have a specific focus on the mind and body connection, relaxation and concentration. Pilates, yoga, Tai Chi, Nia and other similar sessions all use specific techniques to focus the mind and enable meditation/relaxation techniques (moving or static) that can be used to assist with stress management and emotional well-being.

NUTRITIONAL FITNESS

Nutritional fitness is balancing the foods eaten and ensuring foods from all the major food groups (in the appropriate quantities) are supplied in the diet to maintain nutritional and energy requirements (NHS Choices, 2012*a*). The type of food and quantity of food people eat will affect their energy levels and their health and well-being. There are no bad foods per se, just poor diets.

The main food groups are:
- carbohydrates (pasta, potatoes, rice, bread)
- fats (cheese, milk, butter)
- proteins (grains, pulses, meat)
- vitamins and minerals (vegetables and fruit)
- water.

Taking part in regular physical activity can make people more aware of the food they are eating and more conscious of their diet. There are many books devoted to nutrition; some of these are listed as references at the end of this book (see page 264). Some very general guidelines for improving the diet and healthy eating (NHS Choices, 2012*b*) include:

- **Eat less saturated fat**: too much increases the risk of high cholesterol and furring of the artery walls.
- **Eat less sugar (reduce sugar added to tea or coffee or cereal) and eat fewer sugary foods/ snacks (cakes and sweets)**: too much can cause tooth decay and contribute to overweight and obesity.
- **Eat less salt**: too much may elevate blood pressure.
- **Eat more complex carbohydrates**: too little will lower our energy levels.
- **Eat sufficient fibre**: too little may cause constipation and other bowel disorders.
- **Eat more fruit and vegetables** (at least five portions a day).
- **Eat a sufficient calorie intake**: too little will slow down the metabolism and create feelings of lethargy; too much will contribute to weight gain and will be stored as body fat.
- **Drink plenty of water**: too little fluid will cause dehydration and potential heat stroke and place an unnecessary stress on the heart.

- **Eat when feeling hungry**: not eating when hungry or skipping meals may affect blood sugar levels, causing individuals to overeat and/or eat the wrong type of foods to manage their energy and sugar levels. However, some people confuse feeling hungry with other feelings/emotional experiences and can use food to bring comfort. Eating more than is needed to meet energy requirements will contribute to weight gain, which may lead to being overweight or obese.
- **Eat a healthy breakfast**: to rebalance energy and fuel levels e.g. cereal and fruit

Clients with medical conditions will require more specialist nutritional advice and will need to be referred to a dietician who will make the specific recommendations. Some general guidance is provided throughout part 3.

SPIRITUAL FITNESS

An individual's personal development and growth (the type of person they become) can be influenced by their life experiences, belief systems, attitudes and values passed down through generations within families, schools, societies, cultures and religions. Each of these can impact belief systems and mental outlook (how people view themselves and their lives), emotional management (how they respond to their feelings and emotions and to the feelings and emotions expressed by others), their attitude to physical activity (including activity levels and whether they look at exercise as a pleasure or an inconvenience, a pain), their eating behaviour (the type of foods eaten and the size of food portions and plate size), their lifestyle choices (transport, smoking, alcohol, hobbies) and their social relationships (how they relate to others, any prejudices etc.).

From a spiritual perspective, each person is a unique individual with their own life journey and their own life lessons. Each person makes a choice (whether conscious or unconscious) to follow a specific life path and each person has the potential to choose how they respond and grow from life's challenges and the events that contribute to them becoming the person they become. As Van Deurzen (2000:333) suggests: 'some people manage to overcome substantial initial disadvantages or adversity, whereas others squander their advantage or flounder in the face of minor contretemps'.

Illness and experience of death (relatives, friends, world disasters) are particularly significant life events that can awaken the existential search to find answers for being, and can provide an opportunity for spiritual growth, which is a lifelong journey!

Spiritual fitness embraces the inner power all people have to love, create peace and live in harmony and balance within themselves and in the world. Spiritual fitness recognises diversity and difference among people and introduces the possibility that people are all at different stages of growth. It embraces the notion that people make the right choices for themselves, with the knowledge and skills they have at a particular time, from which, together with their unique experiences, they can learn and grow as individuals.

From this perspective, every person has the power to make changes and make a difference in their inner world, which will impact and contribute to their outer world.

MEDICAL FITNESS

Medical fitness is the individual's state of health; it requires the body to be in optimal working order. The evidence reported in chapter 1 (and through part 3) indicates that medical fitness is declining among the population. Regular activity and keeping physically fit can reduce the risk of some diseases and contribute to the management of many of the medical conditions discussed in part 3.

Regular exercise, activity and improved fitness can encourage people to eat a more nutritious diet, maintain a healthy body composition and manage stress more effectively. It can also help them to build social networks and relationships, which in turn may encourage them to cut down or remove habits that have an adverse affect on their health, such as smoking, drinking too much alcohol or eating too many of the less nutritious foods, all of which contribute to an increasing risk to health.

OTHER LIFESTYLE FACTORS
Alcohol and sensible drinking

In moderation (within recommended guidance), alcohol use is not considered a health risk and there is some evidence that small, regular quantities can actually be beneficial for health and can offer some protection against CHD by influencing blood cholesterol and reducing the likelihood of blood clots (*Think About Drink* leaflet, DoH). However, alcohol misuse is becoming an increasing problem throughout the UK and among all age groups (including children and young people).

Too much alcohol can have detrimental effects on health. Drinking more than the recommended levels/units of alcohol (see table 3.1) can increase the risk of liver damage, cirrhosis of the liver and cancer of the mouth and throat. Alcohol is not recommended for certain medical conditions and/or medications that can be affected by alcohol, and caution may be advised.

Safe and unsafe drinking levels are measured by calculating the units of alcohol consumed on a daily basis. See table 3.2 for the units of alcohol in specific drinks and measures. An issue for concern is that the volume/amount of alcohol (ABV) contained in usual pub measures of many beers and wines has actually increased over the years. This means many people may be unwittingly drinking much more than they should be and may be well exceeding the recommended guidelines!

Alcohol may be used to manage the stresses and strains of daily living; it is also a part of many social events (celebrations, parties) and some people may use it to relax and to boost their confidence. Recreational and social use can sometimes lead to habit formation and problem drinking, including misuse, dependence and addiction. Signs that may indicate a risk of alcohol dependence include:

- feeling and thinking 'I have to have a drink' or needing a drink to get going (hair of the dog);
- waking up feeling anxious and with the shakes;
- drinking earlier in the day;
- deterioration in work performance;
- relationships and friendships suffering because of drink;
- drinking in spite of any problems it causes;
- drinking more to get the same effect;
- having drink binges, e.g. consuming all or more of the recommended weekly limits at one sitting.

Individuals with concerns about their drinking habits should seek professional help and be referred to specialist services for support.

Table 3.1	Recommended daily alcohol units	
Units of alcohol and health risk:	**Women**	**Men**
No significant health risks	14 units per week 2-3 units per day At least 2 days a week alcohol free	21 units per week 3-4 units per day At least 2 days a week alcohol free
Increasing risk to health	3 or more units per day on a regular basis Binge drinking (weekly units in one sitting) Regular drinking without the recommended alcohol-free days	4 or more units per day on a regular basis Binge drinking (weekly units in one sitting) Regular drinking without the recommended alcohol-free days

Safe and unsafe drinking levels are measured by calculating the units of alcohol consumed on a daily basis.

Table 3.2	Units of alcohol in specific drinks and measures	
One unit of alcohol		**One and a half (1½) units of alcohol**
• Half a pint of ordinary strength beer, lager or cider – 3-4% alcohol by volume (ABV) • A small pub measure (25ml) of spirits (40% ABV) • A standard measure (50ml) of fortified wine such as sherry or port (20% ABV)		• A small glass of ordinary strength wine (12% ABV) • A standard pub measure (35ml) of spirits (40% ABV)

Adapted from Patient UK (2012)

Stopping smoking

The negative consequences of cigarette smoking on health are well documented. Carbon monoxide and nicotine are the two chemicals in cigarettes that have the most impact on the heart. Carbon monoxide contributes to decreased oxygen being circulated around the body to the tissues. Nicotine stimulates the production of adrenaline, which increases heart rate and blood pressure, causing the heart to work harder. Smoking also damages the lining of the coronary arteries and contributes to atherosclerosis, a building-up of fatty tissue on the artery walls. The tar in cigarettes causes cancer.

Smoking is highly addictive and once started is not easy to quit. Persons who wish to stop smoking should be referred to a local smoking cessation group to receive advice and support to help them quit. Their GP will be able to advise them on services available locally.

Unhealthy habits can sometimes be managed by encouraging the individual to exchange their unhealthy habits (some of the time initially) with some healthier habits. These may include:
- drinking a glass of water;
- eating a piece of fruit;
- going for a short walk;
- practising some breathing exercises;
- practising some short relaxation exercises or mindfulness;
- going to an exercise session.

Summary of the benefits of physical activity and exercise on health and total fitness

- Maintain mobility, flexibility and range of motion
- Improve strength of muscles and bones
- Reduce the risk of osteoporosis
- Manage type 1 diabetes
- Prevent and manage type 2 diabetes
- Improve cholesterol levels
- Reduce the risk of heart disease, high blood pressure and stroke
- Assist with managing blood pressure
- Assist with weight management
- Promote social interaction
- Encourage a healthier lifestyle
- Improve sleep patterns and increase energy levels
- Assist with managing stress, anxiety and depression
- Improve self-esteem and confidence
- Enhance feelings of well-being
- Prevent falls and injuries in older adults
- Manage joint and mobility conditions
- Improve posture and ease movement
- Improve ability to carry out everyday activities and help maintain independence
- Improve overall health

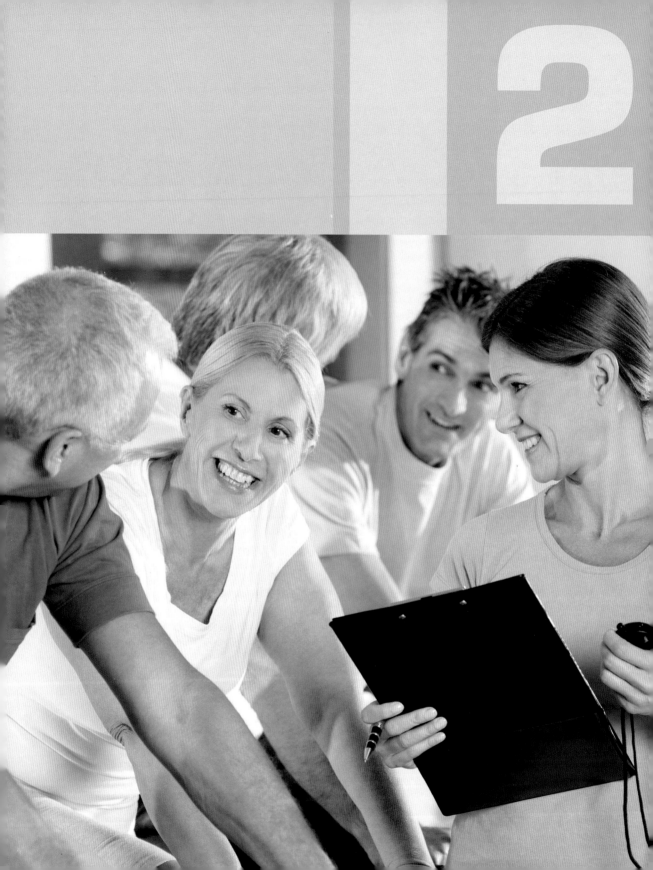

PART **TWO**

PLANNING TO WORK WITH REFERRED CLIENTS

This section of the book discusses considerations for working with referred clients. It includes information on the referral process, screening, assessment, risk stratification, session structure and design, monitoring intensity, and health and safety. Some of the information gathered through the processes and techniques explained through this section can be used to assess, monitor and evaluate a patient's progress, which may also help to inform reports on a scheme's effectiveness at meeting outcomes and targets.

OVERVIEW OF THE REFERRAL PROCESS

Stage 1	Client visits GP with health condition
Stage 2	GP (or practice nurse) clinically assesses client – risk stratify and complete transfer of information and passes forward
Stage 3	Referral manager or co-ordinator receives and checks information and refers forwards (or backwards if incomplete records)
Stage 4	Exercise professional – conducts initial assessment (sometimes co-ordinator role) and works with client for set duration and completes progress checks (mid-term and end) and reports to co-ordinator/GP
Stage 5	Exit strategies identified for client
Stage 6	Follow up checks – 6 month/12 month
Stage 7	Scheme evaluation

THE REFERRAL PROCESS

4

This chapter discusses the referral process and assessment procedures.

THE PURPOSE OF THE REFERRAL AND ASSESSMENT PROCESS

A structured referral system, which includes a comprehensive client assessment, is essential to: assess the appropriateness of exercise/activity as an intervention for specific clients (risk stratification); develop a safe and effective exercise/activity programme, that meets the needs of the individual, for example: cultural needs, social circumstances, exercise capacity, co-morbidities, preferences (likes and dislikes) etc.

The assessment process begins with the client's GP. This initial stage is the key to the referral procedure. For this stage to work effectively it is essential that health professionals are engaged and effective working relationships are established. The scheme will also need the following systems and protocols in place:

- clear inclusion/exclusion criteria;
- well-designed and user-friendly paperwork to transfer information;
- simple referral processes and procedures;
- named medical contact for each patient;

- A named referral contact (scheme coordinator) for each patient;
- clear communication channels.

CLINICAL ASSESSMENT

Before taking part in an exercise programme clients should be clinically assessed by their referring practitioner (GP) to check their suitability. Appropriate patients would usually include inactive individuals with medical conditions (managed) and/or CHD risk factors (2 or more) or mild to moderate mental health conditions (depression, stress, general anxiety) and those needing structured and supported exercise.

The NQAF (DoH, 2001a) states that a referral form/transfer of information record should include the following information:

- relevant current and past health problems;
- details of any medications being taken and their known impact on everyday functional ability;
- standard measures such as blood pressure (BP), heart rate, body mass index (BMI), and lifestyle factors, for example, smoking;
- the possible effects of diagnoses and medications on activities of daily living and, if known, exercise;

- any special considerations or advice given to the patient, for example, a patient with osteoarthritis should be advised to recognise and respect an increase in pain, stiffness or swelling;
- information about any exercise already being undertaken, or for which the patient or the referrer has expressed a preference.

This information should be given in writing, using a transfer of information record (a sample of which can be found in the *BHF Toolkit*, 2010). Information about a change in health status, such as new symptoms or deterioration in an existing condition, should also be communicated to the exercise professional (DoH, 2001*a*). The patient should sign the referral form to agree to the transfer of this confidential information and as part of their informed consent to take part in the referral process.

MEDICO-LEGAL CONSIDERATIONS

It is important for all parties involved in the referral process to be clear about the roles, responsibilities and scope of practice of all clinicians and others involved in the referral process (see table 4.1) and to maintain up-to-date knowledge of the medico-legal aspects. The Medical Defence Union acknowledged the Register of Exercise Professionals (REPs) as a professional body, recognised by the Department of Health (DoH/NQAF, 2001*a*). It was advised that GPs could refer patients to schemes that employed Level 3 exercise referral instructors with qualifications and experience of working with special/referred populations. The current

qualification structure and framework has changed significantly over the last decade and the most up-to-date qualification guidance is outlined in the introduction to this book.

INFORMED CONSENT

An informed consent should be obtained from the patient prior to undertaking the pre-exercise assessment and before commencing an exercise programme (DoH, 2001*a*). This provides an opportunity to discuss the proposed assessment and physical activity programme. An informed consent document should be written and provide the following:

- sufficient information, in accessible language;
- an explanation of the purpose of the exercise assessment and/or programme;
- a description of the components of the exercise assessment and/or programme;
- an explanation of the possible risks, discomforts and benefits;
- clarification of the responsibilities of the patient;
- a reference to confidentiality and privacy;
- an emphasis on the patient's voluntary participation and right to change their mind;
- the opportunity for the client/patient to ask questions (questions and answers can be recorded).

Informed consent is the client's agreement to participate in a pre-exercise assessment and exercise programme. It is not a legal waiver and if someone is not given sufficient information the document is not valid, even if it has been signed (DoH, 2001*a*). Informed consent is part of an ongoing process, so any changes in

Table 4.1	Roles, responsibilities and boundaries	
Role	**Responsibilities**	**Boundaries**
GP or health professional	• Identify and refer patients into a quality-assured scheme • Maintain clinical responsibility for patients • Be responsible for the transfer of relevant and meaningful information (with the patients signed agreement and informed consent) to the exercise professional	Do NOT take responsibility for the delivery of the exercise session(s) Do NOT take responsibility for the administration of the referral programme (NQAF, 2001)
Scheme manager	Responsible for scheme set-up and overall management of operations, which may include: • Building relationships with health professionals and GPs to refer into the scheme • Connecting with commissioning groups • Submitting applications for support and funding • Developing policies and operational procedures to run scheme in line with government policies (health and safety etc.) and to industry standards of best practice • Recruiting appropriately qualified and competent coordinators and exercise professionals to deliver the scheme • Ensuring the scheme operates to industry codes of practice	Are NOT responsible for medical diagnosis Are NOT responsible for delivering sessions (although accountable for staff who do deliver sessions)
Scheme coordinator	Responsible for coordinating operations, which may include: • Receiving information from health professional or GP • Identifying any inappropriate referrals and referring back to GP/health professional • Identifying appropriate referrals and forwarding them to appropriately qualified and competent team members/ services • Conducting the initial client assessment (may delegate this to other exercise professionals within team) • Maintaining client confidentiality • Maintaining accurate records • Having appropriate insurance • Acting professionally • Complying with legislation regarding health and safety, human rights, safeguarding, discrimination, freedom of information, data protection, employment etc.	Are NOT responsible for medical diagnosis and should NOT take responsibility for clients until all relevant clinical information is available (NQAF, 2001)

continued

Table 4.1	continued	
Exercise professional	Responsible for working with clients, which may include: • Initial assessment of patient and informed consent • Refer patient if inappropriate (back to coordinator or GP) or to a specialist service if condition is outside scope of practice • Safe and effective exercise design and delivery • Support and motivate patients and monitor progress • Be members of the Register of Exercise Professionals • Qualified and competent • Have insurance • Knowledge of operational procedures and compliance to all policies and legislation • Report regularly to scheme coordinator • Maintain accurate and up-to-date records • Respectful of inter-professional boundaries and own personal competence	Are NOT responsible for medical diagnosis and should NOT take responsibility for clients until 'all relevant clinical information is available' (NQAF, 2001) Other issues outside of scope of practice and that should be referred to other professionals would include: • Psychological (counsellor role) • Nutritional (dietician role) • Medical – changes to health (GP role) • Contraindications (GP role) • Smoking (cessation team) • Substance misuse (substance addiction service) • Higher risk condition or condition not qualified or competent to deal with (GP, scheme coordinator, qualified Level 4 instructor or clinically supervised activity)

Updated and adapted from Lawrence & Barnett (2006), *BHF Toolkit* (2010)
Professional and Operational Standards for exercise referral, developed by the exercise referral and advisory group (ERAG) 2011 and REPS role descriptor of exercise referral.

an individual's health or exercise programme need to be discussed within the context of this document. Effective communication skills (see part 4) are essential to the informed consent process to enable the client to feel comfortable to ask questions and clarify specific aspects of the assessment or programme.

PRE-EXERCISE SCREENING AND ASSESSMENT

The role of the exercise professional is to provide the appropriate support to enable the client to develop the skills, knowledge and confidence they need to become habitually more active. It is therefore important that they work in partnership with the client, as clients need to be actively involved in the process and in decisions regarding their health (DoH, 2001*a*).

The pre-exercise screening and assessment process provides an opportunity to establish rapport with the client and gather information and take steps as follows:

- personal details (name, address, age, gender, ethnicity, emergency contact);
- informed consent for the assessment process and participation in the programme;
- relevant medical and health information including past medical history and current symptoms;
- medication (what type, how long taken for, any recent changes, effects on exercise);
- past and present activity levels, experience of physical activity (using IPAQ scale – see *BHF Toolkit*, 2010);
- identify and discuss any misconceptions about exercise;
- gather initial monitoring information (height, weight, BMI, waist circumference, blood pressure, pre-exercise heart rate and quality of life measures using EQ-5D – see *BHF Toolkit*, 2010);
- assess client's exercise capacity using appropriate physical assessments, e.g. joint ROM, or other assessments if requested by health professional, such as walk test, Chester step test;
- risk-stratify client using appropriate criteria;
- identify appropriate level of support and supervision;
- lifestyle information (work, habits, stress levels);
- expectations, goals, likes and dislikes (in relation to activity);
- readiness to change and self-efficacy and belief in their ability to make changes;
- personal motivation and desire to make changes;

- any positive strategies already in place (social support, counselling);
- any barriers that exist that may prevent them from making changes;
- mental attitude about their life and medical condition;
- any specific health needs that may require help of a specialist, such as a cardiac nurse or physiotherapist (falls, stroke, cardiac event etc.);
- develop an appropriate exercise programme in partnership with client.

The structure and content of the pre-exercise screening and assessment will also depend on a number of factors including:

- transfer of appropriate information from GP (usually via the referral form);
- local protocols such as inclusion/exclusion criteria;
- resources such as time and appropriately qualified staff.

It is also important to consider the client's feelings and develop strategies to ensure the assessment has a positive impact on her or him. These considerations are discussed further in chapter 15.

Careful planning and preparation for the assessment offers the instructor the opportunity to:

- provide the client with clear written information before s/he attends the session;
- explain what will happen during the initial assessment, with clear instructions about what to wear and what to bring to the assessment;
- prepare the environment to ensure that it meets health and safety requirements and is conducive to the assessment process. For example, images

of older people walking and being active will be more appropriate than posters of young people in trendy sportswear working out;

- prepare for any special needs such as hearing loss or visual impairment;
- ensure privacy and minimise interruptions;
- make sure all the paperwork and equipment is available and accessible;
- have relevant reference books available such as the *British National Formulary* (BNF);
- use effective communication skills;
- provide a non-judgmental, empathic and supportive environment;
- adapt communication style to the needs of individuals, e.g. those with English as a second language, deaf or partial hearing; blind or partial sighted or physical disabilities etc.;
- find out about the client's expectations;
- discuss client's concerns;
- allow sufficient time to carry out the assessment in a meaningful way.

USING THE INFORMATION GATHERED DURING PRE-EXERCISE SCREENING AND ASSESSMENT

It is important to go through the referral/transfer form with the client to confirm the medical information and discuss any changes in health since referral. It is also important to find out the client's perspective about his or her health. How informed are they about their health? How does their health affect their lives? Do they know about the role of exercise in relation to specific health conditions? The information gathered will guide any future work with the client and can also be used to inform reports that monitor and evaluate the effectiveness of the referral scheme for achieving local and national health targets.

Screening and assessment information can be divided into the following eight sections:

1. demographics;
2. reason for referral;
3. current health status and past medical history;
4. cardiovascular disease (CVD) risk factors;
5. current medications and side effects/ implications for exercise;
6. psychosocial factors such as readiness to change, support network;
7. exercise/physical activity history;
8. personal goals.

1. Demographics (age, gender, ethnicity)

This information is collected for basic monitoring purposes. The relationship between age, gender, ethnicity and health is well established and it is important to consider these issues during the assessment process. For example, older people have an increased risk of cardiovascular disease, post-menopausal women have an increased risk of osteoporosis and South Asians living in the UK have a higher than average premature death rate from coronary heart disease (CHD) (British Heart Foundation, 2005c). Information regarding local demographics will also be useful for scheme monitoring and future promotion. For example, is the scheme attracting any specific groups and if not, why not?

2. Main reason for referral

This will usually be indicated on the referral form. There may be a mismatch between the GP's reason for the referral and the client's understanding of why s/he has been referred. This may provide an opportunity to find out more about the client's understanding about the referral and what his or her expectations are, as these factors will influence their engagement, motivation and commitment (including potential for drop out). Engagement (adherence) and drop-outs will also provide useful information for scheme monitoring and evaluation. Motivation and readiness to change are fundamental to long-term behaviour change and need to be central to the assessment process. This is discussed further in chapters 15 and 16.

3. Current health status and medical history

This should include known diseases/conditions with dates (past and present), recent illness/ surgery and current health status including blood pressure, resting heart rate and body mass index (BMI). The quality of information provided on the GP referral form will influence the level of assessment the instructor carries out. For example, just knowing that someone has diabetes is insufficient. If someone with diabetes is referred, it is essential to know the date of onset, the presence of any diabetic complications, the client's experience of diabetes, how well managed the disease is and the last time the client had a hypoglycaemic episode.

If there are any new symptoms or changes to the client's health such as new onset or worsening chest pain, orthopnoea (breathlessness that prevents individual from lying down), shortness of breath on exertion, claudication, palpitations, ankle swelling, dizziness or a recent fall, the instructor will need to refer the client back to the GP prior to exercise. The quality of information transferred can also be monitored and evaluated; it may reflect a need to update and revise scheme protocols and clarify inclusion/criteria.

4. Cardiovascular disease risk factors

This information provides an idea of the person's CVD risk profile and ongoing lifestyle behaviours such as smoking and alcohol consumption. The person may already be classified as at high risk of cardiovascular disease (CVD risk of ≥20 per cent over 10 years) by the GP. It may be useful to have a local health directory with information about services such as smoking cessation clinics, self-help groups and access to health promotion resources. When appropriate, this information can be given to clients to connect them with agencies that can provide more specialised support. Other lifestyle behaviours (smoking and alcohol misuse) are concerns for health promotion, both locally and nationally, so any contribution a scheme can make to help a person make a connection with other support services (even raising awareness of a service's existence) is in part, an achievement of an outcome, albeit small, that can be monitored and reported on.

5. Medications and exercise implications

It is important to know what medications the client is taking because there are those that have implications for exercise. For example, beta-blockers suppress heart rate. The timing of medications may also be relevant for conditions such as diabetes or Parkinson's disease. Any concerns about the client's medication (e.g. you feel the client needs more specific advice about it in relation to exercise, for example, adjusting insulin dose prior to exercise), will need to be discussed with the client's GP and it may be that the client needs to be referred back to their GP. For some clients and some medical conditions, there may be positive outcomes that can be measured and reported, e.g. a hopeful (albeit, ambitious and longer term) outcome would be that the cost of prescriptions could reduce.

6. Social and psychological considerations

Social considerations The Health Education Authority (2000) identified a range of reasons specific to people from ethnic minority groups for not participating in physical activity. These included modesty, avoidance of mixed-sex activity and fear of going out alone. Other factors, such as fear of racism and socio-economic disadvantage, may also affect people's willingness to participate in physical activity in public places.

An isolated older person may prefer to attend a group session aimed at older people where the emphasis is on social support. They may prefer a daytime session, with easy transport links, at a time when they can use their free bus pass; however, this may not be the case and it is important not to make assumptions without checking first.

Any planned activities (current and future) should reflect cultural diversity. Some considerations for attracting broader and more excluded populations may include providing access to exercise professionals from specific groups; connecting with community groups and other services used by these groups and taking activity to them (community centres, day care centres, GP surgeries, church halls etc.); and offering a broader activity provision (not just gym-based programmes) that will appeal to broader populations. Finding out what people want and like is perhaps the first step.

Psychological considerations An individual may be referred because of a mental health condition such as depression. Alternatively, s/he may be referred for another condition but also experience anxiety or depression. People with chronic health conditions such as asthma, chronic obstructive pulmonary disease (COPD), diabetes or arthritis often experience a range of emotions, including worries and fears about the future, frustration at not being able to do the things they used to do and feeling that they have lost control over their lives. These emotions are a common reaction to chronic illness and can lead to increased levels of anger and depression (NHS, 2002). Some exercise referral schemes use questionnaires such as versions of the Short Form 36 (SF 36) or the Dartmouth COOP (a set of charts used to assess health status) to assess quality of life including feelings, social activities, pain, change in health and overall health and social support. Information about the SF 36 and the Dartmouth COOP are available from the Scottish Intercollegiate Guidelines Network (SIGN, 2002). This information can be used to identify people who may require specific support and to monitor changes over a period of time. It is important to use questionnaires that are valid and reliable for specific populations. A quality of life standard measurement tool, recommended for use in the *BHF Toolkit* and Professional Operational Standards, is the EQ5D (Euroqol Group, 2012). Sample questions relate to everyday mobility, self-care, pain and discomfort, health rating and levels of depression.

7. Physical activity history

Previous levels of physical activity It is important to build up a picture of the client's experience of physical activity and/or exercise. The use of open questions can encourage the client to speak more freely and will enable the instructor to find out about what exercise means to the client, how important it is, and her or his personal experience of being sedentary or active. (Questioning skills are discussed further in part 4.)

Current levels of physical activity Measuring a client's physical activity level is an important part of the assessment process and it can be used in the following ways:

- to establish baseline activity level and monitor changes;
- to find out more about the client's current lifestyle;
- to facilitate discussion about the links between physical activity and the client's health;
- to educate the client about the frequency, intensity and type of activity beneficial for health;
- to identify barriers to physical activity;
- to facilitate behaviour change by developing appropriate interventions and support.

There are various subjective and objective methods that can be used to gather this information, including interviewer or self-administered questionnaires, e.g. seven-day recall, diaries and pedometers. The type of methods used will depend on a number of factors. These include:

- availability of local resources;
- the level of information required;
- the aim of the assessment, i.e. to get baseline information to help develop an appropriate exercise programme or to monitor changes over a period of time as part of an evaluation;
- motivation and cooperation of client;
- language and literacy skills.

The methods used will also need to be culturally appropriate and acceptable to the clients. Using more than one method will give you a more accurate picture of an individual's activity levels. The Professional Operational Standards for Exercise Referral recommend the use of the IPAQ.

8. Personal goals

Identifying the individual's personal goals and developing a realistic plan can provide a framework in order to provide focus, motivation and a tool to review and monitor progress. If the client says s/he wants to be fitter, it is essential to try and find out what that means, by asking, for example: 'What sort of things do you want to be able to do? How will you feel?' It often helps to focus on behavioural goals (e.g. I will walk for 10 minutes during my lunch hour for the next week) as opposed to outcome goals (e.g. I will lose 3kg), as these are easier to measure and monitor. Further information on goal-setting is provided in part 4.

SCREENING AND RISK STRATIFICATION

The ACSM (2005a) recommends different levels of screening to help with assessment and decision making. A widely used screening tool is the Physical Activity Readiness-Questionnaire (PAR-Q) developed by the Canadian Society for Exercise Physiology (2002). PAR-Q can be used as a minimum basic screening tool prior to undergoing an exercise test or participation in an exercise programme. A Physical Activity Readiness Medical Examination (PARmed-X), which consists of a physical activity-specific checklist, has also been developed for physicians to use with patients who have had positive responses to PAR-Q. The problem with these tools is that it they are purposely conservative and often screen out people from physical activity if they have a medical condition. Furthermore, these screening tools were developed on expert opinion and are not evidence-based. As a result, the Canadian Society for Exercise Physiologists have recently conducted a review of the evidence in relation to risk and physical activity and has consequently revised the 2002 version of PAR-Q and PAR-Med-X. At the time of publication it is in the final stages of producing revised forms (PAR-Q+ and PAR-Med-X+) and is working in collaboration with the British Heart Foundation National Centre for Physical Activity to adapt the PAR-Q+ for the UK.

EXERCISE CONTRAINDICATIONS

It is important for the referring GP to confirm that the patient exhibits no contraindications to exercise. The following are listed as **absolute contraindications** (BACR, 2005; ACSM, 2005a and *BHF Toolkit*, 2010:93).

- a recent significant change in a resting ECG, recent myocardial infarction or other acute cardiac event;
- symptomatic severe aortic stenosis;
- acute pulmonary embolus or pulmonary infarction;
- acute myocarditis or pericarditis;
- suspected or known dissecting aneurysm;
- BP drop >20mmHg demonstrated during ETT (this will not be evident unless client undergoes an exercise stress test or has exercising blood pressure measured);
- resting systolic blood pressure ≥ 180mmHg/ diastolic BP ≥ 100mmHg;
- uncontrolled/unstable angina;

- acute uncontrolled psychiatric illness;
- acute systemic disease (such as cancers);
- unstable or acute heart failure;
- new or uncontrolled atrial or ventricular arrhythmias;
- other rapidly progressing terminal illness;
- experiences significant drop in BP during exercise;
- uncontrolled resting tachycardia ≥ 100 bpm;
- febrile illness (flu or fever);
- experiences pain, dizziness or excessive breathlessness during exertion;
- any unstable, uncontrolled condition (e.g. diabetes);
- neuromuscular, musculoskeletal or rheumatoid disorders that are exacerbated by exercise;
- unmanaged pain.

RISK STRATIFICATION

As with all activities, there are risks attached to being more active. These may include: condition being negatively impacted or worsening; accidents and emergencies, such as strains, sprains, dizziness, fainting, hypoglycaemia, fractures, falls, exercise-induced asthma, cramps, hyperthermia, dehydration, myocardial infarction etc. However, as highlighted in chapter 1, there is a greater risk to health from being inactive.

The aim of risk stratification is to provide a safe and effective exercise programme at an acceptable level of risk, with appropriate monitoring and supervision. The main purpose of risk stratification is to identify and evaluate people who are at an increased risk of an exercise-related event specific to a disease process and provide appropriate monitoring and supervision. The original model used as a guide for risk stratification was the pyramid model (DoH/

NQAF, 2001*a*) which identified people as high, medium or low risk. In the UK, most exercise referral schemes (set up prior to 2006) developed their own risk stratification tools; however, the NICE review of the effectiveness of exercise referral schemes (NICE, 2006) highlighted a number of inconsistencies in practice, which prompted a review of practice from which the *BHF Toolkit* (2010) and Professional Operational Standards for Exercise Referral (2011) have evolved. The following descriptions broadly classify persons in each risk category:

- **Low**: persons with minor, stable physical limitations or two or less CHD risk factors
- **Moderate**: persons with significant physical limitations related to chronic disease or disability
- **High**: persons needing clinically supervised exercise

However, in reality, people do not necessarily fit neatly into categories. Risk stratification is important, but it needs to be used alongside clinical judgment and in conjunction with other activities, such as client education and observation of the client during the exercise session. For example, a client who is stratified as high risk, is well educated about his or her condition, is able to self-monitor and who complies with their exercise prescription is probably at less risk than a low-risk client who is unable to self-monitor and does not comply with the exercise prescription.

As well as focusing on the medical condition of the client it is important to look at the whole person; for example, the client's behaviour will influence the level of risk during exercise. The skills, knowledge, feelings and thoughts of the client will affect his or her behaviour and may influence the choice of exercise setting and the level of supervision required.

ACSM model

The ACSM model of Risk Stratification Categories (see table 4.2) is designed for use once the following information is known:

- signs and symptoms of cardiovascular disease, pulmonary disease and/or metabolic disease;
- risk factors for coronary heart disease;
- known cardiovascular, pulmonary or metabolic disease.

Irwin and Morgan

The Irwin and Morgan model is the model currently recommended by the British Heart Foundation National Centre for Physical Activity (available in the *BHF Toolkit*, 2010) and the professional operational standards for exercise referral (ERAG, 2011). The model classifies a broader range of conditions, which in some way simplifies the process for both health and exercise professionals. The British Heart Foundation National Centre for Physical Activity are in the process of reviewing and developing the risk assessment tool for exercise referral.

PHYSICAL ASSESSMENTS

It is essential that the exercise professional is qualified and competent to carry out any physical assessments undertaken. It is important to consider both the reasons for conducting the assessment and the appropriateness of the assessment for the client. When conducting the assessment, the aims should be to involve the client as much as possible, provide clear explanations about the assessment

Table 4.2   ASCM risk stratification

Low risk   **Men <45 and women <55 with LESS than TWO of the following risk factors:**

Family history	Cardiovascular event or death before: age 55 (paternal parent or first-degree male relative) or age 65 (maternal parent or first-degree female relative)
Smoking	Current smoker or only recently quit smoking (6 months) or exposed to smoking environment
Sedentary lifestyle	Less than 30 minutes of physical activity a day for last 3 months
Obesity	Male BMI >30 Waist >102cm or 40in Female BMI >30 Waist >88cm or 35in
Hypertension	Systolic >140 Diastolic >90 Confirmed on at least two occasions or medication to manage hypertension
Dyslipidemia	LDL (low density lipoprotein) cholesterol profile >3.37mmol.L HDL (high density lipoprotein) cholesterol profile <1.04mmol.L Total cholesterol 5.18 mmol.L or medication for lowering cholesterol NB: High HDL levels decrease CVD risk; if this reading is high, the risk factor can be removed
Pre-diabetes	Fasting blood sugar levels >5.5mmol.L but <6.93mmol.L Oral glucose tolerance test >7.70mmol.L but <11.00mmol.L Confirmed on at least two occasions

Moderate risk   **Men ≥45 years Women ≥55 years with MORE than TWO of the risk factors listed above**

High risk

Individuals with one or more of the following signs and symptoms:
- Anginal pain or discomfort
- Dizziness or syncope
- Ankle oedema
- Palpitations or tachycardia
- Intermittent claudication
- Known heart murmur
- Unusual fatigue or shortness of breath at rest or with usual activities/mild exertion

Individuals with a known condition (CV, pulmonary or metabolic)
- Cardiac (myocardial infarction, coronary artery bypass surgery, coronary angioplasty, angina)
- Neurological (stroke, transient ischaemic attack)
- Peripheral vascular disease
- Pulmonary (COPD/asthma/cystic fibrosis)
- Metabolic (diabetes type 1 and type 2/thyroid disorders)

Note: Orthopnea refers to breathlessness (dyspnoea) occurring at rest in the recumbent position, which is relieved by sitting upright. Paroxysmal nocturnal dyspnoea refers to breathlessness that usually begins 2–5 hours after going to sleep.

[Adapted from ACSM (2005) and (2010:24)

and provide the client with the opportunity to ask questions.

PHYSICAL MEASUREMENTS

It is important that the exercise professional is qualified and competent to carry out any physical assessments. When conducting assessments, the aim should be to involve the client as much as possible, and provide a clear explanation about what assessments are happening and their purpose and provide the client with the opportunity to ask questions.

Resting heart rate

Measuring a client's heart rate is a first step in checking whether s/he should take part in exercise. It can enable detection of:

- Normal heart rate 60–100 bpm
- Bradycardia (slow heart rate) <60 bpm
- Tachycardia (fast heart rate) >100 bpm
- An irregular heart rate.

A resting heart rate of >100 bpm is a contraindication for exercise and a client presenting this should be referred back to their GP. A client presenting with a slow resting heart rate should be assessed further to check whether they are on medication such as beta-blockers, which affect heart rate. A client presenting with a resting heart rate below 40 or who is experiencing symptoms such as dizziness should be advised not to exercise and referred back to their GP (see chapter 6).

Heart rate is affected by a number of factors, which include medications, stress or anxiety, eating, smoking, caffeine, temperature etc.

Resting heart rate should be taken after the client has been sitting at rest for about five minutes. The most common site for feeling the pulse is the radial artery. It can also be felt at the carotid artery; however, it is essential not to press too hard at the latter point because pressure on the baroreceptors can cause a reflex slowing of the heart rate.

Most clients can be taught how to take their own resting heart rate. However, some clients may find this too difficult due to conditions such as diabetic neuropathy or obesity.

Resting blood pressure

This assessment provides the opportunity to identify:

- hypertension (i.e. persistent systolic blood pressure >140mmHg and/or diastolic blood pressure >90mmHg);
- hypotension (when blood pressure is lower than normal).

If the reading is higher than expected, the instructor should repeat the measurement at the end of the appointment. A systolic blood pressure of >180mmHg and a diastolic blood pressure of >100mmHg is a contraindication for exercise and clients should be referred back to their GP. Hypotension is usually asymptomatic; however, some people may feel dizzy or faint when they stand up. This is referred to as postural hypotension and may be caused by a number of conditions or the effects of medication such as beta-blockers or diuretics. *The British Hypertension Society Guidelines* (2004) recommend taking blood pressure in a standardised way, using a well-maintained, properly validated and calibrated device to ensure accurate and reliable measurements.

Body mass index (BMI)

BMI is used as a practical measure of overweight or obesity; however, it is not an accurate measurement for people who are very muscular or who have a very reduced muscle mass (see chapter 9).

Waist circumference

Central obesity is associated with an increased risk of CHD and other cardiovascular disease. The easiest way to assess central obesity is by measuring the waist circumference (see chapter 9).

Pulmonary function

Spirometry is the method used to measure lung function by measuring the forced vital capacity (FVC) and forced expiratory volume in 1 second (FEV1). The ratio of the two values is then calculated to give an indication of lung efficiency (YMCA, 2004). FEV1 and FVC readings can be compared with normal values based on sex, age and height. Airflow obstruction is defined as:

- FEV1<80% predicted, and
- FEV1/FVC <0.7
  (BTS COPD Consortium, 2005.)

Health professionals who have specific training normally carry out spirometry within Primary Care. Peak expiratory flow (PEF) is a more simple measure than FEV1, and repeat measures can be carried out at home using a hand-held peak flow meter. A normal peak flow is based on a person's age, height and sex and is expressed as a percentage of predicted peak expiratory flow. Clients usually work out a personal best with their GP and use that as a baseline for measurement. The pattern of peak flow measurement is just as important as the actual measurement. A peak flow meter provides a useful tool to support the self-management of asthma; however, it is not a sensitive measure for clients with chronic obstructive pulmonary disease (COPD).

Postural assessment

Posture refers to the alignment between various parts of the body. Optimal posture is important to minimise the stress placed on the body tissues and to ensure safe and effective exercise technique. Over a period of time poor posture may contribute to health problems such as tension headaches, joint problems and back pain. In clients with specific conditions such as Parkinson's disease or COPD, poor posture (kyphosis) can also lead to impaired respiratory function and postural instability. Posture can be assessed using a number of tools such as a standard reference line and a simple checklist to check the position of body parts such as shoulder blade alignment, level of skin creases and asymmetry in muscle bulk. Muscle imbalance contributing to poor posture can be addressed through re-education and strengthening of the postural muscles in conjunction with stretching exercises. Further information regarding postural assessment and improvement is discussed in other texts (Norris, 2000 and Lawrence, 2008).

CLINICAL ASSESSMENTS OF FUNCTIONAL CAPACITY

The Department of Health NQAF (2001a) raised the issue of clinically testing referral patients and recognised that some patients may benefit from a medically supervised exercise test, while acknowledging that exercise testing may not be financially viable and could act as a barrier to promotion of long-term physical activity. Clinical exercise testing is generally recommended for higher-risk patients or individuals undertaking vigorous intensity exercise.

Clients of a low to moderate risk may be able to exercise at a moderate level of intensity without undergoing any specific assessment. Exercising at a moderate intensity minimises the risks associated with high-intensity activity and promotes adherence.

If an exercise assessment is to be included as part of the assessment process, it is essential to ensure that the assessment is individualised to meet the needs of the client, provides meaningful information and is a positive experience for her or him.

Pre-exercise assessments such as sub-maximal exercise tests (while not appropriate for all clients) can be useful to:

- educate the client about her/his current levels of fitness;
- collect baseline information that can be used to develop an exercise programme and tailor advice about activities of daily living;
- monitor progress and help motivate clients;
- assist risk stratification;
- gather useful information about a client's response to sub-maximal exercise including heart rate and rating of perceived exertion (RPE);
- explore difficulties the client has in terms of carrying out the assessment, including following instructions, motor skills and the influence of co-morbidities.

(Adapted from Buckley and Jones, 2005)

KEY CONSIDERATIONS FOR EXERCISE ASSESSMENTS

- Think about what you are assessing and why. Do you want to find out about the client's aerobic fitness, endurance, muscular strength, flexibility, neuromuscular skills or functional performance?
- Ensure the test is appropriate to the needs of the client. For example, a 12-minute shuttle walk test (SWT) may not be appropriate for someone with Parkinson's disease who has difficulties in initiating movement, turning and balancing, and a step test may not be appropriate for someone with an orthopaedic condition.
- Some clients may find the prospect of an exercise assessment anxiety provoking, which could be a barrier.
- If you perform a follow-up assessment, there may be a learning effect, which will influence the results.

ONGOING ASSESSMENT AND REVIEW (MONITORING)

The process of pre-exercise screening and assessment can help to develop a strong foundation for encouraging long-term physical activity behaviour change. It will also enable a more structured exercise programme or exercise prescription to be developed.

However, the assessment process needs to be ongoing when working with referred clients. Before every session it is important to reassess the client's readiness to exercise and monitor (and record) any changes in health status. The assessment may include:

- any other changes in health from the initial assessment or previous session;
- response to previous exercise session such as excessive tiredness or discomfort;
- incidence of chest pain;
- the results/outcomes of any GP appointments and tests.

It can be helpful to plan regular review dates to assess progress, discuss any concerns that the client has and identify ongoing support needs. Most schemes offer an initial assessment, mid-term review (6–8 weeks) and end review (12–16 weeks) depending on the planned duration of the scheme. A structured one-to-one assessment provides the opportunity for the client to discuss any continuing concerns, such as perhaps their frustrations at not losing weight, or difficulties attending the sessions on a regular basis due to other responsibilities. Ongoing assessment enables the instructor to respond to the needs of the client, modify or progress the programme as appropriate and support concordance with their exercise programme. The information gathered can also be reviewed to feed into the evaluation and monitoring for the whole scheme (operations, protocols, achievement of outcomes and targets etc.) and help to maintain the quality assurance and effectiveness.

EXIT STRATEGIES

Exit strategies are signposts to where the client can continue their activity after their supported programme has ended. This may include walking groups, regular mainstream sessions, other specialist sessions or a range of other activities that they have been connected with by the scheme manager and/or coordinator. The staff leading exit sessions should ideally hold the same qualifications as listed for exercise referral instructors. The planned programme may end after a set period due to funding limitations/restrictions etc.; however, the needs of the client (medical condition etc.) often require continued and ongoing specialist exercise professional support.

FOLLOW-UP REVIEWS

Most schemes follow up on client continued progress and adherence after their supported activity has ended. Reviews are usually made after 6 months and 12 months. The information gathered at these intervals is used to monitor the longer term impact of the scheme on behaviour/lifestyle change. Further information on valid and reliable methods (and different research approaches) for monitoring and reviewing the effectiveness of exercise referral schemes is available from the *BHF Toolkit* (2010).

EXERCISE PRESCRIPTION

5

EXERCISE PRESCRIPTION

The aim of exercise prescription is to provide a safe and effective programme, reduce risk factors for chronic disease, increase activity/fitness levels, promote overall health and encourage long-term behaviour change. Individual exercise prescriptions need to be based on the initial assessment process and take into account the following:

- current recommendations for specific conditions (explored in later sections, medical conditions);
- FITT (frequency, intensity, time and type) principles to ensure a safe exercise programme with optimal rate of progression;
- health status;
- functional capacity;
- physical activity level;
- individual limitations, co-morbidity, risk stratification;
- interaction of medications and exercise;
- personal goals and preference;
- response to exercise (physiological and psychological);
- feedback from client.

A flexible and responsive approach to exercise prescription will ensure that the programme is adapted to meet the changing needs of the client, e.g. a client with Parkinson's disease may have daily fluctuations in their health status. Exercise prescription becomes increasingly complex with people with multiple co-morbidities and may require the input of a range of health professionals (dietician, GP, counsellor etc.). Guidelines and limitations/considerations for each specific condition are outlined in part 3.

PROGRESSION OF EXERCISE

The initial goal is to engage the client in a regular exercise programme and rate of progression will be highly individual with any changes introduced conservatively, emphasising frequency and/or duration before intensity. Ongoing monitoring and feedback from the client will be important to ensure the progression is well tolerated, e.g. there is no increase in pain or tiredness. If there is a change in health status the client may be unable to exercise, e.g. if the client has a chest infection. When s/he returns to exercise the programme will need to be modified to take into account any loss of training adaptations due to inactivity (methods of progression are outlined in chapter two).

CARDIOVASCULAR EXERCISE INTENSITY

The aim of setting cardiovascular exercise intensity is to ensure that the client exercises safely and effectively. If the intensity is too high, there is an increased risk of complications during exercise; if it is too low, the physiological adaptations associated with cardiovascular fitness will not occur. Ideally, exercise intensity should be based on the results of a functional capacity test carried out as part of the initial assessment, using a standardised step, cycle or walking protocol. These tests will provide baseline measurements such as heart rate, rating of perceived exertion (RPE) and estimated metabolic equivalents (METs), which can then be used to guide exercise intensity. See ACSM (2005a) for detailed information on sub-maximal exercise tests.

In the absence of a functional assessment, you will have to base exercise intensity on subjective information about the individual's past and present levels of physical activity, along with their past medical history and current health status. You will need to start the client on a very conservative programme using heart rate, RPE, observation and client feedback to ensure an appropriate workload. Over a number of exercise sessions you can observe and record the client's response to specific workloads using different exercise modes, for example bike, treadmill or elliptical trainer, and use this as a baseline for developing the exercise programme. The methods most commonly used in the health and fitness setting for prescribing and monitoring cardiovascular exercise intensity include heart rate (HR), rate of perceived exertion (RPE) and metabolic equivalents (METs).

HEART RATE

Heart rate is widely used as a marker of exercise intensity. This is because of the linear relationship between heart rate and the oxygen demands of the muscles (VO_2) during sub-maximal exercise (ACSM, 2005b/2010). To calculate a target or training heart rate zone you need to know the maximal heart rate (HRmax); however, this requires an exercise stress test, which is impractical in a community setting. Alternatively, you can calculate HRmax based on the formula shown in the box below.

Calculating HRmax

Age adjusted maximal heart rate (HRmax)

220 – age = age-adjusted HRmax

Example: Client who is 55 = 220 – 55 = 165 HRmax

Age adjusted maximal heart rate for individual on beta blockers

220 – (age) – 30 = age-adjusted HRmax

Example: Client who is 55 and on beta-blockers = 220 – 55 – 30 = 135HRmax

The age-adjusted HRmax should only be used as a guide as there is standard deviation (SD) of plus or minus 10–12 beats. This means that an individual may have an actual HRmax of 20 beats per minute higher or lower than the age-adjusted calculation, so relying on this formula to guide exercise intensity could potentially lead to an unsafe or less effective exercise prescription. Medications such as beta-blockers can affect heart rate and this needs to be taken into account when calculating HRmax

Methods for calculating target heart rate zone

The two most common methods for calculating target heart rate range include:

1. percentage of heart rate max (HRmax);
2. Karvonen formula or heart rate reserve (HRR).

1. Percentage of maximal heart rate (%HRmax)

This method is based on the percentage of HRmax and is calculated using the actual or age-adjusted maximum heart rate. For example (see box below), if the target heart rate range is 60–75 per cent HRmax:

Step 1: Calculate age-adjusted HRmax
220 − age

Step 2: Calculate target heart rate range
HRmax × 0.6 = 60% HRmax
HRmax × 0.75 = 75% HRmax

2. Karvonen formula or heart rate reserve (HRR)

The Karvonen formula calculates the heart rate reserve (HRR) to determine a target heart rate zone. The heart rate reserve is the difference between the HRmax and the resting heart rate and corresponds to the VO_2 reserve, e.g. 50–70 per cent HRR corresponds to 50–70 per cent of VO_2 reserve. VO_2 reserve is the difference between VO_2 max and resting VO_2. Where possible use an actual HRmax and an actual resting heart rate (ACSM, 2005*b*).

To calculate 50–70 per cent HRR:

Step 1: Calculate HRR
HRmax (or age-adjusted HRmax) − resting heart rate = HRR

Step 2: Calculate training heart rate (e.g. 50–70% of HRR)
(HRR × 0.5) + RHR = 50% HRR
(HRR × 0.7) + RHR = 70% HRR

For example, Client X is 55 years old, his resting heart rate is 60 and his actual HRmax is unknown.

Percentage of maximal heart rate

To find 60–75% HRmax for 55 year old client:

Step 1:
220 − 55 = 165

Step 2:
165 × 0.6 = 99
165 × 0.75 = 123.75

60–75% HRmax = 99–124

The HRR method

To find 50–70% HRR for 55-year-old client/ resting heart rate 60bpm:

Step 1:
220 − 55 = 165

Step 2:
165 − 60 = 105

Step 3:
105 × 0.5 = 52.5 + 60 = 112.50 (50% HRR)
105 × 0.7 = 73.5 + 60 = 133.50 (70% HRR)

Monitoring heart rate response to exercise

It is difficult for people to take their own pulse during exercise and heart-rate monitors are recommended for pulse monitoring (SIGN 2002). Coded heart-rate monitors enable people to work in close proximity with other people wearing heart-rate monitors, without interference. Heart-rate monitors do not detect irregular heart rates so it may be appropriate to use manual palpation with some clients. Heart-rate monitoring can be used alongside other methods of monitoring, such as RPE. Once clients are familiar with RPE and competent at using the scale they may not need to continue using a heart-rate monitor.

RATING OF PERCEIVED EXERTION (RPE)

A perceived exertion scale can be used to quantify the subjective intensity of exercise (SIGN, 2002). The participant is encouraged to focus on the sensations of physical exertion such as feelings of breathlessness, strain and fatigue in muscles and then to rate his or her overall feelings of exertion using a scale such as the Borg scale. The more experienced a client becomes at detecting and rating sensations, the more closely the ratings correlate with the exercise intensity. Borg developed two scales, the RPE 6–20 and the CR10 scales. The 6–20 scale (see table 5.1) is designed for rating overall feelings of exertion and is generally used for steady state aerobic activity, while the CR10 scale is designed for rating more individualised responses such as breathlessness and pain. The CR10 scale is more commonly used with clients with health conditions such as chronic obstructive pulmonary disease, where the rating of breathlessness is more relevant than overall feelings of exertion. Alternative rating scales are suggested for specific conditions such as angina and claudication (ACSM, 2005a).

Guidelines for effective use of RPE scale

- Allow enough time to teach the scale to clients so it can be used as a safe and effective tool to monitor intensity.
- Measure RPE at varied work rates and using different exercise modes to confirm relationship between heart rate and workload.
- Ensure all staff are teaching and using RPE in a standardised way.
- Get client to anchor the lowest and highest level of exertion to known sensations.
- Encourage clients to practise using the scale outside the exercise environment.
- Use RPE throughout the session including the warm-up and cool-down.
- Use the scale when people are exercising, not between or after exercises.
- Ensure the RPE chart is clearly visible at each exercise.
- Encourage client to focus on sensations throughout the session.
- Be aware of factors which may influence RPE such as anxiety, depression, preconceptions of activity, activity mode, mood and distractions such as loud music.
- Ensure client can reliably estimate ratings of perceived exertion (estimation mode) before you hand the client the responsibility of self-regulating her or his exercise intensity (production mode).

(Adapted from Buckley et al, 1999)

Table 5.2 provides a useful classification of exercise intensities with corresponding description for, RPE, %HRR or VO_2R, and %HRmax.

Table 5.1	Borg rating scales		
Perceived sensations	**CR10 scale** **Individual sensation**	**RPE scale** **Overall sensation**	**Component**
Nothing at all	0	6-7	
Extremely light/weak	0.5	8	
Very light/weak	1	9	Warm up / Cool down zone
Light/Weak	2	10-11	
Moderate	3	12	
Somewhat hard/strong	4	13	
	5	14	
Hard/Strong	6	15-16	Aerobic zone
Very hard/strong	7	17	
	8	18	
Extremely hard/strong	9	19	Intervals – anaerobic zone
	10		
Maximal/highest possible	11	20	

Table 5.2	Classification of exercise intensity for cardio-respiratory endurance		
Intensity	**RPE**	**% HRR or VO_2R**	**% HRmax**
Very light	<10	<20	<35%
Light	10–11	20–39	35–54%
Moderate	12–13	40–59	55–69%
Hard	14–16	60–84	70–89%
Very hard	17–19	>85	>90%
Maximal	20	100	100%

Adapted from ACSM (2005b)

METS (METABOLIC EQUIVALENTS)

METs provide another method for guiding exercise intensity. One metabolic equivalent is defined as the amount of oxygen the body uses at rest:

1 MET = 3.5ml of oxygen per kilogram of bodyweight per minute

METs are used to express the energy cost of physical activity as a multiple of the resting metabolic rate. During activity the oxygen demands increase to cope with the additional energy demands placed on the body. Activities are classified according to their oxygen requirements as multiples of the resting metabolic rate (1.0 MET). See table 5.3.

METs can be used to give advice about a range of activities, based on their known MET value, which the client can carry out within a safe exercise level. For example, if a client can walk at 3mph (3.5 METs) at 70 per cent of their HRmax at 12–13 on the RPE 6–20 scale, one can prescribe a range of exercises equivalent to 3.5 METs and give them appropriate advice about activities of daily living and leisure activities.

Physical activity of <3 METS is classified as light intensity, 3–6 METS is moderate intensity and >6 METs is vigorous activity. For some activities other factors such as environmental effect or individual technique will increase the MET value of an activity, e.g. windy weather or poor swimming technique. For further information about using METS to prescribe exercise, see ACSM (2005).

Table 5.3	Activities and metabolic equivalent (MET) and intensity	
Activity	**Metabolic equivalent**	**Intensity**
Washing face and hands	2.0	Light
Cleaning and dusting	2.5	
Light gardening	3.0	
Walking (strolling) at 2.5mph (1 mile in 24 minutes)	3.0	
Painting and decorating	3.0	
Vacuuming	3.5	
Cycling (stationary bike) 50W, very light effort	4.0	
Walking at 3.5mph (1 mile in 17 minutes)	4.0	
Heavy gardening	4.0	Moderate
Golf (walking and carrying clubs)	4.5	
Tennis – doubles	5.0	
Cycling (stationary bike) 100W, light effort	5.5	
Swimming leisurely	6.0	
Walking at 4mph (1 mile in 15 minutes)	6.0	
Mowing lawn (hand mower)	6.0	
Aerobic dancing	6.5	
Swimming (crawl, slow moderate or light effort)	8.0	
Running 5mph (12 min/mile)	8.0	Vigorous
Running 8mph (7.5 min/mile)	13.5	

Adapted from Ainsworth et al (2000); DoH (2004) and (2012)

MONITORING EXERCISE INTENSITY

Effective monitoring of exercise intensity is a key safety factor in exercise. Exercising above a prescribed intensity level increases the likelihood of complications during exercise (AACPVPR, 2004). It is important to educate clients about appropriate exercise intensity and teach them how to monitor exercise. Referring to the risks and benefits discussed within the informed consent can be a useful reminder for clients who do not adhere to their programme.

MONITORING RESISTANCE TRAINING

It is more difficult to determine appropriate intensities for resistance training. A common method for guiding intensity uses a percentage of 1 repetition maximum (1RM), which is the maximum weight that can be lifted once by a particular muscle group, e.g. 40–60 per cent of 1RM. Determining 1RM is impractical for referred clients and a conservative approach is more often used to find a weight that a client can lift comfortably for a set number of repetitions, e.g. 8–12. The ACSM (2005a) defines intensity as the effort required, or how difficult the exercise is. A resting muscle represents minimal effort and momentary muscular failure or fatigue in the concentric phase of contraction represents high intensity. For clients with high risk of cardiovascular disease or other chronic conditions, the ACSM (2005a) recommends stopping an exercise as the concentric phase of the exercise becomes difficult (RPE 15–16), while maintaining good technique (specific recommendations and considerations are described for different conditions in part 3).

A low initial workload will reduce the risk of orthopaedic, musculoskeletal problems or elevated blood pressure response to training. The initial training period provides the opportunity to familiarise the client with resistance equipment and teach correct exercise technique with an emphasis on developing the client's competence and confidence in the safety of the exercise environment.

OBSERVATION

Observation is an equally important method for the instructor to assist detection of any changes in the client. Observation can be used to monitor:

- excessive breathlessness and changes in levels of breathlessness;
- sweating;
- pallor and changes in skin colour;
- anxiety in relation to the exercise response;
- loss of coordination and exercise technique.

Ideally, a combination of methods (heart-rate monitoring, RPE and observation) should be used to monitor exercise intensity.

SESSION STRUCTURE

All sessions should include a warm-up, conditioning section and cool-down, and a comprehensive programme should include all the components of physical fitness. However, it may not be appropriate to target all components of fitness in every session for all clients. When working with referred populations, specific considerations and adaptations need to be made to accommodate the presented medical condition(s) and other factors that relate to the individual (age, medication, current fitness and activity levels). For some medical conditions it may be more appropriate to focus more specifically on a particular aspect of fitness, such as postural and functional movement for persons with back pain, or mobility activities to manage arthritis.

As a general guideline, with most referred populations the warm-up and cool-down components will need to be longer and of a lower intensity than for an apparently healthy individual, and the main workout (cardiovascular and muscular fitness) will need to be tailored (intensity, type, duration) to accommodate the specific needs of the individual(s). Specific considerations for each condition are discussed in part 3.

THE WARM-UP

The aim of the warm-up is to prepare the body and mind for the activity to follow, to reduce the likelihood of injury or any adverse effects and to increase the effectiveness of the exercise session. A beneficial warm-up will increase body temperature, enabling the muscles to contract and relax more efficiently and the joints to move more freely. The warm-up also provides an opportunity to practise or rehearse movement patterns specific to the activity to follow, for example, performing a pressing action with the arms in preparation for a wall press-up or chest press using resistance equipment.

Components of a warm-up

- **Pulse raising** which consists of low-level aerobic activity to warm the body and gradually raise heart rate. A gradual increase in intensity will decrease the likelihood of abnormal changes to heart rate and heart function.
- **Mobilising major joints** by taking them through a full range of movement, taking into account the range of movement required during the main workout.

- **Stretching major muscle groups** after active warm-up to elevate muscle temperature. Evidence about the role of stretching within the warm-up is inconclusive and you may want to consider the appropriateness of maintenance stretching or full-range mobility activities for your client within the warm-up.
- **Rehearsal of movement patterns**, specific to the activity to follow, to develop skill level and enhance performance.

As a general guideline, with most referred populations the warm-up and cool-down components will need to be longer and of a lower intensity than for an apparently healthy individual.

MAIN WORKOUT OR CONDITIONING SECTION

This section generally includes both cardiovascular and resistance training, however, with referred clients it may not be appropriate to include both fitness components within one session. For example, a client who has had a stroke may benefit from a focus on resistance and neuromuscular (e.g. balance and coordination) training in one session and cardiovascular training in a separate session.

Main considerations for referred clients

- Decide on use of interval approach v. continuous activity: clients with a limited exercise capacity may benefit from an interval approach with active rests.
- Select appropriate activity taking into account orthopaedic limitations, postural instability, etc.
- Choose level of impact, e.g. minimal impact for people with orthopaedic problems.

- Decide on level of support, e.g. when getting on or off equipment.
- Consider implications of medications, e.g. beta-blockers which suppress heart rate.
- Consider use of fixed machines and/or chair-based options if there are balance, stability or orthopaedic conditions.
- Floor-based activities may be inappropriate for some clients, e.g. those who are unable to get up and down without assistance, or have postural hypotension.
- Consider an emphasis on functional activities that will help clients perform activities of daily living (ADLs).

Refer to chapter 2 for adaptations for referred clients.

THE COOL-DOWN

As with all exercise sessions, the cool-down needs to return the body physically and mentally to an appropriate pre-exercise state. A gradual reduction in exertion intensity is required to maintain adequate venous return and enable the heart rate to return to near resting levels. Stretches to maintain and, where appropriate, develop flexibility can be included, along with breathing and relaxation exercises (see pages 252–256.

Referred populations may need to spend longer on the cool-down section. For example, older clients have an increased risk of blood pooling and also of hypotension (low blood pressure) following exercise. Specific considerations for medical conditions are provided in part 3. With higher-risk clients a period of post-exercise observation may be important to ensure people are feeling well before they leave the exercise area.

For many clients the post-exercise period (refreshments and chatting or tea and talk) provides the opportunity to develop social networks. This is especially important for people who may be socially isolated, such as older adults.

HEALTH AND SAFETY

6

When working with clients it is important to ensure a safe exercise environment. People who are suitably trained or who have the appropriate knowledge and skills can carry out risk assessment. There is usually someone within an organisation who is designated health and safety lead, however, it is the responsibility of all employees to identify risks and carry out appropriate action. A risk assessment involves identifying any significant risks or hazards present in the working environment or arising out of work activities.

The Health and Safety Executive (2003) offers a five-step guide which provides an introduction to carrying out a risk assessment in the exercise environment. The steps are outlined in table 6.1.

Table 6.2 provides examples of hazards and control measures in the exercise environment.

The risk assessment must be tailored to the specific exercise environment, such as the client's home, a local park or a community venue. It is important to ensure your exercise environment is accessible to disabled people. Under the Disability Discrimination Act (1995), which aims to end discrimination against disabled people, and related legislation, service providers have a duty to give disabled people access to everyday services and to consider making reasonable adjustments to

Hazard:
A hazard is something that has the potential to cause harm; this could include faulty equipment, a slippery floor surface, teaching too many people in a confined space.

Risk:
A risk is the likelihood of potential harm arising from the hazard.

the way they deliver services so as to make that possible (Directgov, 2005).

MANAGEMENT OF PROBLEMS AND EMERGENCIES IN THE EXERCISE ENVIRONMENT

Before every exercise session it is important to pre-screen clients to find out if there has been any recent change in health, including:

- change in symptoms, e.g. worsening symptoms of asthma, or onset of chest pain;
- new symptoms, e.g. pain in calf when walking;
- change in medications, e.g. beta-blockers, insulin;
- the results of any tests or investigations;

Table 6.1	Risk assessment	
Step	**Actions**	**Considerations**
Step 1	Identify the hazard	Concentrate on significant hazards. Ask other people involved in the activity. Use own knowledge and experience (and some common sense). Hazards may relate to equipment, environment, individuals, behaviour, self (what you do and don't do) etc.
Step 2	Who might be harmed	Who might be at risk? • Client • Exercise professional • Other users
Step 3	Evaluate the risk	What is the *likelihood* of the risk occurring – low, moderate or high likelihood? How *severe* is the risk – low, moderate or high severity? For example: Using the treadmill. *Likelihood*: One risk would be falling off. It doesn't happen that often, but it can happen. *Severity*: May depend on how fast the person is walking or running, where the treadmill is positioned etc. However, the risk may change depending on who is using the equipment and how etc. The likelihood and severity of risk would be much higher for a frail older person with poor balance and coordination, than for a young healthy adult with good balance and coordination. Safeguards need to be put in place to reduce the potential for the risk and to reduce the severity of the risk. These may need to be checked by the HSE officer at the specific work location. If in doubt, leave it out!
Step 4	Record your findings	Use a risk assessment report to record all hazards and controls that you put in place to manage risks.
Step 5	Review and revise	Set a review date. If there are any changes to working practice, e.g. new equipment, changes to venue, or new client group, the risk assessment will need to be updated and amended.

Table 6.2	Examples of hazards and control measure in the exercise environment
Hazard	**Control measures**
Equipment For example, injury associated with faulty equipment or inappropriate use	• Check equipment is in good working order • Conduct regular maintenance and calibration checks • Ensure all users are fully inducted to use equipment (induction should be tailored to meet specific needs) • Provide appropriate levels of supervision
Confined space For example, collision with equipment or other people	• Ensure adequate space for activity and number of clients • Remove any obstacles (bags, water bottles) • Plan appropriate activities for the space • Use effective teaching skills
Slips, trips and falls For example, injury as result of fall	• Check area is safe for use, e.g. no spillages, no trailing leads, no slippery floors • Advise clients about appropriate footwear and clothing • Assess clients to identify risk of falling • Adapt exercises to meet client needs, e.g. slower speed and longer transition time, simpler step and movement patterns, appropriate equipment
Temperature For example, dehydration	• Check temperature • Adapt or postpone activity if needed • Ensure drinking water available
Fire	• Check emergency exits are well signed, clear and unlocked • Point out exit doors and fire points to new clients • Ensure adequate staff training
Exercise-induced complications For example, hypotension, hypoglycaemia, angina, cardiac arrest	• Ensure protocols in place for management of incidents • Ensure adequate staff training (first aid and life support) • Know location of duty first aider, first aid equipment and nearest emergency contact point – must be available and easily accessible • Assess and risk-stratify clients • Ensure inclusion/exclusion criteria adhered to • Tailor exercise programmes for specific needs and risk stratification • Maintain up-to-date client records • Provide appropriate client education, e.g. self-monitoring of exercise intensity and medical condition symptoms (angina etc.) • Verbal pre-screen check at start of all sessions • Appropriate level of supervision and observation

- exacerbation of existing joint problems;
- new joint problems, e.g. knee or back problems;
- feeling unwell, e.g. sore throat or cold;
- any other health-related concerns, e.g. increasing fatigue, low mood, depression.

The pre-exercise assessment is an important aspect of minimising risk and reducing the likelihood of adverse incidents during exercise. It also provides the opportunity for ongoing client education, for example, reminding clients to check blood glucose levels. The information gathered can be used to inform decision making about exercise participation and provide an appropriate intervention. These decisions may include:

- postponing exercise until client feels better, e.g. after cold or sore throat;
- referring back to GP for reassessment;
- modifying exercise session, e.g. avoiding upper-body resistance exercise if there are problems with a shoulder joint;
- exercising with increased level of monitoring, e.g. if a client has slightly elevated blood glucose levels and is asymptomatic, it may be appropriate to advise him or her to begin exercise, then monitor blood glucose levels to check response.

Clients with any symptoms or conditions that are contraindicated should not be allowed to exercise until they are resolved (contraindications are listed in chapter 4).

If a deterioration in the client's functional capacity is noticed, this should prompt the instructor to ask further questions about other factors, such as concordance with their home-based exercise programme or medication. If there is no apparent reason for the deterioration in functional capacity, the client should be referred back to her or his GP. A standard GP letter indicating clear reasons for referral can facilitate this process. Before a client can resume exercise, confirmation from the GP that it is appropriate for the client to continue with a structured exercise programme is required. The client's consent is required when additional medical information is requested from GPs. These issues are discussed in chapter 4.

It is important to document any changes in health, including type of symptoms, any change in pattern or relevant factors in client notes, along with any action taken. An incident or accident book should be used to report any adverse events.

In spite of carrying out a risk assessment and pre-screening clients before exercise, there is always the potential for the development of complications before, during and after exercise. An action plan outlining the main problems likely to be encountered provides a useful framework for managing medical problems and emergencies within the exercise setting. The action plan in table 6.3 gives some examples of medical problems which may occur along with appropriate actions. Action plans need to be developed in line with local protocols and will be informed by the exercise setting and level of staff training, e.g. whether staff are trained in the use of automated external defibrillators (AEDs). Follow-up procedures might include:

- reporting of incident/accident in line with local protocols;
- updating of client records;
- review of procedures and risk assessment;
- dissemination of any changes to procedures or risk assessment to other team members;
- debriefing – the opportunity to discuss any feelings associated with the incident;
- reassessment of client and review of exercise programme if appropriate.

Table 6.3	Management of problems and emergencies in the exercise environment

After any problem or emergency, follow reporting procedure, update client records and if appropriate review risk assessment.

Event/problem	Signs and symptoms	Immediate action	Further action
Angina	Pain in the chest, arm, throat, neck, back, shortness of breath. (In some cases people have non-typical pain or there may be no symptoms at all)	Stop exercising and sit down Assess client If client uses GTN advise to take 2 puffs spray or 1 tablet GTN. Repeat at 5 minutes intervals up to 3 doses. If pain relieved after one or two doses, wait 5 minutes. If appropriate resume exercise at lower intensity. If the symptoms of angina continue after third dose of GTN call 999 and inform of suspected MI. If angina is different or more severe than usual call 999 and inform of suspected MI. Monitor client and respond to any changes, reassure client, reassure other class members, provide paramedics with relevant information, contact relative/emergency contact If pain relieved after 15 minutes remain with client while they rest. Do not resume exercise. Arrange escort home if appropriate.	Refer to GP re symptom control Liaise with GP
Change in pattern of angina In pre exercise assessment client reports a change in pattern of angina since last exercising	Including: • worsening angina • angina on minimal exertion • angina at rest • sudden severe chest pain at rest	Do not exercise. This may indicate unstable angina, which is a contra-indication for exercise. If left untreated unstable angina may lead to a myocardial infarction. Ask client to see their GP soon. Advise client to call 999 if they experience sudden severe chest pain at rest.	Refer to GP

Event/problem	Signs and symptoms	Immediate action	Further action
Myocardial Infarction (MI)	Pain in chest, radiating to arm, throat, neck and back pain. Prolonged, severe pain, not relieved by GTN. Pale, sweaty, nausea, vomiting, dizziness (Clients may experience severe symptoms, have mild chest pain or generally feel unwell)	Assess client Call 999 and inform them of suspected MI Ask client to adopt a half sitting position with head and shoulders supported and knees bent (W position) Encourage client to take their medication for angina, monitor client and respond to any changes in condition, reassure client, reassure other class members, provide paramedics with relevant information, contact relative/ emergency contact	Liaise with GP
Cardiac arrest	Absence of pulse and respiration	Call 999 Commence basic life support (BLS) Reassure other class members Provide paramedics with relevant information Contact relative/emergency contact	Liaise with GP
Collapse	A sudden faint or loss of consciousness. Pale, sweaty, rapid pulse	Assess client (*Consider diabetes, epilepsy or hypotension*) If unconscious, breathing with a pulse, place in recovery position and call 999 Monitor client and respond to any changes in condition Reassure other class members Provide paramedics with relevant information Contact relative/emergency contact If consciousness regained consider GP or 999 as appropriate	Liaise with GP regarding cause of collapse

Event/problem	Signs and symptoms	Immediate action	Further action
Arrhythmias *Tachycardia*	Heart rate >100bpm	Assess client and check BP If new onset or client is symptomatic refer to GP or call 999 as appropriate Check for any change in medication	Refer to GP
Bradycardia	Heart rate<60 bpm	Assess patient and check BP Check whether client is on beta-blockers If asymptomatic client can exercise unless <40 bpm	Refer to GP
Irregular		Assess client Check BP Check whether new onset If symptomatic e.g. feels faint, dizzy or lethargic refer to GP or call 999 as appropriate Monitor and reassure client Provide paramedics with relevant information If treated and client is asymptomatic monitor weekly	Refer to GP if new onset
Hypotension	Dizziness, faint	Assess client Check BP and heart rate Lie client flat and elevate feet Check for any change in medications Ensure recovery before travelling home and arrange escort home if appropriate	Refer to GP
Hypertension	Usually no symptoms, however may be detected on BP check	If BP unusually high for individual recheck after resting for 5 minutes If still higher than usual modify exercise programme and monitor Do not exercise if systolic >180mmHg and diastolic >100mmHg Discuss concordance with medication	Letter to GP Refer to GP

Event/problem	Signs and symptoms	Immediate action	Further action
Hyperglycaemia Hyperglycaemia is more likely to occur in individuals who take insulin. In adults symptoms usually develop over 1-2 days	Blood glucose levels > 13 mmol/l before exercise Confused, nauseous, headache, thirsty, abdominal pain and vomiting, hyperventilation	Do not allow to exercise if signs and symptoms of hyperglycaemia or if blood glucose levels > 13mmo/l and rising. If appropriate test for ketones. If ketones are elevated do not exercise, due to increased risk of diabetic ketoacidosis. Advise client to contact healthcare team immediately to discuss appropriate action or call 999 as appropriate If unconscious and breathing, with a pulse place in the recovery position and call 999. Monitor client and respond to any changes in condition, reassure other class members, provide paramedics with relevant information, contact relative/ emergency contact	Refer to GP/ diabetes healthcare team Liaise With GP
Hypoglycaemia Blood glucose levels < 4 mmol/l or sudden drop in blood glucose levels *Clients with Type 2 diabetes who are not on insulin or hypoglycaemic agents are very unlikely to have a hypo	Blood glucose levels < 4.00mmo/l before exercise or a sudden drop in blood glucose levels 5 – 6mmo/l before exercise Pale skin colour, palpitations, muscle tremors, confused, unreasonable behaviour, cold, clammy skin, sweating, pallor, weakness, fainting or hunger, tingling lips Deteriorating level of response	Do not exercise Consume sugary snack (10–15g) for light to moderate exercise and ensure blood glucose levels rise before commencing exercise. Increase intake according to the intensity and duration of the activity Stop exercise and sit client down Give sugar e.g. a glass of fruit juice, not diet drink, three glucose sweets, followed by a starchy snack such as a sandwich, biscuits or bowl of cereal If unconscious and breathing, with a pulse place in recovery position and call 999. Monitor client and respond to any changes, reassure other class members provide paramedics with relevant information, contact relative/emergency contact	Refer to GP/ diabetes healthcare team

Event/problem	Signs and symptoms	Immediate action	Further action
Asthma	Client needs to use inhaler more than once a day, is having difficulty sleeping or their peak flow reading has fallen below normal	Do not allow client to exercise, as asthma control needs to be improved Encourage client to take 2 puffs or more of reliever straight away, preferably using a spacer	Refer to GP to discuss asthma control/ check inhaler technique
	Asthma attack Typical symptoms include: Wheezing Coughing Chest tightness Shortness of breath	Encourage client to keep as calm and relaxed as possible • **Get client to sit down and rest hands on knees for support** • **Try and get client to slow down breathing to conserve energy** Wait 5 – 10 minutes Do not resume exercise	As above
	Life threatening symptoms The reliever medicine is having no effect on symptoms Too breathless to talk or eat Too tired to breathe normally Confused or irritable Looking pale or blue in colour	If the reliever has no effect and/or client has life threatening symptoms, call an ambulance Encourage client to continue using reliever every few minutes until help arrives Monitor client and respond to any changes Reassure other class members Provide paramedics with relevant information Contact relatives	Liaise with GP
COPD	Excessive breathlessness People with COPD may have an increased risk of CHD therefore important to be aware of symptoms of angina during exercise. (See section on angina)	Encourage client to stop, adopt a comfortable position, either seated or standing and allow breathing to return to normal Use inhaled medication as appropriate	Refer to GP if worsening of symptoms

Event/problem	Signs and symptoms	Immediate action	Further action
Stroke	Facial weakness, drooping mouth or eye Arm weakness, inability to raise both arms Speech problems, inability to speak clearly or understand what you say	Stop exercise immediately Sit client down Call 999 and inform of suspected stroke Reassure client and monitor Provide paramedics with relevant information Contact relative/emergency contact	Liaise with GP
TIA	Symptoms same as stroke but effects last 24 hours or less and may pass within a few minutes	Stop exercise immediately Treat as a medical emergency even if symptoms subside after a few moments. Treat as suspected stroke as above	Liaise with GP
Accident or incident	Strains, sprains, falls, etc.	Ensure safety of both casualty and other participants Monitor client as appropriate Access appropriate services	Liaise with GP

(BACR 2000, Asthma UK 2005, Diabetes UK 2004, Stroke Association 2005)

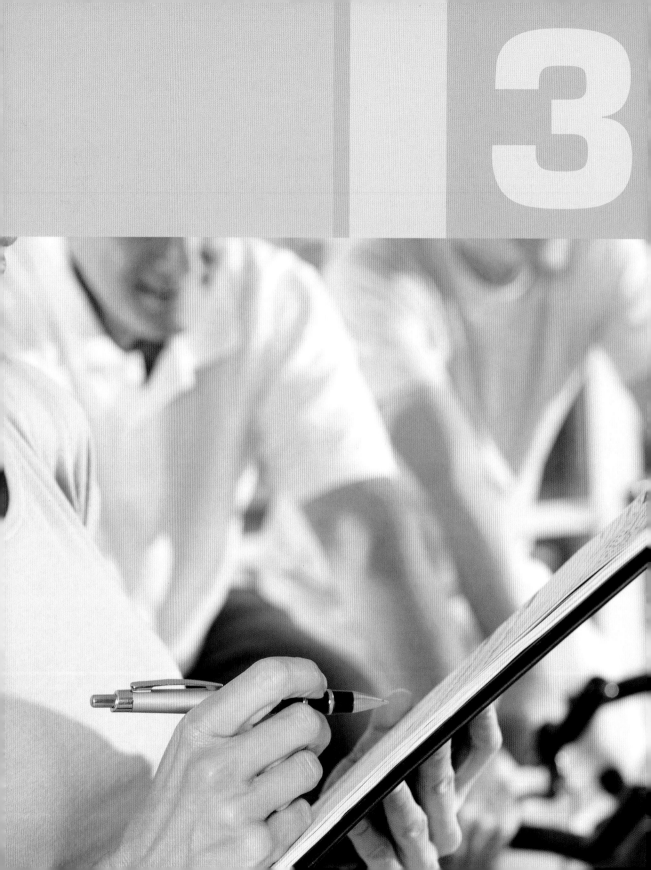

PART THREE

MEDICAL CONDITIONS, MEDICATION AND EXERCISE GUIDELINES

This section of the book discusses specific medical conditions and the exercise guidelines and considerations for working with persons with these medical conditions. It should be noted that most referred clients present with a combination of conditions and therefore the guidelines and considerations in relation to each condition need to be explored and adapted to work with the specific individual, with guidance from, and collaboration with, the referring health professional.

The specific conditions that are named and included within the Level 3 Diploma in exercise referral include:

- Hypertension
- Hypercholesterolaemia
- Chronic obstructive pulmonary disease (COPD)
- Asthma
- Obesity
- Diabetes type 1 and 2
- Osteoarthritis
- Rheumatoid arthritis
- Osteoporosis
- Depression
- Stress
- Anxiety
- Simple mechanical back pain
- Joint replacement

Many conditions now form part of the level 4 qualifications (see qualification structure, in the introduction to this book). It should be noted that a combination of some of the conditions listed in this section, may elevate the client's risk stratification. Level 3 instructors are only qualified to manage clients who are considered to be of low to moderate risk. See chapter four for risk stratification guidance currently used.

Level 4 qualifications and conditions include:

- Mental health (eating disorders, psychosis, substance misuse etc.)
- Stroke
- Chronic respiratory disease
- Cancer rehabilitation
- Falls prevention
- Back pain
- Obesity and diabetes
- Cardiac Disease
- Long Term Neurological Conditions (multiple sclerosis, cerebral palsy, motor neurone disease, spinal cord injury etc)

MENTAL HEALTH CONDITIONS

7

Mental health problems are among the most common health conditions. They reportedly affect 1 in every 4 people (one quarter or 25 per cent of the population) in any one year and it is estimated that 450 million people worldwide have a mental health problem (Mental Health Foundation, 2009:7). Mental health conditions include a range of conditions from eating disorders, schizophrenia and bipolar to substance misuse and personality disorders. The conditions discussed in this chapter are limited to:

- Depression
- Stress
- Anxiety

There is no clear, single boundary that creates a defining point between what is considered mental health and what is considered mental ill health or illness. A psychiatrist generally diagnoses a 'mental illness' when there is a clear range of signs and symptoms present (referred to as a syndrome) and where there is a distinct deterioration in the person's functioning (Daines et al, 1997).

However, an individual's mental well-being may be at risk without the diagnosis of a mental health condition (e.g. stress). Mental well-being refers to the extent to which an individual's thinking, perception, responding, behaving, personality, intellect and emotion (aspects of functioning that are not related to a bodily system e.g. gastrointestinal) are healthy (functional) or unhealthy (dysfunctional) (Daines et al, 1997). For example, an individual may have a diagnosed mental health condition, but may be coping and managing effectively; alternatively, another individual may not have a diagnosed mental health condition and yet may not be coping or managing their life effectively.

A person's behaviour and response to specific life events and circumstances is highly impacted by the cultural and social group to which s/he belongs. What is considered normal by one culture or social group (including families) can often be seen as abnormal by another culture and social group. With this in mind, it is suggested that the notion of similarity and difference between different groups needs to be explored and embraced before any classification is made regarding what is considered 'normal'. Persons interested in reading further into this area are referred to the ideas and viewpoints expressed by Fernando (1988), Gross and McIlveen (1998:562–613), Lago and Thompson (2003), Mindell (1995) and Rack (1982).

Each of the major models that contribute to the study of human psychology and behaviour: *medical*, *biological*, *psychodynamic*, *behavioural*, *cognitive*, *humanistic* and *social*, have their own theories regarding how mental, emotional and behavioural disturbances can occur and how they should be treated. The most influential model has been the medical model, which identifies collections of signs and symptoms that lead to diagnosis of specific mental conditions against the classificatory systems (DSM-IV, APA, 2000). The medical model tends to focus on biological and medical factors; hence, treatment plans tend to rely heavily on medication. An introduction and overview of the classificatory systems is provided in Gross and McIlveen (1998).

However, the Mental Health Foundation (2000) suggests 'most mental health problems result from a complex interaction of biological, social and personal factors'. With this in mind, while diagnosis of a specific condition can guide the planning of medical treatment, other contributory factors, such as social support systems, impact of stressful life events etc. should also be considered for guiding care and treatment plans. As Daines et al. (1997:68) suggest, 'no single model can provide all the answers, so an experienced psychiatrist learns the value of eclecticism of working as part of a team' within both primary care (GP, practice nurse, counsellor) and secondary care (psychologist, social worker).

DEPRESSION

Depressive disorders are conditions that embrace a wide range of signs and symptoms (see table 7.1) that adversely impact the body (physical and behavioural), thinking (mental) and mood (emotional). It is not the same as a passing low mood, as it can cause more serious problems that impact daily living (how a person eats, sleeps, thinks and feels about themselves and the world and how they cope) and in severe instances it can lead to suicide. Of all the psychological disorders, it is the one that is most commonly seen by GPs. The World Health Organization ranks depression as one of the leading causes of years lived with a disability worldwide, and places it second only to ischaemic heart disease in developed countries.

CAUSES

Many people believe that depression is a condition for the weak, however, this is far from the truth. Many great world leaders have experienced depression, including Abraham Lincoln and Winston Churchill (who named the condition 'his black dog') and in recent years a number of celebrities (comedienne Ruby Wax and actor Brad Pitt) and sporting heroes (cricketer Andrew 'Freddie' Flintoff and footballer Stan Collymore) have spoken about their experience of depression. People who experience depression are usually those who are trusted and whom others would turn to in a crisis. Their strength is sometimes taken for granted and people are often surprised when they announce they are ill (Cantopher, 2003:6).

There are various theories regarding the causes of depression (Cantopher, 2003; Elverton, 2004; Davies & Craig, 2009). These include:

- biological (changes in brain chemicals, serotonin, dopamine, norepinephrine, which are influenced by stress);
- genetic disposition (heredity);
- socio-economic factors (deprivation, long-term stress, financial problems, relationship

problems, illness, bereavement, loss of job, life transitions, etc.);

- psychoanalytic (early developmental experiences, i.e. loss of a care giver);
- cognitive-behavioural (distorted thinking patterns and focusing on fear);
- humanistic (low self-worth and self-esteem);
- family systems (relationships and roles within the family).

As Strock (2000) suggests, a combination of these factors can contribute to onset of the condition and later episodes may be 'precipitated by only mild stresses, or none at all'.

PREVALENCE

Depression reportedly affects 8–12 per cent of UK population and 121 million worldwide in any one year and the World Health Organization (WHO) forecast that by 2020 it will be second only to coronary heart disease as the leading contributor to the global burden of disease (MHF, 2007:10).

It is reported that 'one in four women and one in ten men will experience an episode of depression serious enough to require treatment at some point in their life' (MHF in Halliwell, 2005: 13). Therefore, the ratio of women to men experiencing depression is 2:1 (Strock, 2000). This may be due to hormonal factors that affect women (menstruation, pregnancy, birth etc.) and/or other responsibilities (caring for children and/or elderly relatives, work). Alternatively, Strock (2000) suggests that depression in men may be 'masked by alcohol and drugs' and that men are less likely to admit to feeling depressed. She also suggests that depression in men tends to be displayed as irritability and anger and that men may be less inclined to ask for help.

It is estimated that over 20 per cent of individuals with major depression never seek help nor are seen by their GP and that 40 per cent of those with depression are not recognised by their GP because they present with another, physical, illness (Daines et al, 1997). Approximately 15 per cent of severely depressed adults commit suicide after only one month of a first episode.

SIGNS AND SYMPTOMS

A clinical episode of depression is diagnosed when at least two out of three of the core symptoms and three other symptoms (see table 7.1) are experienced for most of the day, nearly every day, for a minimum of two weeks (Davies & Craig, 2009).

Table 7.1	Signs and symptoms of a depressive episode

Core symptoms

- Low mood
- Reduced interest, pleasure and enjoyment in life
- Reduced energy and fatigue

Other symptoms

- Feelings of guilt, worthlessness, self-reproach
- Recurrent thoughts of suicide
- Reduced concentration and attention
- Low self-esteem and self-confidence
- Pessimistic views of the future
- Decrease in sexual drive
- Continuing state of worry and apprehension
- Disturbed sleep (insomnia or hypersomnia)
- Disturbed appetite (poor appetite with weight loss or increased appetite with weight gain)
- Physical inactivity or hyper-activity
- Thoughts of self-harm or suicide (with or without intent)

Other reported symptoms include:

- **Emotional** Persistent sad, anxious or empty mood, feelings of hopelessness, pessimism, helplessness, irritability (Strock, 2000; Davison & Neale, 2001).
- **Mental** Negative outlook on life, self and environment, inability to make decisions (Strock, 2000; Davison & Neale, 2001).
- **Behavioural** Deterioration in relationships, withdrawal from supportive relationships, increased smoking and/or use of alcohol, change in work or academic performance (Strock, 2000; Davison & Neale, 2001).
- **Physical** Decreased motivation, lethargy, fatigue, persistent physical symptoms that do not respond to treatment (headaches, aches and pains, gastroenteritis), which mask the psychological symptoms (Strock, 2000; Davison & Neale, 2001).

The severity of diagnosis (mild, moderate or severe) is determined by the intensity of the symptoms presented (MHF, 2007). A clinical depressive episode can occur only once, but more frequently occurs more than once during the lifespan. Without treatment, the symptoms can last for months or years (Strock, 2000).

OTHER TYPES OF DEPRESSION

Bipolar disorder or manic depression is less prevalent than other types of depression, affecting 1 in 100 people (MHF, 2007). It is characterised by extreme mood swings that range from extreme highs and euphoria (during the manic phase) to severe lows (during the depressive phase). Diagnosis involves the experience of one or more manic/mixed episodes accompanied by a major depressive episode. During the depressive phase

the signs and symptoms listed in table 7.1 may be present. During the manic phase, symptoms may include: abnormal or excessive euphoria/elation; decreased need for sleep; increased libido; grandiose notions; increased energy; irritability; rash and inappropriate social behaviour; racing thoughts and speech (Strock, 2000; Davison & Neale, 2001).

There are different types of bipolar disorder and this condition is considered to be outside of the scope of practice for a Level 3 exercise referral instructor. Other types of depression include cyclothymia and dysthymia, seasonal affective disorder and post-natal depression (Lawrence & Bolitho, 2011).

TREATMENT

There are numerous treatments for depression, depending on the severity of the diagnosis, and often a combination of treatments will be prescribed. The treatments favoured by most GPs (55 per cent) are the counselling and talking therapies (MHF, 2007), which include a variety of approaches ranging from relational, integrative, psychodynamic, humanistic and cognitive behavioural approaches and many others. One of the most widely used approaches in the UK (favoured by the NHS and National Institute for Health and Clinical Excellence – NICE) is cognitive behavioural therapy (CBT). Further information on the range of talking therapies is available from the British Association for Counselling and Psychotherapy (BACP) website http://www.bacp.co.uk/

However, counselling waiting lists are often too long (usually at least six months) for a person in crisis, so the more readily available antidepressant medication (e.g. selective serotonin reuptake inhibitors, SSRIs) is often prescribed (by 55 per cent of GPs). Medication is not recommended by NICE as the first line of treatment for mild depression, due to the side effects (weight gain, dizziness, increased blood pressure and heart rate) (MHF, 2007).

Exercise is only prescribed by 5 per cent of GPs, however, 81 per cent of persons experiencing depression who tried exercise reported that it was effective (MHF, 2007).

Medication

A variety of drugs can be used in the treatment of depression. The cost of anti-depressant prescriptions alone has risen rapidly since the early 1990s. In England, this increase amounts from an estimated cost of £18.1 million in 1992, to an estimated £400 million in 2005 (MHF, 2007).

Antidepressants These are the most commonly prescribed drugs to treat depression. In particular, SSRIs (selective serotonin reuptake inhibitors) are prescribed as they have fewer side effects than other medications. They affect neurotransmitters (dopamine and norpinephrine). MAOIs (monoamine oxidase inhibitors) and tricyclic antidepressants are used less frequently because of adverse interactions with other drugs and more frequent side effects, which may include sleep disturbance, dizziness, gastrointestinal disorders, headache, restlessness, agitation, oedema, confusion, dry mouth and postural hypotension. Antidepressants help to reduce the symptoms of depression and boost motivation (Strock, 2000).

Anti-anxiety drugs or sedatives These are sometimes prescribed alongside antidepressants to assist with anxiety and promote sleeping. They are not effective for treating a depressive disorder if taken alone (Strock, 2000). The most commonly used is the benzodiazepine (BDZ) group. They produce effective short-term benefits but are highly addictive and therefore not recommended for long-term use (see treatments for anxiety, pages 90–91, for more information on these medications).

Psychological 'talking' therapies (counselling and psychotherapy)

There are a number of talking therapies that can be used to assist with the treatment of depression. The most common is probably CBT (cognitive behavioural), which focuses on retraining thinking patterns that contribute to low moods. Humanistic or person-centred approaches focus on listening and building an empathic, non-judgmental, congruent relationship where the individual can discuss her or his problems. Psychodynamic treatments tend to work at deeper levels to resolve inner conflicts and are usually only introduced when the depression has significantly improved. There are also a whole range of self-help books and strategies to assist with personal management of depression (see Lawrence & Burns, 2011b).

Alternative/complementary therapies

There is a wide range of complementary therapies that can be used to assist with treatment of depression. These include: nutrition (reducing stimulants, such as coffee, sugar and alcohol); herbal medicine, such as St John's Wort (Strock, 2000 cites some ongoing research); and specific meditation and relaxation techniques to alleviate stress and anxiety. At this time, there is comparatively limited research evidence to support the use of these treatments. There is a greater evidence base to support medication intervention.

Nutritional

Many of the mental health charities report on the impact that diet can have on mood, well-being and mental health (MHF; Mind). Some foods have a negative effect, and are referred to as stressors and others have a positive effect and are referred to as supporters (see table 7.2). It is important to eat regular meals to manage blood sugar levels, which may contribute to fluctuations in mood. Any specific dietary advice should be provided by a dietician.

Table 7.2	Food stressors and supporters
Food stressors	
sugar	
coffee	
sugary drinks	
chocolate	
alcohol (is a depressant, see chapter 3)	
dairy	
processed foods containing additives and saturated fat	
cakes and sweets	
Food supporters	
water	
seeds	
nuts	
fibre	
wholegrain foods (bread, rice, pasta)	
oily fish	
fruit and vegetables	
protein (fish, lentils, meat, cheese)	

From: Mind, 2009 in Lawrence & Burns (2011b)

EXERCISE RECOMMENDATIONS

There is ongoing research and increasing evidence to support the use of exercise and activity as part of the treatment of mild to moderate depression (Biddle et al, 2000; Halliwell, 2005; NICE, 2009). The guidance suggests that persons with depression 'should be advised of the benefits of following a structured and supervised exercise programme of typically up to three sessions per week of moderate duration (45 minutes to one hour) for between 10 and 12 weeks' (Halliwell, 2005; NICE, 2009).

However, the specific type of exercise recommended is dependent on a number of factors. Exercise professionals working with this population should conduct a detailed screening assessment and work with other healthcare professionals to identify ways of supporting the person. The severity of the condition is a primary consideration as some clients with depression are totally demotivated and even regular daily activities, such as getting out of bed and housework, are too much. In these instances, it may well be worth their seeking counselling support to discuss and learn to manage the thoughts and feelings that may contribute to this state prior to embarking on an exercise programme. Other considerations include the side effects of specific medications on exercise and also the treatments of any other coexisting medical conditions (which can be varied). It may be that depression occurs in response to another medical condition (rheumatoid arthritis, heart disease, cancer), in which case the exercise and activity plan would need to be different from if depression presented as an isolated condition. Each of these issues should be considered prior to making any

Table 7.3	Exercise guidelines for depression			
Training guidelines	Cardiovascular	Muscle strength	Flexibility	Functional
Frequency	3–5 days a week	2 days a week	5 days a week	Promote ADL
Intensity	RPE 11–14	50–70% of 1RM	To position of mild tension, not discomfort	Related to daily activities e.g. walking etc.
Time	20–30 minutes	1–2 sets 8–12 repetitions	15–30 seconds 2–4 repetitions	Move more often
Type	Large muscles, walk, swim, cycle	Whole body approach 8–10 exercises	Whole body approach	Gardening Housework Walking etc.

Adapted from Durstine & Moore (2003:318)

exercise prescription or recommendations. As a guideline, Durstine and Moore (2003:317) recommend following the ACSM prescription for the general population with a more conservative approach in relation to intensity, as inactivity, high body fat and low self-esteem may be more common in this population (see table 7.3 for exercise guidelines).

The client's age, fitness and current activity levels will also affect the exercise recommended. As a starting point, the *General Activity Guidance* (DoH, 2011) can be offered as a preliminary target guideline for building activity to a level that can assist with the maintenance of health and promote general feelings of well-being (see chapter 1, table 1.2, page 16).

The appropriateness of specific types of activity will be dependent on the individual and the existence of other medical conditions (obesity, high blood pressure etc.). For example, an overweight individual would be advised to perform lower impact and non-weight-bearing activities, whereas an individual with osteoporosis or osteoarthritis would need to follow specific guidelines that account for these other conditions.

Cardiovascular exercise can contribute to the feel-good factor (release of endorphins), which can motivate the individual to take on other activities.

Muscular strength and endurance activities assist with muscle tone and shape, which can contribute to increased physical self-esteem.

Flexibility and mobility exercises assist with efficiency of movement, making daily tasks easier. Stretching also assists with relaxation and can improve posture, which in turn can have an impact on increasing confidence.

EXERCISE IMPLICATIONS

The main implications when working with depressed clients include:

- Low levels of motivation will require sensitivity and patience on the part of the trainer. When people feel depressed, they are often unmotivated. A supportive, encouraging and empathic approach is essential.
- Energy levels may also be low and the person may feel tired a lot of the time, therefore, intensity needs to be lower with the possibility of rests within the session or an accumulative approach to activity taken.
- The positive benefits of exercise need to be reinforced and the person must be praised for small efforts, which can make a big difference to their overall health.
- Medication can have an effect on heart rate, blood pressure and energy levels and may contribute to weight gain. All of these must be accounted for prior to recommending any specific exercise programme.
- Enjoyment, fun and pleasure should be emphasised in the activity plan and, where possible, opportunities for socialisation included to reduce isolation, for example, group exercise where participants can encourage and support each other.
- The inclusion of specific relaxation techniques that the client can practise at home is useful for managing depression and anxiety.
- Specific techniques that promote positive self-talk and affirmations are also useful to assist with the development of a positive attitude that can carry over into other areas of life.
- Frequency, intensity, time and type of activity will be determined by other individual factors already discussed.

STRESS AND ANXIETY-RELATED DISORDERS

Stress is not considered to be a mental health condition in its own right, however, it is often linked to both depression and anxiety (MHF, 2007:14). Anxiety-related conditions are listed as mental health conditions and include:

- general anxiety disorder (GAD);
- post-traumatic stress disorder (PTSD)
- panic attacks;
- phobias.

Stress is something that most people recognise, yet it is hard to define. Stress levels are often influenced by an individual's perceived ability to balance the demands of their environment (work, relationships, health etc.) with their internal and external coping resources (positive mental attitude, physical fitness, friends, family, finances etc.). Unhealthy stress levels occur when a person feels unable to cope, and when s/he perceives a situation as applying an abnormal pressure that taxes and exceeds their internal and external resources (Lawrence, 2005; Lawrence & Bolitho, 2011c).

General Anxiety Disorder (GAD) This is the most common of the anxiety-related conditions. It is diagnosed when an individual has experienced extreme tension, increased fatigue, trembling, restlessness, muscle tension, worry and feelings of apprehension about everyday problems on most days for the previous six months. The person will be anxious in most situations and there is no known trigger for their experience. GAD is commonly diagnosed with at least one other mental health condition, most frequently depression, but also other conditions e.g. alcohol and substance misuse (MHF, 2009:14).

Panic attacks These are characterised by a sudden and overwhelming sense of fear, which brings on panic and apprehension. The person may experience laboured breathing, hyperventilation, palpitations, sweating, giddiness and nausea. Learning to breathe calmly when feeling an attack coming on can reduce most of the physical symptoms and bring back a state of calm.

Post-traumatic stress disorder (PTSD) is brought on by exposure to a stressful experience that is considered outside the normal range of life events, for example, being the victim of or witnessing abuse, torture, accidents and/or disasters that involve death and traumatic human suffering. Persons experiencing PTSD will relive the traumatic experience through repetitive thoughts or dreams, which cause the physical, mental and emotional responses brought on by the original event to be re-experienced. Learning to relax and reframing the experience (e.g. reducing self-blame) are key methods of treatment. Medication can sometimes be used to manage symptoms and social support can provide a sense of belonging and care that will ease the pain.

Phobias Davison and Neale (2001:128) describe a phobia as a disrupting fear and avoidance that is out of proportion to the danger posed by the feared object/situation and which is recognised by the person as groundless. Common phobias include: heights, animals, injections, blood, flying, lifts, open or closed spaces.

PREVALENCE

While not listed as a mental health condition in its own right, stress actually affects a large number of people and can lead to more serious mental and physical health problems. In 2003/4, half a million individuals in the UK reported they were experiencing work-related stress that was making them ill (HSE, 2005) and between 2007/8, it was estimated that 13.5 million work days were lost through stress-related absence (HSE, 2012).

Over 12 million people visit their GP each year for mental health problems and most are diagnosed as suffering from anxiety and depression that is stress related (Daines et al, 1997). Mixed anxiety and depression is reported to affect approximately 9 per cent of the population (MHF, 2007) and it is reported that around 254,000 people first become aware of work-related stress, anxiety or depression in the 12 months prior to actually reporting it (HSE, 2005)!

CAUSES

There are numerous theories regarding the causes of stress and anxiety – these include those listed for depression (see causes of depression above). Often, it may be a combination of factors that can make an individual more vulnerable and an episode of stress and anxiety may be triggered by social and environment factors, which may include:

- **Work**: Change of job, unemployment, redundancy, promotion, retirement
- **Relationships**: Marriage, divorce, birth of child, arguments with partner
- **Financial**: Mortgage, loans
- **Life events**: Death of relatives, partner or friends
- **Family**: Moving house, holidays, trouble with relatives
- **Health**: Changes in health status, diagnosis of medical condition

Table 7.4	Signs and symptoms of stress		
Physical	Mental	Emotional	Behavioural
Spots	Irrational thoughts	Sadness	Eat more or less
Shoulder tension	Mental fatigue	Depression	Drink more or less
Skin disorders	Poor decision making	Helplessness	Smoke more
Chest pain	Low self-esteem	Anger	Swearing
Increased heart rate	Low self-worth	Fear	Aggression
Nervous indigestion	Inability to listen	Panic	Violence
Fast, shallow breathing	Procrastination	Irritability	Crime
Upper back hunched	Excessive self-criticism	Boredom	Crying
Yawning/sighing	Egocentricity	Loneliness	Increased or decreased sexual libido
Increased blood pressure	Accident prone	Jealousy	Excessive talking
Abdominal pain	Making more mistakes	Resentment	Foot tapping

SIGNS AND SYMPTOMS OF STRESS/ANXIETY

There are numerous signs and symptoms of stress and anxiety, which can manifest in different ways (see table 7.4).

In instances where stress is prolonged, for example, being out of work for a long time or experiencing the effects of a debilitating condition (e.g. rheumatoid arthritis), the body has to find additional ways to cope. In such times the pituitary gland and adrenal cortex system play a greater role to ensure energy is managed to meet the extra demands. The impact of longer-term stress on the body is outlined in table 7.5.

TREATMENT

Many of the recommended treatments used for depression are prescribed and recommended for stress and anxiety, including cognitive behavioural therapy (CBT), for which there is a strong evidence base (NICE in Davies & Craig, 2009:28), medication and self-help strategies.

Medication

Medication may be prescribed to assist with the management of both depressive and anxiety-related symptoms. The medications for depression would be prescribed to manage the depressive symptoms (SSRIs – see medications for depression, page 85). These would also be used as the first-line treatment for GAD, panic disorders and social phobias (Davies & Craig, 2009:28).

Table 7.5	Some of the longer-term effects of stress and anxiety
Hormonal system	The pituitary-adrenal cortex system is more dominant in terms of long-term stress. Cortisol levels are increased to supply the energy to meet these demands. Excessive levels of cortisol suppress the immune system, which increases susceptibility and vulnerability to other illnesses.
Immune system	Suppression of the immune system increases vulnerability to colds and flu and diseases that affect the immune system itself, such as some cancers.
Sex hormones	The sex hormones increase when we feel more secure. Testosterone (and the female version androstendione) levels can increase when feelings of power, control, dominance and success are experienced. Sex hormones can also play a significant role in social behaviour and relationships (support systems). Suppression of the reproductive system can lead to cessation of menstruation in women, impotence in men and the loss of libido in both genders.
Respiratory system	The effects of long-term stress on the respiratory system may be to induce and increase the symptoms of asthma and other conditions.
Digestive system	Suppression of the digestive system may lead to diseases such as constipation, diarrhoea and irritable bowel syndrome (IBS).
Heart and circulatory system	Excess blood sugars contribute to clog the arteries (athersclerosis) and increase the risk of CHD.
Other systems	Long-term stress can affect blood sugar levels and is linked to adult onset diabetes.

Anxiolytic medication (benzodiaepines) may also be prescribed to reduce the physical symptoms of anxiety and provide a sedative and relaxing effect. However, they should not usually be used beyond 2–4 weeks (Davies & Craig, 2009:29). Beta-blockers may also be prescribed, but usually as a second line of treatment. There are numerous side effects to the medications. Side effects of anxiolytics include daytime drowsiness, dizziness, unsteadiness, muscle weakness, reduced alertness, confusion, blurred vision and slower reactions, and side effects of beta-blockers include hypotension, bradycardia, fatigue, SOB/wheezing, gastrointestinal disturbances, lethargy, sleep disturbance, peripheral vasoconstriction, cold extremities, leg pain and cramps.

Self-help

There are numerous self-help books available to assist with management of stress, anxiety and panic and also depression. Some self-help strategies (positive thinking, relaxation techniques, goal-setting, time management, assertiveness) are discussed in *The Complete Guide to Exercising*

Away Stress (Lawrence, 2005) and *Exercise Your Way to Health: Depression* (Lawrence & Burns, 2011*b*).

Breathing

When anxious and stressed, there is a tendency towards shallow and rapid breathing, using mainly the upper thorax or chest (where the upper chest and shoulders lift and lower as we breathe). Poor breathing habits such as these can contribute to further anxiety and panic, and are more common in people who are sedentary (see chapter 17, page 252 for breathing exercises).

Ideally, the whole of the ribcage and abdomen should be used during breathing (diaphragm and abdominal breathing). Focusing on deeper and slower breathing and allowing the lower ribcage to expand and the tummy to rise and fall during inhalation and exhalation respectively can help to return the body to a more natural and calmer state.

Counselling and psychotherapy

The therapies listed for depression are appropriate for exploring stress and anxiety-related conditions. CBT is usually recommended as the first-line treatment for PTSD, rather than medication (Davies & Craig, 2009:29). The BACP or UKCP would list the names of accredited therapists.

Alternative therapies

The alternative therapies listed for depression would help with the management of stress and anxiety-related conditions and include nutrition, massage, homeopathy and acupuncture (see treatments for depression, page 85).

Relaxation

Learning to relax and release tension from the body and mind can be important for persons with anxiety and stress and other mental health conditions. There is a growing evidence base to support the practice of mindfulness (MHF, 2007). Some simple relaxation exercises with scripts are provided in chapter 17.

EXERCISE RECOMMENDATIONS

Specific training recommendations for frequency, intensity, time and type (FITT) should be prescribed and considered in relation to the individual, and consideration should be given to each of the following:

- the existing fitness level and activity levels of the individual;
- the severity and length of experience of their stress-related condition;
- personal circumstances and support systems;
- previous and current medical history;
- existence of other medical conditions that may be medicated;
- medications.

The activity guidance in chapter 1 would be the starting point for building activity levels for those who are inactive with low fitness.

EXERCISE IMPLICATIONS

The main implications when working with clients experiencing stress or anxiety may be similar to those for clients with depression (see page 87). One of the key factors is for the exercise professional to be empathic and understanding when working with clients and give consideration to other co-morbidities.

Table 7.6	Exercise guidelines for stress and anxiety	
Exercise modality (type)	**Exercise aims (goal outcome)**	**Frequency** **Intensity** **Time**
Aerobic/cardiovascular Large muscle groups e.g. walking, cycling, jogging	Improve aerobic and cardiovascular capacity Progress frequency, intensity and duration as appropriate	3–5 days a week 20–30 minutes 55–85% of age predicted heart rate (APHR) max
Muscle strength Fixed resistance machines Dumbbells Body weight exercises	Improve posture and strength of postural muscles Whole body approach Progress resistance, frequency and repetitions remain constant	8–12 repetitions 1 set @ 60–85% of 1RM 2 days a week 8–10 separate exercises
Flexibility Stretching for all major muscles	Increase/maintain ROM Stretch to point of mild discomfort	Following each session At least 3–5 days a week and ideally every day stretch for 15–30 seconds

Adapted from Hand, Jaggers & Dudgeon in Durstine & Moore (eds) (2009:384)

MUSCULAR AND SKELETAL CONDITIONS

8

Muscular and skeletal conditions are those that affect the muscular system and/or skeletal system and contribute to a reduction in mobility, bringing about physical limitations that effect daily functioning. The conditions discussed in this chapter are:

- Osteoporosis
- Osteoarthritis
- Total hip replacement
- Rheumatoid arthritis
- Low back pain.

OSTEOPOROSIS

Osteoporosis quite simply means 'porous' bones. It occurs when the bones suffer a loss in calcium and other mineral content, which contributes to their becoming thinner, more porous and as a consequence more brittle. This makes the bones more susceptible to breaking (fractures) when put under even the minor stress of an everyday bump or fall, which would not affect a person with a healthy bone mass.

The definitions used for clinical diagnosis are those used by the World Health Organization (WHO) who differentiate between osteopenia and osteoporosis by defining them as follows:

- Osteopenia: Bone mineral density >1 standard deviation below young normal values
- Osteoporosis: Bone mineral density >2.5 standard deviation below young normal values (Smith, Wang & Bloomfield in Durstine & Moore, 2009).

PREVALENCE

The National Osteoporosis Society (2011) reports that one in three women and one in twelve men over 50 will fracture a bone due to osteoporosis. They also report that by the time some women

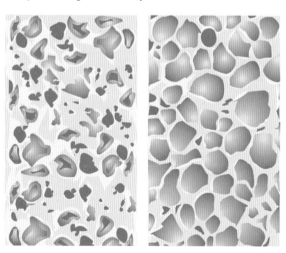

Figure 8.1 Healthy and unhealthy bone mass

reach the age of 70 they have lost anything up to 30 per cent of their bone. The Chief Medical Office report (2004:54), suggested that there are 'around 60,000 osteoporotic hip fractures in the UK each year' and that '15–20 per cent of those people with fractures will die within a year from causes related to the fracture'.

CAUSES

Loss of bone density, or mineral mass, is to some extent a process that is related to the unchangeable and natural process of ageing. Bones stop growing in length in the late teens, between the ages of 16 and 18 years. However, the thickness or density of bones continues to develop and builds to a peak mass until the age of 30. Bone growth (construction and deconstruction) usually stabilises for a few years and then after the age of 35 it steadily begins to deteriorate at a rate of approximately 1 per cent per year, which can be variable and dependent on other genetic and lifestyle factors; many of which can be avoided or minimised to reduce risk.

Some of the genetic and lifestyle factors which contribute to bone density (McArdle, Katch & Katch, 1991:54; Smith, Wang & Bloomfield in Durstine & Moore, 2009:271) include:

- **Gender**: Females have smaller bones and are more susceptible than men. They also experience more significant hormonal changes throughout the lifespan. Women develop bone loss more quickly than men: approximately three times faster. This rate increases during the menopause, when there is an evident reduction of the hormone oestrogen, which influences their bone mass.
- **Age**: Loss of bone density increases with seniority; men are less susceptible to clinically

significant changes before the age of 70, but other lifestyle factors may impact this.
- **Hormones**: women who experience an early menopause (before age 45) are more susceptible due to a reduction in the hormone oestrogen. Men with low testosterone levels are also more at risk. The worst combination for bone health is late onset of menstruation combined with early menopause (CMO, 2005:54).
- **Heredity**: Women with a maternal parent experiencing osteoporosis are more susceptible. In addition, a family history of fractures will also pose an increased risk.
- **Diet**: Diets lacking a sufficient intake of calcium rich foods (yogurt, cheese, sardines, salmon, cereal, almonds, spinach and broccoli) and vitamin D-rich foods (salmon, mackerel, sardines, pilchards, spinach, watercress, liver, soya) will increase risk; diets with an excessive intake of caffeine, protein, alcohol (three or more drinks per day), and carbonated drinks will also increase risk, as these will reduce calcium absorption.
- **Body type**: Slender and lean body frames and individuals with a low body mass index (BMI); and low body weight (who weigh less than 58kg) are more susceptible.
- **Sedentary lifestyle**: Inactivity or lack of weight-bearing exercise contributes to the rate at which the skeleton ages. Muscles pull on bones; this increases blood flow and the delivery of nutrients (calcium). Inactivity and lack of use of specific muscles will affect the density of the specific bones in the less-used areas. Persons with lower muscle mass and lower muscle strength are at risk of lower bone density.
- **Smoking**: Smoking effects the calcification and consequently the mineral content of bones.

- **Prolonged amenorrhoea (pre- and post-menopause)**: Interruptions to monthly cycles (periods) affect hormone levels and bone density.
- **Ethnicity**: Caucasian, Hispanic/Latino and Asian women are more susceptible. African and Caribbean people have a lower risk, as their bones tend to be stronger.
- **Medication**: Some medications contribute to losses of bone density; these include: corticosteroids and anticonvulsants; some treatments for breast cancer (aromatase inhibitors) and treatments for prostate cancer (which affect the production or action of testosterone); some injectable progestogen contraceptives; some medications used to treat psychosis. A GP will consider and discuss the risks prior to prescribing medication.
- **Certain diseases**: Eating disorders (anorexia and bulimia nervosa), asthma, coeliac disease, rheumatoid arthritis and cystic fibrosis all increase the risk of osteoporosis (Smith, Wang & Bloomfield in Durstine & Moore, 2009).
- **Nulliparity**: Women who have never ex-perienced a pregnancy are also more at risk, since hormone levels rise during pregnancy.

SCREENING AND DIAGNOSIS:

There is no national screening programme in the UK, at present. Woman over 50 who have gone through the menopause and have several risk factors may be referred for a DEXA scan (Dual Energy X-Ray Absorptiometry) which uses special X-rays to check bone density. Another test is a DXR (Digital X-Ray Radiogrammetry), which uses less sensitive equipment, but may be offered to individuals who have broken a wrist after a fall.

SIGNS AND SYMPTOMS

Osteoporosis can develop steadily and progressively over several years without any observable signs or symptoms. Osteopenia and osteoporosis are both becoming more prevalent, therefore some conscious awareness raising of the risk factors (via health education and promotion) associated with the condition is essential for persons to identify both their potential risk(s) and the appropriate lifestyle changes they can make to prevent deterioration becoming more rapid. The National Osteoporosis Society (NOS) provides a range of valuable and downloadable resources to support health promotion and public awareness.

In most instances the first indication of osteoporosis is a fracture to a bone (often the wrist) that occurs as a result of a falling accident, which would not occur in a younger person with a healthy bone density who has experienced the same fall or accident. Healthy bones should be able to withstand a fall from standing height without breaking. Typical areas of breakage are the wrist, hip and spine:

- Fractures of the wrist (Colles' fracture), usually occur in middle-aged women who put their arm out in an attempt to break a fall.
- Fractures of the hip joint usually occur in later life (between ages 70 and 80) as the result of a fall, recovery from which can be challenging and can impact independence.
- Fractures of the spine may occur when the condition is in a progressed stage.

In more severe cases of osteoporosis, there may be evidence of changes to the spinal curvatures, in particular of the thoracic spine (but also the lumbar spine). As the vertebrae lose density they crumble, which leads progressively to a decrease in height and contributes to an increased kyphotic curve of the thoracic spine, giving a hunchback appearance (kyphosis). This occurs because of an increased anterior pressure on the vertebrae, which contributes to a wedge-shaped crushing. Kyphosis reduces the mobility in that area of the spine and may also contribute to breathing problems, as the ribs attach with the thoracic spine, and it is the contraction of the intercostal muscles (attached to the ribs) and the diaphragm muscle (lying underneath the ribcage like a hammock) that assists breathing. These factors may also contribute to fractures occurring to the ribs and vertebrae in response to coughing (in severe cases). An extreme kyphotic posture can also increase the risk of falls, because the rounding forward of the spine creates a change in the centre of gravity, which affects the person's balance, stability and coordination.

TREATMENT

Treatment and management of the condition will be dependent on its progression and severity. The condition may be in early stages and undiagnosed (low risk), diagnosed (moderate risk) or in a progressive stage (higher risk). Individuals who present with a more progressed condition may need to be referred to falls prevention services for a specialised and supervised activity programme.

Alternative therapies

There is no substantial evidence base to support the use of alternative or complementary therapies (they are not subject to the same testing as drug interventions). However, many people do find these helpful as part of their treatment plan (NOS, 2011*b*). Therapies may include: massage, acupuncture, herbal medicine, aromatherapy, reflexology, homeopathy, osteopathy and alternative exercise therapies, such as: Tai Chi, Alexander technique, yoga, Pilates and relaxation (see chapter 17, page 252 for an example of the Benson relaxation method).

Nutritional

Eating a healthy diet has an important role in bone health. In addition to following the guidance offered by the DoH (*The Eatwell Plate*), the following guidance is also recommended (Lawrence & Sheppard, 2011 and NOS, 2012):

- Reduce intake of caffeine and carbonated drinks
- Reduce intake of salt
- Increase intake of fruit and vegetables
- Adequate intake of vitamin D-rich foods (salmon, herring, sardines, watercress, spinach, kale, almonds, orange juice etc.)
- Adequate intake of calcium-rich foods (sardines, tofu, almonds, baked beans, boiled spinach, broccoli, kale, oats, whole milk and dairy products)
- Healthy alcohol consumption
- Maintenance of a healthy weight
- Plentiful intake of water.

Exercise professionals should refer clients to a dietician for specialist information and advice.

Medication

There are a number of medications that may be prescribed for the treatment of osteoporosis when diagnosed. Once medication is started, it is likely that it will need to be continued for life. As with any medications, there are often side effects, so medical professionals will consider different needs before making their prescription.

Table 8.1	Medications for osteoporosis
Bisphosphonates (alendronate, risedonate)	These are the most widely used. They are non-hormonal medications. They work by slowing down the cells which break down (deconstruct) bone (osteoclasts) and enable the bone-building (constructing) cells (osteoblasts) to work more effectively.
Calcium and vitamin D supplements	Calcitonin may be prescribed for those at high risk of osteoporosis and for whom bisphosphonates are unsuitable. These are especially beneficial to older people as they can reduce the risk of hip fracture. They are also effective for people who are not very active and may not be getting enough calcium in their diet.
Hormone replacement therapy (HRT)	HRT is less commonly used. HRT uses oestrogen replacement and is prescribed for women during the menopause, as it can help maintain bone density and reduce fracture rates while it is being taken. It can also help diminish some of the side effects of menopause. However, HRT may not be suitable for all women and carries the risk of breast cancer, stroke or thromboembolism (BMA:105).
Selective estrogen receptor modulators (SERMs) (raloxifene)	This acts in a similar way to oestrogen by helping to maintain bone density and reduce the risk of vertebral fractures. It has less risks than HRT and may be prescribed for women who cannot use HRT.
Testosterone	This is prescribed to help maintain bone density for men with low testosterone levels.

EXERCISE GUIDANCE (RECOMMENDATIONS AND LIMITATIONS)

Smith, Wang & Bloomfield in Durstine & Moore (2009:277) offer the exercise guidelines listed in table 8.2. However, any specific exercise recommendation would need to take the following into account:

- the existing fitness level and activity levels of the individual;
- the progressive stage of the condition (severity and longevity of the condition may have an impact on psychological well-being and contribute to depression or anxiety);
- personal circumstances and living/support systems;
- previous and current medical history;
- existence of other medical conditions (co-morbidities) that may be medicated and may present further considerations regarding exercise type and intensity;
- the exercise setting (gym, studio, pool, community centre, residential or care home for the elderly);
- individual factors: age, gender, lifestyle and other associated risk factors (smoking, diet, alcohol etc.).

The general aims of exercise as an intervention for the treatment of osteoporosis would be to maintain bone density, reduce the progression of the condition, strengthen around fracture sites

Table 8.2	Exercise guidelines for osteoporosis	
Exercise modality (type)	**Exercise aims (goal outcome)**	**Frequency** **Intensity** **Time**
Aerobic/cardiovascular Large muscle groups (type of activity depending on BMD and client needs)	Improve or maintain aerobic and cardiovascular capacity Maintain bone mass	3–5 days a week 30–60 minutes 40–70% peak HR, METs
Muscle strength Fixed resistance machines Dumbbells Body weight exercises	Improve posture and strength of postural muscles Maintain bone mass Decrease risk of falls Improve strength of trunk, upper and lower limbs, emphasise strengthening of hip musculature	8–12 repetitions 2 sets @ 75% of 1RM 2–3 days a week for 20–40 mins
Flexibility Stretching Chair-based exercises	Increase/maintain ROM especially hip, knee and pectoral muscles	At least 5 days a week and ideally every day Prolonged hold (30 seconds, as tolerable)
Functional E.g. brisk walking, chair sit to stand, balancing exercises	Increase or maintain ADL Improve balance Decrease risk of falls	3–5 days a week

Adapted from Smith, Wang & Bloomfield in Durstine & Moore (eds) (2009:277)

(hip, wrist and spine), maintain mobility and functioning, improve balance and reduce potential risk of falls.

Individuals in the lower risk grouping can generally participate in mainstream exercise programmes depending on their current fitness and activity levels etc. Individuals in the moderate group risking would need a more carefully considered programme and would be eligible to use exercise on referral. Individuals in a higher risk category will most often be referred to a specialist and/or falls preventions services (see tables 8.3 a–c).

OTHER TYPES OF EXERCISE AND ACTIVITY
Tai Chi
Tai Chi is one of the ancient Chinese martial arts and it uses slow controlled movements, breathing and relaxation (a moving meditation). Tai Chi can improve mobility, assist balance and will provide weight bearing (if standing); it can also be adapted for a seated group. (See chapter 17 – Chiball®, a method which uses components of Tai Chi, as well as other alternative exercise approaches).

Table 8.3a	Risk level and treatment aims: Group 1 (low risk)
Group description and treatment aims	**Exercise and activity aims**
Persons with healthy bone mass or mild changes (osteopenia) with other lifestyle factors that may contribute to reduction in bone mass Prevent deterioration of bone health Reduce the lifestyle risk factors associated with loss of bone density, to include: • reduction of (ideally stopping) smoking; • reduction of alcohol and caffeine intake; • improving diet and eating more calcium and vitamin D-rich foods; • drinking less carbonated drinks; • being more active; • moving more often. Maintain and where possible increase the density of the bone and prevent premature deterioration Raise activity levels to promote maintenance of bone density Activity and exercise can be managed through mainstream activity and exercise sessions	Improve posture to reduce risk of kyphosis through: • spine mobility (trunk rotation); • stretching pectorals, upper trapezius and anterior deltoid; • strengthening lower trapezius (reverse flyes). Consider Pilates/yoga for postural and balance gains Strengthen and increase weight-bearing around potential fracture sites (wrist, hip and spine) e.g. resistance weights or body weight **Upper body**: Chest press, press-ups, dips, shoulder press, biceps curls (wrist extensors/flexors fixate) **Lower body**: Hip abduction, adduction (side leg raises or total hip), extension (gluteal raises), hip flexion (knee raises), squats, leg press, calf raises **Trunk**: Back extension and trunk curls/abdominal hollowing Consider Pilates/yoga for core strengthening and balance benefits **Cardiovascular:** Activities appropriate to current fitness and progress to recommended levels e.g. walk, CV machines, group exercise Some high-impact activities may be appropriate **Activities for daily living**: Climbing stairs, gardening, DIY, walking

Pilates

Pilates focuses on posture, strengthening, mobility, stability and balance. The exercises of the original method have been modified and adapted by some schools, and in their adapted form would be suitable for referred groups.

Chair-based sessions

These are excellent for persons with lower exercise tolerance and higher risk. The focus in these sessions is on improving mobility, flexibility and strength, while the opportunity to take a rest is easily available. These sessions can include activities that relate to daily functions, such as getting up and down from a seated position,

Table 8.3b	Risk level and treatment aims: Group 2 (moderate risk)
Group description and treatment aims	**Exercise and activity aims**
Persons with a clinical diagnosis of osteoporosis without a history of fracture	Improve posture to reduce risk of kyphosis through:
Similar to that of the first group with sensitivity and consideration to medical interventions, especially for post-menopausal women	• spine mobility(trunk rotation); • stretching pectorals, upper trapezius and anterior deltoid; • strengthening lower trapezius (reverse flyes)
Reduce the risk of further deterioration of bone health	Consider Pilates/yoga for postural and balance gains
Reduce the lifestyle risk factors (as table 8.3a)	Promoting balance and maintenance of stability may be a key
Check with GP prior to becoming more active	Strengthen and increase weight-bearing around potential fracture sites (wrist, hip and spine), e.g. with resistance weights or body weight (see table 8.3a for some exercise examples)
Exercise prescription should be offered with greater sensitivity to individual needs, the progressive state of the condition and the increased risk of fractures and falls	Offer greater sensitivity to exercise position, resistance and repetitions and use more care getting into and out of positions
See functional circuit plan as a guideline (pages 245–247)	**Cardiovascular**: Activities of lower impact (walking, cycling, rowing, stepping) with consideration to coordination
	Any balance issues – use more CV machines (e.g. recumbent cycle)
	Activities for daily living: Climbing stairs, gardening, DIY, walking

reaching down to the side to lift something from the floor while seated, and wrist-strengthening exercises with exercise bands to assist with unscrewing jars or buttoning shirts/blouses. A further benefit of these exercises is that they also target key potential fracture sites (wrist, spine and hip). One example of a chair-based activity session is provided in chapter 17.

Exercise in water

Exercise in water offers a supportive exercise environment (once in the pool) and can assist with improvements in mobility, flexibility, strengthening and cardiovascular fitness. Different types of session may include water walking, water running, deep water exercise, aerobics, circuits etc.

Table 8.3c	Risk level and treatment aims: Group 3 (higher risk)
Group description and treatment aims	**Exercise and activity aims**
Persons with advanced changes in bone density with a history of fracture, most commonly the frail and elderly population	Exercise prescription for this group would need to be more considerate of postural and balance changes, lack of mobility and strength and the comparatively low fitness level and tolerance to exercise
The primary aim is to reduce the risk of falls, improve balance and maintain levels of mobility and bone and muscle strength	Risk of falls and fear of falling would also need to be considered
Reduce the lifestyle risk factors (as table 8.3a)	Gentle mobility (include smaller joints – fingers etc.) and postural and balance work to reduce risk of falls and maintain coordination
Check with GP prior to becoming more active	Mobility of the thoracic spine and the mobility and flexibility of the upper body are appropriate (trunk rotations, side bends, shoulder girdle retractions, abdominal hollowing)
This group will need to be managed by more specialist and supervised activity (Level 4)	However, the range of motion may need to be reduced and the speed of movement slowed down; in some instances there may be no or very little range of movement (e.g. spine rotation) and so care must be taken, especially if the person presents with kyphosis that is due to bone deterioration
Hip protectors can be used by those who have a fear of falling	
See seated circuit plan as a guideline (pages 245–247)	**Strengthening** • Can be chair-based and adapted by using resistance bands • Strengthening of the back extensors is particularly important, so they can act as a splint to the crumbling spine • Seated back extensions and spine rotations, or simply sitting upright in a chair
Specialist training to work with frail older adults, persons at risk of falling, Parkinson's Disease and stroke is provided by Later Life Training (www.laterlifetraining.co.uk)	Gentle lateral breathing exercises (as used in Pilates) can also help to improve mobility of the thoracic area
	Functional movement should be promoted (sit to stand, opening jars, buttoning cardigans and shirts)
	Floor exercises are likely to be inappropriate (especially supine lying)
	Cardiovascular: Low exercise tolerance will be an issue, as will balance issues. If able: walking (can be with a stick) or using supportive CV machines (e.g. recumbent cycle) or exercise in water (only if appropriate, which may be highly unlikely for very frail groups)

Exercise in water is less effective for improving bone density because it is non-weight-bearing, however, the muscles still have to pull on bones and this will still have some strengthening effect.

The water should be warm to prevent chilling and the exercise performed at chest depth to maximise buoyancy and promote flotation, which contribute to relieving weight-bearing and can assist with easing and improving range of motion.

Some considerations would be that the hydrostatic pressure of the water could press against the ribcage and make breathing more conscious. This may create an additional risk for persons with breathing and respiratory problems (e.g. asthma, COPD).

EXERCISE CONSIDERATIONS AND IMPLICATIONS

- Avoid forward flexion performed alone or combined with twisting movements as this may contribute to vertebral fractures.
- Avoid high-impact work with clinically diagnosed osteoporotic clients (these may cause fractures) (NOS, 2011:25).
- Avoid dancing movements which may contribute to trips/falls (e.g. crossing legs).
- Avoid ballistic and bouncing movements.
- Control neck movements and avoid rolling the neck backwards (NOS, 2011:25).
- Ensure appropriate and supportive footwear.
- Take care with excessively vigorous exercise.
- Include breathing exercises and pelvic floor exercises.
- Prone and supine lying positions may be inappropriate for persons susceptible to vertebral fractures; use standing and seated alternatives.
- Persons with extreme kyphosis may be able

to walk only with support (to prevent falls) so alternative modes of cardiovascular training, such as a recumbent cycle, may be more appropriate, as this offers some support to the body.
- Ensure environment is free of obstacles to reduce anxiety about falling.
- If weight-bearing exercise is not possible, select chair-based or water-based exercise programmes.
- Target fracture sites (hip, wrist, spine).
- Certain medications may cause uncomfortable side effects and these should be considered prior to making specific exercise recommendations to the individual.
- Any further doubts or concerns should always be discussed with the client's physiotherapist.
- Be aware of other medical conditions (CHD etc.) in more sedentary and senior clients.
- Teach clients correct lifting technique to assist daily functioning.
- Teach clients how to move safely from standing to floor positions and floor to standing using the support of a chair.
- Promote activity in daily living – walking, instead of using the car, gardening, dancing, golf, bowls, standing or sitting with correct posture.
- See also tables 8.3a–c.

OSTEOARTHRITIS

Osteoarthritis is a degenerative condition of the joints that is most commonly brought on by the natural wear and tear associated with daily living and moving. It can also be brought on as a result of an injury or other joint-related condition (NHS Choices, 2012c).

The articular cartilage in the affected joints becomes roughened and eventually thinner (worn down), which makes joint movement less easy and sometimes painful. As the condition worsens, the body attempts to compensate for this thinning: first, the outer edges of the bones thicken and change shape, and bony outgrowths called osteophytes form at the outer edges. Then the membranes lining the joint can become inflamed. This makes movement more uncomfortable, increases pain further and can lead to inflammation and swelling around the joint. In severe cases, calcium can be laid down in the cartilage (calcification), hardening it further.

The primary joints affected are the weight-bearing joints of the body, which include:

- Knees
- Hips
- Lumbar area of the spine
- Wrists and hands

PREVALENCE

Osteoarthritis affects an estimated 8.5 million people in the UK and is more common in women than in men (NHS Choices, 2012d). The National Institute of Arthritis and Musculoskeletal and Skin Diseases (2002) suggests it is more common in men before the age of 45 and more common in women after the age of 45. This may be influenced by a higher participation in sporting activities by men or maybe the types of activities they take part in (contact sports, such as rugby, football and boxing), which, while not exclusive to men, do tend to be male-dominated. NIAMS (2002) also suggests it is a frequent cause of disability among the adult population.

CAUSES

The causes of arthritis are not yet known (NIAMS, 2002). However, it is believed that the following are all contributory factors:

- Ageing brings the culmination of natural wear and tear and is a primary cause and risk, although there are cases of osteoarthritis in younger age groups.
- Being heavily overweight or obese increases the stress on the joints and can contribute to deterioration.
- Injury to the joints makes highly active sportspeople more susceptible.
- Overuse of the joints, including excessive and repetitive joint movements or positions (such as excessive kneeling), may make it more prevalent in specific types of occupation.
- A family history of osteoarthritis increases the risk.

SIGNS AND SYMPTOMS

A combination of examinations would need to be performed for clinical diagnosis and may include a physical examination, clinical history, X-ray, etc. The signs and symptoms of osteoarthritis (including number of symptoms and severity) will vary from one person to another, but can sometimes include:

- damage to the cartilage;
- bony growths around the edge of the joints;
- steady or intermittent pain in the affected joints;
- discomfort or stiffness when moving the joints;
- reduction and limitation to range of motion;
- inflammation and tenderness of the tissues in and around the joint;

- a crunching or creaking feeling when moving the joints;
- joint instability and weakness in surrounding muscles;
- joint deformity.

The impact of the condition on lifestyle and limitations to mobility can also contribute to feelings of helplessness, anxiety and depression.

TREATMENT

There is no cure for osteoarthritis; prevention or reduction of the factors that may contribute to arthritis is the first line of treatment and includes: maintaining an ideal body weight; being active to maintain a wide range of motion in joints and maintain strength of surrounding muscles to assist joint stability; avoiding extremes of activity where the joint(s) may be overstressed, such as prolonged kneeling or excessive impact, or some sports; wearing shock-absorbing insoles in shoes or trainers. Other treatments include medication, physiotherapy and sometimes surgery (NHS Choices, 2012*d*). In severe cases, using a walking aid assists with weight bearing.

Medication

There is a range of medications used to treat osteoarthritis. These aim to reduce pain and limit deterioration in the joints, maintaining their functionality. GPs may prescribe in the first instance a pain reliever such as paracetamol and in some cases stronger painkillers such as co-codamol or co-dydramol, which are a combination of paracetamol and codeine.

If the joint becomes inflamed, non-steroidal anti-inflammatory drugs may be prescribed (NSAID), such as ibuprofen. These medications have anti-inflammatory and analgesic properties to reduce pain, swelling and stiffness in the joints. However, these can sometimes cause side effects, which include indigestion, diarrhoea and gastrointestinal bleeding. These medications could also trigger an asthma attack in asthmatics.

In more extreme cases where the joint(s) become very painful, localised corticosteroid injections can be effective for reducing pain and swelling. However, Minor and Kay (2003) suggest that these injections should not be administered too frequently as they can cause tissue destruction. The type and intensity of activity after an injection would also need to be considered. In some instances, no exercise should occur for two weeks following an injection. Corticosteroids are not usually recommended on a long-term basis because they have serious side effects, which include weight gain, increased risk of osteoporosis, muscle weakness, thinning of the skin, and can worsen conditions such as diabetes (NHS Choices, 2012*d*).

Surgery

In extreme cases, surgery can be used as a treatment. The NHS in England and Wales performs over 140,000 hip and knee replacement operations every year (NHS Choices, 2012*d*). Hip replacements are usually effective for about 10 years and can bring about improved mobility and pain reduction. Knee replacements are more complex, but again can eventually improve mobility and reduce pain. As with all surgery, there are risks associated that are similar for most major surgical procedures.

Exercise

Although certain types of exercise may be contraindicated, it is generally recommended to keep the joints moving. Mobility and flexibility exercises will help to maintain and improve range of motion. Muscular strength and endurance activities will help to strengthen the muscles around the joints, to maintain or improve joint stability. These exercises can also assist with reducing pain. Cardiovascular activities are important to maintain fitness of the heart and lungs and prevent coronary heart disease etc., which can lead to further disability. The type of activity selected will be dependent on the severity of the condition and other factors specific to the individual, for example, age, previous exercise and activity levels, other medical conditions and medications etc. A general recommendation would be for cardiovascular activities to be non-weight-bearing for the specific affected joint(s).

EXERCISE GUIDANCE (RECOMMENDATIONS AND LIMITATIONS)

Some general guidelines for working with persons with osteoarthritis include:

- **Mobility and flexibility exercises** will maintain joint mobility and range of motion. The range of motion, speed and repetitions for each movement will need to be adapted for the specific individual, to accommodate the severity of the condition. These exercises can be performed in a weight-bearing position if comfortable, or can be performed on a chair to reduce weight bearing. They can also be performed in a non-weight-bearing environment, such as a swimming pool. Exercising in chest-depth water offers the body buoyancy, supporting its weight and making movement of the joints much easier and more comfortable, thereby allowing joint movement to be increased while in the water. Exercise in water can also help to reduce swelling around the joint (Lawrence, 2004a).

- **Strengthening exercises** It is essential to condition the muscles sufficiently in order to maintain joint stability. Muscle conditioning work is also essential before increasing the workload of any other activities, although again this will be dependent on the individual and factors specific to him or her (current fitness and activity levels etc.). Weight-bearing exercises do not have to be excluded, but consideration must be given to the severity of the condition. For example, the performance of squatting movements (as in sit to stand) may be comfortable for some people if the speed of the movement is controlled, repetitions limited, and the individual works to a range of motion that is comfortable for them with correct alignment. A benefit of this type of exercise is that it is functional and relates to activities the person would need for daily living. However, this type of exercise may be totally inappropriate for a person with more progressive arthritis in the knee joint, and an alternative strengthening exercise such as leg extensions (using fixed resistance machines or bands or trainer resistance) may be more appropriate. Additionally, it may be worth starting with isometric exercises (no or small range of movement) and progressing to isotonic exercises (full range of movement), increasing the repetitions gradually (one repetition at a time) and monitoring any increase in pain occurring after exercise (>2 hours). If weight-bearing activities are too uncomfortable, chair-based strengthening exercises can be an alternative; so too can specific water-based strength exercises.

- All exercise and activities used should be low impact in nature as high-impact work increases stress on the joints. In addition, the repetitions of specific joint movements need to be reduced to avoid overuse and repetitive strain. The speed of exercise and range of motion should always be adapted to suit the individual's ability.

- **Cardiovascular activities** It is important to maintain cardiovascular fitness (health of the heart and lungs) and prevent associated conditions (high blood pressure, CHD etc.). The exercises and activities should be low impact, such as walking, cycling, swimming or exercise in water. However, care must be taken to avoid over-repetition. Thus, it may be advisable for some to accumulate activity over the day and follow the activity guidelines suggested in chapter 1, table 1.2 (see page 16).

EXERCISE IMPLICATIONS

- High-impact activities and contact sports should be avoided.
- Use correct footwear and shock-absorbing insoles for any weight-bearing activities.
- Excessive repetitions of same joint movement, particularly weight bearing (step machines, high repetition resistance training) should also be avoided. In some instances, excessive cycling can aggravate the condition, and cross training methods are more effective to vary joint stress.
- Prolonged activities in the same exercise position, such as kneeling or resting on all

fours, should be avoided. If these activities are included, regular rests should be offered. Alternatively, a hand weight with a flattened edge can be held to support the all-fours position to maintain wrist alignment, as opposed to resting on the palms of the hands.

- Avoid activities where direction changes are excessive or fast.
- Reduce intensity and duration of exercise and/ or use a different activity mode (e.g. exercise in water) if joint pain or swelling appears or continues.
- Side effects of any medications should be considered prior to making specific exercise recommendations to the individual.
- Other medical conditions, such as depression or CHD in cases of prolonged inactivity, would also need to be considered.
- See also implications for rheumatoid arthritis (page 111).

Any further doubts or concerns should always be discussed with the client's GP.

TOTAL HIP REPLACEMENT

A hip replacement or other joint replacement is a surgical procedure used to replace a joint (partially or fully) where disease (e.g. osteoarthritis) has worn down the joint tissue. Total hip replacement can be effective in relieving pain and improving function of the joint for approximately 10 years (Prodigy 2005*d*).

A new joint will be unstable and more susceptible to dislocation for a few weeks after the operation, thus great care must be taken when moving. During the post-operative phase, patients will be guided by a health professional regarding

Table 8.4	Exercise guidelines for arthritis	
Exercise modality (type)	**Exercise aims (goal outcome)**	**Frequency** **Intensity** **Time**
Aerobic/cardiovascular Large muscle groups (depending on client needs) Swimming, water-based, dance, walking, cycling, rowing	Improve or maintain aerobic and cardiovascular capacity and endurance	3–5 days a week 5–10 minutes and building to 30 minutes 60–80% peak HR
Muscle strength Fixed resistance machines Free weights Isometric exercises Body weight exercises Circuit training	Improve strength around affected joints Increase repetition maximum Increase repetitions and resistance	2–3 and building to 10 repetitions 1 or more sets 2–3 days a week
Flexibility Stretching May be chair-based exercises	Increase/maintain ROM especially around affected joints Reduce joint stiffness	At least 5 days a week and ideally every day Before aerobic or strength activities
Functional E.g. brisk walking and other ADLs	Increase ADL Improve balance	Not specified

Adapted from Minor, M and Kay, D in Durstine & Moore (eds) (2009, 264)

the type of activity and movement needed to assist their rehabilitation. Most people are back to normal functioning within six months, provided that no other complications present.

EXERCISE RECOMMENDATIONS

- Walking;
- gentle cycling;
- low range of motion in all hip movements;
- low resistance;
- progress steadily;
- strengthen muscles around hip joint: hip flexors, hip extensors (gluteus maximus), adductors and abductors;
- exercise in water (deep water).

EXERCISE LIMITATIONS AND CONSIDERATIONS

- For hip replacement, only limited abduction will be possible.
- Avoid adduction across the midline of the body.
- Hip flexion should be encouraged only to hip height (not more than 90 degrees).

- Avoid breaststroke leg action when swimming.
- Seated exercises can be performed in a chair where the buttocks are positioned slightly higher than the knees (a more comfortable joint angle at the hip).
- Static contractions to strengthen abductors can be appropriate (seated outer thigh exercise using resistance band or hands to resist movement).

RHEUMATOID ARTHRITIS

Rheumatoid arthritis is an auto-immune disease that causes chronic inflammation. Auto-immune diseases occur when the antibodies produced by the body's immune system, which normally fight foreign substances such as viruses and bacteria, attack other tissues in the body because they identify them as foreign tissue. Rheumatoid arthritis is also referred to as a systemic disease because it affects multiple organs in the body, not just the joints.

The joints most affected are the smaller joints of the wrists, hands, fingers and toes, although as a systemic condition, it can occur anywhere in the body. In some instances the chronic inflammation can destroy other joint tissues such as cartilage, bone, ligaments and tendons, which causes the joints to become swollen, painful, stiff and sometimes deformed.

PREVALENCE

Rheumatoid arthritis is less common than osteoarthritis, but is more severe. In the UK, the disease affects around 400,000 people. It is three times more common in women than men and can begin at any age, although it most commonly occurs between the ages of 40 and 60 (NHS Choices, 2012d).

CAUSES

The causes of rheumatoid arthritis are unknown, however, it is suspected that certain infections or triggers in the environment may cause the body to attack its own tissues.

SIGNS AND SYMPTOMS

When the body tissues are inflamed (flare-up) the condition is considered to be active and when inflammation subsides the condition is considered to be in remission. During a flare-up the symptoms can include:

- fatigue;
- loss of appetite;
- muscle aches;
- fever;
- joint stiffness after periods of inactivity (particularly in the morning);
- red, swollen and painful joints, which in severe cases can become deformed.

Rheumatoid arthritis is a systemic disease and is not isolated to the joints. It can cause inflammation of other tissues around the eyes and other vital organs of the body such as the heart, lungs, etc.

It is essential to be aware of emotional and mental symptoms in addition to the physical symptoms. The disability and deformity that can be caused by the condition can impact daily activities (work etc.) quite significantly and can contribute to feelings of emotional distress, hopelessness, anxiety and depression.

TREATMENT

The main goal of any treatment is to:
- reduce joint inflammation and pain;
- prevent destruction and deformity of the joints;
- maintain joint functionality.

Treatment usually involves a combination of medication, joint strengthening exercises and mobility and rest. In severe cases surgery can be used to restore joint mobility, repair damage to joints and sometimes replace joints with artificial materials. The use of support groups and counselling can also help individuals to manage the emotional stress, discuss problems associated with changes to their physical condition and provide education about their illness.

Medication

Painkillers such as paracetamol or co-codamol may be prescribed for pain relief. Aspirin and ibuprofen (NSAIDS) are the fast-acting first line of treatment to reduce swelling and relieve stiffness and pain. Corticosteroids may also be prescribed. The side effects of corticosteroids (see osteoarthritis, page 105) include thinning of the skin and bone (which adds the risk of osteoporosis), weight gain (which can place further stress on the joints, if unmanaged) and easier bruising. Disease-modifying anti-rheumatic drugs (DMARDS) are the slower acting second line of drug treatment, which aims to prevent the progressive destruction to the joint tissues and, if effective, promote the remission phase of the condition. Side effects of DMARDS include sickness, diarrhoea, mouth ulcers, hair loss or thinning and skin rashes (NHS Choices, 2012e).

Exercise

Regular exercise plays an important role in maintaining joint mobility and strength of the muscles around the joint. However, the degree of joint destruction will affect the type of exercise that can be performed. Painful joints should be rested and not exercised during a flare-up, but once pain eases, stretching and mobility exercises, gentle weight-training to increase muscle strength and cardiovascular activities such as swimming and cycling can be performed. Exercise in water is particularly beneficial as water offers support to the body and the increased buoyancy minimises stress on the joints. Water also adds a resistance to movement that can be utilised to increase muscular strength and cardiovascular gains. Managing body weight and losing excess weight can prevent additional stress on the joints.

EXERCISE RECOMMENDATIONS

The most essential point is that *no* exercise should be performed on the affected joints when the condition is active (in a flare-up phase) because this may worsen the damage (the exception may be some gentle warming and stretching exercises, as suggested by Minor and Kay, 2009). During a remission phase, exercise and activity can resume with a focus on maintaining joint mobility and range of motion and maintaining or increasing strength of the muscles around the joint. However, the speed of movement, range of motion, repetitions and any resistance must be adapted to suit the individual's ability. In most cases, the intensity (repetitions, rate, ROM, resistance) of any exercise will need to start low and progress gradually.

The exercise guidelines offered for osteo-arthritis can be applied to rheumatoid arthritis (see table 8.4, page 108). Again, particular consideration needs to be given to the severity of the condition and limitation of movement in damaged or deformed joints before recommending any specific exercise or activity.

EXERCISE LIMITATIONS AND CONSIDERATIONS

- Never exercise the affected joints during a flare-up as this may cause further damage to the joint structure.
- Be considerate to any past damage to the joints as this may affect the intensity, range of motion and speed of movement that is achievable.
- During remission periods work on maintaining strength of muscles around the joint and working through full range of motion.
- Avoid high-impact activities or contact sports.
- Avoid stop and start actions (Minor & Kay, 2009:264).
- Avoid stair climbing (Minor & Kay, 2009:264).
- Avoid activities using a prolonged one leg stance (Minor & Kay, 2009:264).
- Avoid activities that cause pain.
- Avoid excessive repetitions of same joint movement.
- Reduce workload if pain or swelling occurs.
- Some exercise positions may not be appropriate, for example resting on all fours will be uncomfortable for wrists.
- Avoid over-stretching and hypermobility.
- Avoid fast-paced movements and/or quick changes of direction.
- Advise exercise in the afternoon or evening to avoid morning stiffness.
- Reduce intensity and duration of exercise and/or use a different activity mode (e.g. exercise in water) if joint pain or swelling appears or continues.
- Side effects of any medications should be considered prior to making specific exercise recommendations to the individual.
- Recommend cross training to vary joint stress.

- Allow an accumulated approach to activity.
- Stretching and warm up activities may be performed daily even during a flare-up (Minor & Kay, 2009:263).
- Use a combination of weight-bearing, non-weight-bearing (exercise in water) and partial weight-bearing activities.
- Emotional and stress-related conditions, such as depression, that may occur in response to the condition should be considered.
- Expect some post-activity discomfort (Minor & Kay, 2009:264).
- The risk of CHD in cases of prolonged inactivity should be considered.
- An occupational therapist or physiotherapist may use splint supports to assist performance of some movements. Sometimes devices to assist with lifestyle activities, such as jar grippers and toilet-seat lifters, are used to assist with daily activities.
- See also implications for osteoarthritis (page 107).

Any further doubts or concerns should always be discussed with the client's GP.

NON-SPECIFIC LOW BACK PAIN (SOMETIMES REFERRED TO AS SIMPLE LOW BACK PAIN)

Non-specific low back pain (LBP) is described as back pain for which the exact cause is not known, but which can usually be attributed to problems with the structures of the spine (NICE, 2009; Patient UK, 2012). LBP can be either acute (less than six weeks) or chronic (more than twelve weeks).

Low back pain can contribute to a significant restriction in movement that makes daily activities uncomfortable, painful and sometimes more difficult and may also lead to psychological distress (stress, depression). The pain can vary from severe and long term, to mild and short-lived. Low back pain will usually resolve within a few days or weeks for most people; however, episodes can be recurrent.

Although most LBP is not due to any serious disease, there are some instances of LBP that are caused by more serious conditions (fractures, cancer or infections). A GP's advice should always be sought. See 'red flags' listed in signs and symptoms (page 114).

STRUCTURES OF THE LOWER BACK

The lower back (lumbosacral area) is between the bottom of the rib cage and top of the legs and comprises of the following structures:

- Five irregular bones (the lumbar vertebrae) with inter-vertebral discs between each bone and spinous processes at the back of the vertebral bones that form the attachment points for all the muscles.

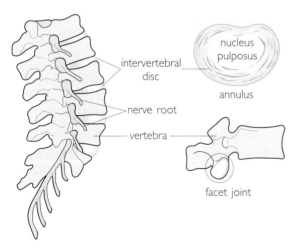

Figure 8.2 Lower back vertebrae and discs

- The inter-vertebral discs, with a strong fibrous external layer and a gel-like pulp in the centre. These allow the spine to be flexible and act as shock absorbers (Patient UK, 2012*a*).
- The spinal cord and nerves, which run through the centre of the vertebral column and are protected by the bony structures of the spine. The nerves transmit messages to and from the brain.
- Strong ligaments, which attach to adjacent vertebral bones, giving support and stability.
- Various muscles, surrounding the spine, which move (mobilise) and help to stabilise the spine (transversus abdominus, multifidus, internal and external obliques, rectus abdominus, erector spinae and other stabilisers of the pelvis which will also affect posture).

PREVALENCE

Low back pain is very common, affecting eight out of ten (80 per cent) of people in the UK at some point in their lives (CMO, 2004; NICE, 2009), with an estimated 150 million working days being lost each year due to low back pain. It occurs equally between men and women and most commonly between the ages of 30 and 50 and accounts for approximately 4 per cent of visits to the GP (Prodigy, 2005*c*).

CAUSES

A number of lifestyle factors may contribute to the risk and trigger an episode of LBP (many of which relate to poor static and dynamic posture). These include:

- manual handling – the lifting and carrying of heavy loads, which includes lifting people and also resistances that are positioned awkwardly or too heavy;

- sustained awkward postures and repetitive movements, which include bending, twisting, over-stretching and sustained static postures (driving, standing or sitting for long periods of time); poor positioning of desks, slouching in chairs (including crossing of the legs when seated, which contributes to pelvic misalignment) and at work stations or while driving, all of which contribute to postural misalignment and may lead to atrophy of some of the spine stabilisers (e.g. multifidus);
- whole body vibration (which can occur when truck driving or drilling);
- heavy physical work (building and labouring);
- heavy sporting activities (weight-lifting) can have an adverse effect on the spine
- other medical conditions: sciatica, whiplash, frozen shoulder, ankylosing spondylitis, slipped disc etc.;
- damage or wear and tear to the spinal structures;
- overweight/obese – the increased weight creates pressure on the spine;
- pregnancy – during the antenatal period the weight of the baby can increase the strain on the spine, contributing to postural misalignment and pelvic instability. During the post-natal period, relaxin levels may continue to affect pelvic stability and new mothers will need to be mindful of their posture when lifting and carrying;
- smoking, which may be due to tissue damage or because smokers tend to lead less healthy lifestyles;
- stress – due to increased tension in the muscles;
- psychological factors (lack of self-esteem, self-worth, satisfaction, confidence etc.);

- some medications, such as corticosteroids, which weaken bones.

(Adapted from NHS Choices, 2010; Patient UK, 2012a)

Consultation with a GP is essential to identify potential causes and associated problems, so that appropriate treatment and management can be recommended.

SIGNS AND SYMPTOMS

Symptoms include pain, discomfort, tension and soreness in the lower back with about 70 per cent of people reporting the experience of a dull and poorly localised referred pain to the legs and buttocks, and some people reporting pain in the shoulders and neck (Prodigy 2005c, NHS Choices, 2010).

With appropriate management most people are pain free and able to resume normal activities within a few days or weeks. However, low back pain can vary in the intensity of pain experienced and is usually recurrent. Table 8.5 gives a list of questions that can be used in clinical practice to assess the severity of back pain (mild, moderate, severe) and the feeling/sensation of the pain, which people may describe in various ways: throbbing, tingling, stabbing, spasm-like, spider-like, pins and needles etc., see also red flags on page 114.

TREATMENT AND MANAGEMENT

The primary guidance recommended by NICE (2009) is for individuals to be educated and learn how to self-manage and also take part in structured exercise.

Medication

Medication may be offered to relieve pain but cannot cure the condition. Paracetamol is

Table 8.5	Questions for assessing the severity of back pain
Does back pain limit you?	**Standard limits:**
Standing	Standing in one place for less than 30 minutes
Walking	Walking less than 30 minutes or 1–2 miles
Travelling by car or bus	Travel less than 30 minutes
Socialising	Miss or curtail social activities (excluding sport)
Sleeping	Sleep disturbed by pain at least twice a week
Sex life	Sexual activity reduced or curtailed
Dressing	Help required to put on footwear

Adapted from Prodigy (2005)

Red flags

Signs that may indicate a more serious condition (NHS Choices, 2010/Patient UK, 2012) include:

- A fever of 38°C (100.4°F) or above
- Unexplained weight loss
- Pain that is higher in the back behind the chest
- Swelling of the back
- Drug use
- HIV
- Constant pain that does not ease after lying down
- Pain or weakness in the lower legs
- Loss of bladder or bowel control
- Numbness around buttocks, back passage or genitals, incontinence (equine syndrome)
- Pain that worsens at night
- Back pain following a fall or trauma.

usually the first choice because side effects are low. NSAIDs (ibuprofen) are another option, however, long-term use is not recommended for lower back pain (as this medication can have adverse effects on other conditions, such as asthma, hypertension, etc.). Stronger painkillers, like codeine, are a further option and sometimes a combination of medications can be offered. If pain relievers are ineffective or if muscle spasms are experienced, then muscle relaxants (such as diazepam) may be recommended but only in short courses due to the risk of dependency/addiction (NHS Choices, 2009).

Functional activity

Keeping moving is essential. The spine is designed to move, so bed rest does not promote recovery and can actually prolong pain and disability. During an episode of back pain, most activities need to be adapted and modified slightly, but the focus should be on getting on with life.

Positive mental attitude

Mental attitude has a strong influence on recovery. People who cope and get on with it and who are involved and committed to self-management of the condition (correcting posture, lifting correctly, etc.) usually recover much more quickly and have less long-term trouble. People who are frightened of the pain, fearful of further injury, who avoid activity and rest a lot hoping the pain will go away tend to suffer for longer and increase their risk of becoming more disabled by the condition.

Hot or cold treatments

Hot or cold treatments can be used to provide relief of pain and relax the muscles, e.g. a hot water bottle on the affected area or a hot bath or application of ice packs (dependent on the patient). Specific guidance from a physiotherapist should be sought and followed regarding the application of these treatments.

Massage

A professional massage by a qualified practitioner (chiropractor, physiotherapist, osteopath) can help to soothe pain and relax muscles.

Relaxation and breathing

A usual response when people experience pain is to tense up – this makes the pain worse! Learning to relax and using breathing to promote relaxation can assist with management of pain. Breathing and relaxation activities are explained in chapter 17.

Lifestyle

Work stations/desks Assessing the height and positioning of chairs and desks used at home or work and getting up and moving around and stretching regularly to avoid stiffening up is recommended. A back support can be used when driving and, when possible, regular breaks from driving to stretch out the body should be encouraged.

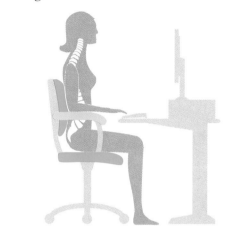

Figure 8.3 Correct work station set-up

Lifting Correct lifting should be practised when moving equipment and/or shopping (ideally, a wheel trolley should be used for shopping).

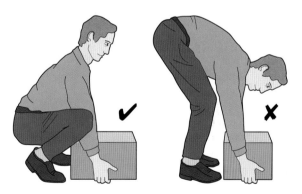

Figure 8.4 Correct and incorrect lifting set-up

Sleeping Sleeping on a firm mattress that supports the body weight sufficiently is important and sometimes changing the sleeping position can help. Side lying sleepers can raise their knees slightly towards their chest and place a pillow between their legs. Back lying sleepers can place a pillow under the backs of the knees, to help maintain a normal spinal curve.

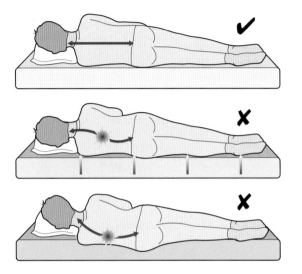

Figure 8.5 Good and bad sleeping set-up

Posture awareness

Prolonged muscle imbalance by holding an incorrect posture will lead to increased muscle tension and tightness and may contribute to low back pain. In addition, poor posture, maintained and uncorrected for long periods of time, can also lead to permanent postural problems, for example lordosis (hollow back) can be a cause of low back pain, and also a hunched back posture (kyphosis) can contribute to the risk of falls in later life. Exercises to open and align posture can help to alleviate a build-up of muscular tension and can also enhance the functioning of inner organs (e.g. diaphragm). Pilates and yoga-based programmes focus on posture, mobility, flexibility and breathing. Learning to stand and sit correctly can be essential as part of self-management.

Abdominal and pelvic floor engagement

It is important for the individual to learn how to use the abdominal muscles and pelvic floor muscles to help support the spine (a selection of pelvic floor exercises are described in chapter 14).

For abdominal engagement, the first step is to find the neutral spine position – the midway point between full extension (hollow back) and flexion (flat back); where the natural curve of the spine is allowed. This can be found in either a standing or seated position (as described in table 8.6) or it can be found on all fours.

All fours abdominal hollowing is achieved as follow:
- Place the hands under the shoulders and the knees under the hips.
- Have your shoulder blades sliding down towards your buttocks, so that the shoulders are away from the ears.
- Engage the abdominals so that the spine rounds upwards slowly.
- Relax slowly down from the position so the back hollows.
- Find the mid-point between the two ends of the movement range.
- Engage the abdominals without changing the spine position.

Engagement is feeling the abdominals lightly pull inwards from all directions (like tightening a corset). Once abdominal hollowing has been achieved, then the next stage is to look at abdominal bracing, where engagement of the inner obliques helps to stabilise the spine further.

Table 8.6	Correct postural alignment	
Standing posture	**Seated posture**
Stand with feet hip-width apart, feet parallel	Sit on a chair with buttocks on the front third of the chair. Feet hip-width apart and parallel. Knees over ankles
Distribute weight between heel bone, big toe and little toe (three-point weight distribution)	Distribute weight evenly between heel bone, big toe and little toe (three-point weight distribution)
Spread toes	Spread toes
Align second toe with knee and hip	Align second toe with knee and hip
Find neutral pelvic position (pubic bone and hip bones in line to ensure minimal forward or backward tilt of pelvis)	Lift out of sitting bones to find neutral pelvic position (pubic bone and hip bones in line to ensure minimal forward or backward tilt of pelvis)
Lengthen torso and neck	Sit upright and lengthen spine; lengthen torso and neck
Engage the deeper abdominal muscles (so that the contraction can be maintained)	Engage the deeper abdominal muscles (so that the contraction can be maintained)
Look forwards – chin parallel to floor	Look forwards – chin parallel to floor
Shoulders relaxed and down	Shoulders relaxed and down
Shoulder blades squeeze down	Shoulder blades squeeze down
Arms relaxed, hands by the side of body	Arms relaxed, hands by the side of chair

EXERCISE RECOMMENDATIONS

Ideally, any specific exercises should be designed in consultation with the client's health professional (GP, physiotherapist). The following are suggested for guidance.

Specific exercises to strengthen the abdominal and back muscles

- Abdominal hollowing (all fours, prone lying, seated or standing)
- Pilates-based abdominal exercises: supine lying heel slides, heel raises, knee raises, lying pelvic tilts, reciprocal reach (progressing from cat peddles, pin point arms, then legs before both, adapted side plank etc.)
- Adapted curl-ups such as McGill sit-ups, to working towards more complex postures such as one knee bent and one extended, and back extensions
- Bridge to strengthen gluteals and assist mobility.

Gentle mobility of the spine

- Side bends (seated or standing)
- Gentle rotations (seated or standing)
- Pilates-based mobility exercises for the spine (spine rotations, pelvic tilts, shoulder bridge, knee drops, etc.).

Flexibility exercises

- Hip flexors
- Erector spinae
- Upper trapezius
- Hamstrings
- Piriformis
- Abductors
- Obliques.

Pelvic floor exercises

See chapter 17 for examples.

Core ball exercises

Maintaining correct seated posture while sitting on a core ball can assist in strengthening the abdominals. However, the individual should have sufficient strength to perform on a stable surface before progressing to using an unstable surface. Some gentle core ball exercises may include:

- seated pelvic tilts;
- seated heel raises;
- seated leg extensions;
- seated resistance exercises (bicep curls, shoulder press, lateral raise, etc.).

Exercise in water

Exercise in water can be an effective exercise medium for people with low back pain. It provides support to the body weight and may enable exercises to be performed for longer periods. The water provides a massaging effect, which can help to release muscle tension. Also, those who are fearful of hurting their backs can be assured of the additional support offered by exercising in water.

Correct posture and engagement of the abdominals to assist stability must be reinforced when exercising in water as buoyancy can affect both balance and posture.

Swimming may be performed, although care must be taken as some swimming strokes may aggravate low back pain (e.g. breaststroke). See table 8.7 for exercise guidelines.

EXERCISE LIMITATIONS AND CONSIDERATIONS

- Correct posture and technique should be a focus.
- Teach spine sparing strategies at start of programme (lifting, moving from floor to standing, rolling on mats or bed).
- Encourage a longer warm-up to allow for gentle mobilisation and increase the circulation of blood. Morning sessions may need a longer warm-up as the back may be more vulnerable. ROM needs to be built gradually.
- The cool-down should emphasise lengthening tight muscles and promoting relaxation (comfortable positions are needed and may require the use of blankets and pillows to assist relaxation).
- Ensure engagement of abdominals for all exercises.
- Avoid high impact as this may be jarring.
- A postural assessment may be useful to identify and make provision for any muscle imbalances.
- Avoid heavy lifting (weight training).
- Avoid jerking and jarring movements (gyrating movements at rapid speed/some dance styles).
- Avoid trunk exercises during episode of back pain (focus on abdominal hollowing).
- Avoid repetitive bending movements.
- Ensure correct lifting techniques.
- Avoid fast twisting or bending movements of the spine.

Table 8.7	Exercise guidelines for low back pain	
Exercise modality (type)	**Exercise aims (goal outcome)**	**Frequency** **Intensity** **Time**
Aerobic/cardiovascular Large muscle groups (depending on client needs)	As per general populations (see chapter 2) unless other specific co-morbidities present	See chapter 2 General guidance for healthy adults, but may need to adapt type of exercise to accommodate specific needs
Muscle strength Core muscle focus	Increase abdominal strength Increase lumbar extensor strength	Under 50: 10–15 reps Over 50: 8–12 reps >2 days a week
Flexibility Stretching that does not increase LBP	Increase/maintain ROM, especially trunk and hip flexor and extensor	2 min/muscle groups 30-second hold Point of mild tension without loss of technique
Functional E.g. brisk walking, sit to stand, correct lifting	Increase and maintain ADL	Brisk walk 3–5 days a week Chair sit to stand for 1 minute, 2–3 days a week

Adapted from Simmonds & Derghazarian in Durstine & Moore (2009:268)

- Avoid exercises that apply a heavy load to the spine, e.g. double leg raising, straight leg sit-ups, straight leg dead lifting.
- Avoid staying in one position for too long.
- Gentle mobility and stretching activities for the spine can be performed (adapted Pilates) and modifications to ROM can be made to suit client needs.

- Contraindications for any other co-existing medical conditions should also be considered.

Please note: There is a Level 4 qualification for exercise professionals who would like to work specifically with persons with back pain. This chapter provides basic guidance for Level 3 Exercise Professionals.

// OBESITY

9

Obesity can be defined as a significant excess of body fat that presents an increased risk to health (WHO, 2012). Obesity is generally measured using the body mass index (BMI; see box). A BMI of 25 or more would classify a person as being overweight and a BMI of 30 would classify a person as obese (see also table 9.1).

> ## Calculating body mass index
>
> BMI = Weight (kg) ÷ Height squared (m²)
>
> **For example**: For an individual who weighs 70kg with their height being 1.75m.
>
> The calculation would be:
> 70kg ÷ 1.75m x 1.75m = 22.9 BMI

Over a decade ago, Waine (2002:2) suggested that obesity was 'the major nutritional disorder facing westernised civilisations'. It is currently being reported as the fifth leading risk for global deaths (WHO, 2012), with at least 2.8 million adults dying each year as a result of being overweight or obese. In addition, while it was once believed to be a condition affecting only countries with high income, it is now being reported as an increasing problem in low- to middle-income countries, particularly in urban settings (WHO, 2012).

Obesity and being overweight are also risk factors for other, more serious health conditions, such as CHD, respiratory conditions, type 2 diabetes, joint problems (osteoarthritis), hypertension (high blood pressure), hyperlipidaemia (high cholesterol), stroke and some cancers (Waine, 2002; Wallace, 2003; McArdle, Katch & Katch, 1991; WHO, 2012). It can also create an additional hazard and complications for individuals during pregnancy and/or for individuals undergoing surgery. Its contribution as a risk for other medical conditions means that it is fast becoming a major economic burden for the healthcare services in most developed countries (Waine, 2002).

In addition to the physical and medical problems, the psychological impact of the condition should also be seriously considered: social discrimination (prejudice and bullying), which includes being picked on at school or work, being labelled, being judged or being called names, all contribute to wounding an individual psychologically. In addition, the struggle that many individuals face with experiences of dieting and trying to lose weight may contribute to feelings of distress, hopelessness, powerlessness, lowered self-esteem and depression. Obesity therefore has serious implications for an individual's overall health (physical, medical, mental, emotional and social) and overall well-being.

However, the paradox of obesity is that while the medical profession has been willing to recognise and treat the complications of obesity, it has been much less willing to treat obesity as a 'disease in its own right and devote it the time and attention that it deserves' (Waine, 2002:27).

As indicated above, the most common measure to define obesity is the BMI (body mass index). The key advantage of this measure is that it is non-invasive. However, one disadvantage of the BMI calculation scale (see table 9.1) is that it does not distinguish the actual percentage of body fat, for example, a bodybuilder with low body fat

and a high muscular weight might be classified as obese when calculating their weight in relation to their height.

Another key disadvantage of using the BMI scale is that it fails to distinguish between general obesity and truncal (central) obesity (storage of fat in the trunk area of the body, which represents the apple-shaped rather than the pear-shaped body, storage of fat around the hips and thighs). Truncal obesity is associated with other risk factors that include insulin resistance, hyperinsulinaemia, decreased glucose tolerance, decreased HDL (high-density lipoproteins) cholesterol, elevated LDL (low-density lipoproteins) cholesterol and triglycerides, and hypertension (high blood pressure); this combination of symptoms is often known as 'syndrome X' (Waine, 2002:5).

Table 9.1	BMI/waist circumference measurements and health risk				
BMI	Classed as	Waist circumference			
		Men 94–102cm	Men >102cm	Women 80–88cm	Women >88cm
<18.5	Underweight	No increased risk	No increased risk	No increased risk	No increased risk
18.5 to 24.9	Ideal Healthy weight	No increased risk	Increased risk	No increased risk	Increased risk
25 to 29.9	Overweight	Increased risk	High risk	Increased risk	High risk
30 to 39.9	Obese	High health risk	Very high health risk	High risk	Very high health risk
> 40	Very obese	Very high health risk	Very high health risk	Very high health risk	Very high health risk

Adapted from Prodigy (2003); NOO (2009)

Taking a waist measurement can give a further guide to risk. The waist circumference indicators combined with BMI measures (see table 9.1) are suggested to offer a more accurate indicator of health, especially in older people and people from South Asia. These recommended indicators are those endorsed by NICE (WHO, 2012). People from South Asia are prone to carrying excess truncal or central fat and should therefore be aware of the risk attached to obesity health risks at a lower BMI and potentially lower waist circumference levels (see table 9.2).

In addition, central adiposity measurements have been shown to predict future ill health, independently of BMI (NOO, 2009). The waist circumference measurement is the most common tool used in public health to assess risk because it is simpler than other measures (e.g. hip:waist ratio or waist:height ratio), with less potential for inaccuracy of measure (e.g. one measure rather than two and limited calculations needed). However, there is some evidence to suggest the other measures are superior, but this is inconclusive (NOO, 2009).

PREVALENCE

Worldwide obesity rates have more than doubled since 1980. In 2008, 1.5 billion adults were reported as being overweight and of these 200 million men and 300 million women worldwide were obese (WHO, 2011).

It was reported in 2008, that 25 per cent of adults over the age of 16 (in England alone) were obese and 32 per cent of women and 42 per cent of men were overweight. It is predicted that by 2025, 50 per cent of men and a third of women will be obese. Obesity is also increasing in children, and affects one in every six boys and one in every seven girls, with a reported one in every seven children being overweight (NHS Choices, 2012).

The number of prescriptions to treat obesity has risen ten-fold since 1999, from 127 thousand to 1.28 million in 2008 and the number of bariatric surgery treatments has also increased from 1951 between 2006/7 to 4221 between 2008/9, a more than 50 per cent rise in a two-year period (Health and Social Care Information Centre, 2012).

CAUSES

There is no conclusive evidence as to what specifically causes obesity, and it is not simply a result of gluttony and over-eating, which is a common belief. Most people will put on weight if the energy they put into their body (food and drink) exceeds their energy output (activity and exercise). However, there are a number of other multi-level factors that may contribute as causes for obesity, including:

- environmental and social factors (eating patterns, changes in technology, media, social class, education, marketing of food, food packaging, the diet industry, exercise and activity promotion, levels of inactivity, junk food, increased TV and computer games and/ or computer-based work);
- genetic factors (having parents who are obese, which may be linked more with learning poor eating habits, although it may be that other genetic factors such as hormones and chemicals that control appetite may be faulty);
- physiological factors (metabolic rate, body type, fat cells);
- psychological factors (body image, eating patterns in relation to mood, trauma, abuse, comfort eating etc. Many people with mental health conditions often have obesity as a

Waist (men)	Waist (Asian men)	Waist (women)	Waist (Asian women)	Health risk
94cm (37in)		80cm (32in)		Increased health risk
102cm (40in)	>90 cm (36in)	88cm (35in)	>80cm (32in)	High health risk

Table 9.2 Waist circumference and health risk

Adapted from Prodigy (2003); Diabetes UK (2004); NICE (2006); International Diabetes Association recommendations in NOO (2009)

co-morbidity; as weight gain is a side effect of some medications);

- medical factors (less than one in 100 obese people have a medical cause, such as underactive thyroid. Some medications can contribute to weight gain, such as antidepressants and steroids).

These factors are to some extent intertwined, and each one will have an impact on another (Waine, 2002:12; McArdle, Katch & Katch, 1991:657; Prodigy, 2005f).

However, the impact of decreasing activity levels in response to an increasing reliance and dependence on technology, e.g. motorised transport (inactive travel), energy-sparing devices, lifts, escalators, video games, television and central heating; and changes in dietary habits over the last half-century, e.g. eating higher-fat diets and snacking, which can reduce the conscious recognition of food being eaten (non-mindful eating) and satiety are recognised as being high contributory factors (Waine, 2002:13; Durstine & Moore, 2003:149).

Obesity often starts in childhood and this factor increases the prevalence of adult obesity at a ratio of approximately 3:1 in comparison to children of a normal body mass (McArdle, Katch & Katch, 1991:656).

SIGNS AND SYMPTOMS

The major sign of obesity is obvious: obese people 'wear their problem for all to see at all times' (Waine, 2002:2). The psychological signs and symptoms, however, are usually much deeper and less observable. The impact of social prejudices and ignorance that begin in childhood in the playground can have long-lasting effects on the individual's self-esteem and self-worth, which will also impact their levels of motivation and self-efficacy, which are key factors for engaging with (and sustaining) lifestyle change.

TREATMENT

The aim of any treatment should be focused on managing rather than losing weight and measures of success need to be focused around effects of changes made to the individual's overall health and well-being, rather than changes to their body weight per se. Even minor weight losses (5–10 per cent) can assist with the reduction of other risk factors/conditions such as high blood pressure, high cholesterol, diabetes, osteoarthritis, respiratory disorders, etc.

OBESITY

Weight management and lifestyle interventions

NICE (2006*a*) guidance for adults (without other medical conditions) is to follow a reputable (based on best practice) weight loss programme (e.g. commercial or self-help groups, books or websites). Best practice guidance indicates the programme should be based on the following principles:

- A balanced diet (see nutritional guidance)
- Recommends no more than 0.5–1 kg as a weekly weight loss
- Encourages regular exercise

People with other specific medical conditions (e.g. type 2 diabetes, heart failure, uncontrolled hypertension or angina) should check with their GP's surgery or hospital dietician before starting a weight loss programme (NICE, 2006*a*).

Nutritional guidance

NICE (2006*a*) offer the following guidance for individuals:

- Base meals on starchy carbohydrate foods such as potatoes, bread, rice and pasta (ideally wholegrain).
- Limit calorie/energy intake from fats.
- Eat plenty of fibre-rich foods, such as oats, beans, peas, lentils, grains, seeds, as well as wholegrain bread, brown rice and pasta.
- Increase consumption of fruit and vegetables, as well as legumes, whole grains and nuts.
- Eat as little as possible of fried foods, drinks and confectionery high in added sugars and other food and drinks high in fat and sugar, such as some take-away and fast foods.
- Eat breakfast.
- Monitor portion size of meals and snacks, and how often you are eating.

- Avoid taking in too many calories in the form of alcohol.

NICE (2006*a*) also highlights the responsibility of the food industry, workplace and schools in promoting healthy eating, which includes:
- making a range of nutritious foods accessible, available and affordable;
- responsible marketing;
- reducing the salt, fat and sugar content within processed foods.

Medication

Medication should only be prescribed if diet and exercise have been tried (without success), and only when the risks and benefits of taking medication have been fully discussed. Support for lifestyle change should also be continued (NICE 2006*a*).

The only medication that is currently prescribed is Orlistat and the side effects may include flatulence, abdominal pain, fatty or oily stools and discharge from rectum, and needing the toilet urgently and more frequently (NHS Choices, 2012*f*).

Surgery

Surgery would usually only be considered for people who are severely obese and have tried all other options. For people with body mass index over 50kg/m2 surgery can be a first-line treatment (NICE, 2006*a*).

Patient-/client-centred working

A patient-centred approach that emphasises compassion and appropriate use of communication skills, intimacy and relational skills (Waine, 2002:47) is essential for helping individuals to manage obesity. Patient-centred working can be described as being:

- empathetic as opposed to unconcerned;
- unbiased as opposed to judgmental;
- supportive as opposed to dismissive;
- accepting as opposed to fault-finding;
- optimistic as opposed to being skeptical.

Treating the individual with respect and an understanding and empathy towards the problems they face can impact the success of any weight-loss interventions. In particular, discussion regarding the individual's commitment is essential for assessing his or her readiness to make changes, which will ultimately impact the success of any interventions made. So too is the ability to establish realistic targets in relation to weight loss etc. The almost impossible goal of achieving their ideal body weight should be avoided with obese individuals. A more realistic and achievable target of making small and progressive increases to their physical activity levels and small weight losses, with the emphasis being on the benefits of these losses on overall health, should be aimed at.

Hughes and Martin (1999) offer a range of suggestions for consideration when designing a weight-management programme. These include:

- raising the profile of exercise;
- support of GPs and health professionals to promote the benefits of exercise and activity;
- including a clinical psychologist in the team to assist with lifestyle and behaviour change;
- treating depression before making any attempt to start a weight-loss programme;
- assessing the individual's readiness and commitment to make changes;
- dietary recommendations that are aimed at

the whole family, implemented gradually, and negotiated rather than imposed, which assists with compliance;

- the use of food diaries to assess current eating and drinking patterns;
- a combination of dietary advice and exercise is more effective than either intervention offered in isolation;
- group activities that are dependent on attendance at a facility to enhance support, motivation and monitoring of progress are more effective than attempting to go it alone (Waine, 2002).

Counselling

Counselling can sometimes be useful for exploring the individual's relationship to food and eating patterns and choice of food (including any other underlying psychological struggles/issues). Being able to discuss struggles and issues openly and honestly in a non-judgmental and supportive environment can increase the confidence of the individual and assist with their motivation towards making changes to improve health. Specific strategies that can help the individual can also be explored, for example:

- keeping a food diary and becoming more conscious of eating behaviour;
- identifying healthier food options that are lower in fat and calories;
- recognising and managing stress or mood triggers that promote snacking or eating for comfort;
- eating more slowly (mindful eating);
- having smaller meals;
- discussing relapses and exploring strategies to overcome these;
- positive self-talk/affirmations.

EXERCISE RECOMMENDATIONS

The actual exercise and activity recommendations suggested will be dependent on a number of factors, which include the individual's:

- level of obesity and its duration (how long have they been overweight/obese);
- current level of activity;
- age;
- other lifestyle factors that contribute to health (smoking etc.);
- other medical conditions (CHD, diabetes, depression);
- associated problems (joint pain, arthritis, high blood pressure, etc.);
- medication.

The benefits of exercise and activity are numerous and include improved fitness, reduced risk of CHD, stimulation of fat oxidation, improved lipid profile, improved energy levels, decreased blood pressure, increased metabolic rate, improved psychological well-being, and potential appetite suppression (Waine, 2002:60).

An excellent starting point is to encourage the individual to become more active in their daily life. These smaller but more achievable activity goals will contribute to the individual's ability to tolerate other exercise and activity interventions. Examples include:

- walking more frequently to replace short journeys in the car or on public transport;
- walking for a short duration during work lunch breaks;
- walking up escalators or stairs rather than using lifts (even for a few floors, and progressing the number of floors climbed);
- doing the housework a little more vigorously and maybe more frequently;

- washing the car;
- taking up an active hobby (gardening, swimming, rambling, walking group);
- moving around more in the house (playing music and dancing, climbing stairs more frequently, etc.).

General mobility exercises Even when seated, short bouts of chair-based mobility, stretching and strengthening exercises can be performed. Again, these can be used to build the individual's tolerance for more sustained activity. They can also develop a habit and routine (see chapter 17 for chair-based/seated activities).

Cardiovascular activities are essential as part of a weight-management programme. The disadvantage for the obese individual and other individuals who may be aiming to lose weight is that the exercise needs to be sustained for a considerable duration and frequently to make an impact on body weight. A pound of body fat is equivalent to 3,500 kilocalories and a significant amount of exercise would need to be performed to burn this number of calories. An obese individual is already carrying extra weight around with them and therefore may not be able to tolerate some activities for long durations. Activity needs to start off at a much lower intensity and for a shorter duration and progress steadily. This may make their progress slower, which can be disheartening. It is therefore essential to highlight all the positive steps and changes they make to self-manage their condition and highlight any positive changes to their health, even if this is quite simply feeling better about themselves. Each step the person makes towards increasing their activity throughout the day also needs to be acknowledged and validated as a personal contribution for improving their overall health, whether weight loss is or is not achieved.

Walking is an excellent low-impact activity. However, for the obese individual, long periods of time bearing their body weight (even just standing up for the heavily obese) can be highly demanding (comparatively high intensity) and can place a lot of stress on the joints and other bodily systems.

Low-weight-bearing cardiovascular machines such as exercise bikes and/or rowing machines may also be appropriate. However, the individual's ability to get on and off the machines will determine whether they can be used. Sensitivity is paramount as the individual will feel very self-conscious and these feelings will be heightened if the gym is busy and other people are watching. These factors may also affect the person's adherence to the programme. Tolerating feelings of shame and embarrassment is not easy and most people (obese or not) would choose to avoid these feelings! Therefore, environmental factors, such as the time of the session (gym-based programmes) and the empathy of the trainer are essential to promote the person's comfort and confidence.

Group exercise A specialist group exercise programme, which is much slower and lower in impact and intensity, may be appropriate. Once again, sensitivity to the individual's confidence should be considered, although group exercise can provide many social and motivational benefits. There is also evidence to show that obese people prefer to exercise with other obese people and that programmes that encourage the participation of friends and partners are recommended (Hughes & Martin, 1999).

Exercise in water can be effective for obese people. First, it provides a support to the body weight and may enable exercises to be performed for a longer duration without placing unnecessary or excessive stress on the joints (non-weight-bearing). Second, the support of the water will also enable exercises that could not be done safely on land (jogging, jumping, etc.) to be performed. As explained previously, being able to maintain and sustain performance of an activity for an extended duration is crucial for managing weight; therefore, exercise in water can contribute to this. Water also covers the body, so any self-conscious feelings pertaining to body image would be less apparent than if exercising in a more exposed environment (i.e. exercise studio or gym).

See also table 9.3.

EXERCISE LIMITATIONS AND CONSIDERATIONS

- The individual's functional capacity will need to be considered as this will affect whether they are able to perform certain activities. For example: how easily can they get out of a chair (sit to stand)? Are they able to get on and off specific exercise equipment? Are they able to get up and down from the floor? Are they comfortable lying or sitting in certain positions? Does body bulk prevent them from performing certain exercises and stretches?
- Activity should be low impact and where possible non-weight-bearing.
- The intensity will need to be comparatively low.
- Thermoregulation will need to be considered.
- Adequate hydration is essential.
- Exercise at cooler times of day.
- Loose fitting clothing should be worn.
- The duration of the activity should be built progressively.
- Sensitivity should be given to overuse injury risk and precautions taken.

- Care with exacerbating any existing joint problems should be taken.
- Lower resistance must be used for any cardiovascular and muscular training as the body weight is already adding to the resistance being moved.
- Body bulk may restrict range of motion.
- Speed of exercise should be slower to compensate for extra weight being carried.
- Music speed (if used) must be much slower.
- Transitions and moving from one exercise to another will take longer.
- Becoming more active and building activity into daily life is an excellent starting point for developing a positive habit.
- Other medical conditions and medications must be taken into account and exercise guidelines and specific activities adapted accordingly.
- Maintaining levels of motivation by offering support and encouragement and regular assessments can help adherence and management of any relapses.

- A sensitive and empathic approach from the instructor is essential.
- Community-based programmes may be more effective at attracting this group, as walking into a gym or leisure centre for the first time can be intimidating and most people would choose to avoid the feelings of humiliation and shame that can be triggered from past memories (e.g. playground taunting) and experiences of prejudice and bullying. Exercising in an environment with other similar individuals (peers) can provide support and assist with building self-confidence.
- Keeping an activity and exercise diary can be useful to monitor activity.
- The use of a pedometer to measure steps taken in a day can also be a motivational tool and a way of monitoring progress.
- Encouraging the person to become involved in creating their own ways of becoming more active will promote adherence.

Table 9.3	Exercise guidelines for obesity	
Exercise modality (type)	**Exercise aims (goal outcome)**	**Frequency** **Intensity** **Time**
Aerobic/cardiovascular Large muscle groups, e.g. walking, cycling, exercise in water, rowing	Reduce body weight Reduce risk of CHD Increase functional performance Build exercise tolerance	5 days a week or more 30–60 minutes 40–60% of VO_2 max Emphasise duration rather than intensity Minimise weight bearing
Flexibility Stretching for all major muscles	Increase ROM Stretch to point of mild discomfort	Daily At least 5 sessions per week Can be chair-based or seated
Functional	Increase ADLs Build physical confidence	Posture Climbing stairs Sit to stand Walking
Muscle strength Fixed resistance machines Dumbbells Body weight exercises	Improve posture and strength of postural muscles Whole body approach Progress resistance, frequency and repetitions remain constant	10–15 repetitions 1–3 sets @ 40–50% of maximal voluntary contraction 2 days a week 8–10 separate exercises Circuit approach

Adapted from Wallace & Ray in Durstine & Moore (eds) (2009:384); Wallace in Durstine & Moore (eds) (2003:212)

ENDOCRINE // CONDITIONS

10

DIABETES (TYPE 1 AND TYPE 2)

Diabetes comprises a group of disorders that are characterised by having too much glucose in the blood (DoH, 2001c, NHS Choices, 2012f). Diabetes occurs when there is a lack of the hormone insulin and/or the body is unable to respond to the action of insulin.

The two main hormones responsible for controlling blood glucose are insulin and glucagon.
- Insulin is produced by beta cells in the pancreas.
- Glucagon is produced by alpha cells in the pancreas.

In the absence of diabetes these two hormones work in partnership to maintain a healthy level of blood glucose, between 4 and 7 millimoles of glucose per litre of blood (mmol/l). When levels of blood glucose increase (e.g. after a meal) insulin levels rise to facilitate the uptake of glucose by the body cells. When blood glucose levels fall (e.g. skipping breakfast) glucagon is released. This converts glycogen in the liver back to glucose, resulting in increased blood glucose levels.

Insulin is produced by the pancreas and enables the cells of the body to use glucose, which is stored in the muscles and liver as glycogen. Glucose is broken down from the food we eat and is needed as a source of energy by most body tissues, including the brain and skeletal muscles. If there is insufficient insulin, no insulin, or the cells of the body are resistant to insulin action, the levels of blood glucose will increase. The cells of the body begin breaking down fat and protein as a source of energy and the kidneys produce extra urine to try and remove the excess glucose from the blood. This affects the way the body functions and results in hyperglycaemia (raised blood glucose levels) and the symptoms of diabetes (see table 10.3).

TYPE 1 DIABETES

In type 1 diabetes the pancreas no longer produces insulin. The insulin-producing beta cells in the pancreas have been destroyed by the body's immune system and there is no insulin to enable the blood glucose to move out of the bloodstream into the body cells. Glucose levels build up in the blood and are excreted in urine (DoH, 2001c).

Type 1 diabetes can develop at any age but usually develops at a much younger age than type 2, often in childhood. Once developed, this condition is lifelong and the person will need to use insulin daily to survive. It cannot be cured, but can be controlled through daily insulin and eating a healthy diet.

There is currently no evidence that exercise improves blood glucose control in type 1 diabetes, as measured by HbA1c (AACPVR, 2004). The main role of exercise in type 1 diabetes is to modify risk factors for cardiovascular disease and improve overall health.

TYPE 2 DIABETES

In type 2 diabetes the beta cells in the pancreas are not able to produce enough insulin for the body's needs, and/or the cells in the body become 'insulin resistant' and are unable to use insulin properly. Insulin resistance refers to how sensitive the organs and cells of the body are to the action of insulin.

Type 2 usually develops later in life, although it is being increasingly diagnosed in children and adolescents. In the past it has been known as late-onset or non-insulin dependent diabetes mellitus (NIDDM); however, insulin may be part of an individual's treatment.

Unlike type 1 diabetes, type 2 is preventable and can be delayed by a change in lifestyle.

Research has demonstrated that an increase in physical activity along with dietary changes can prevent or delay the onset of type 2 diabetes in people at risk of the disease (ADA, 2004).

PREVALENCE

Over 2.8 million people in the UK are diagnosed with diabetes, and 90 per cent of these are diagnosed with type 2. It is believed that a further million people in the UK have undiagnosed type 2 diabetes (Diabetes UK, 2004*b*; NHS Choices,

2012*f*). There is also evidence (DoH, 2001*c*) that shows:

- Diabetes is increasing in all age groups.
- Type 1 is increasing in children, particularly children under 5.
- Type 2 diabetes is increasing across all groups, and particularly among people from black and ethnic minority groups.
- Type 2 diabetes is more prevalent among less affluent populations and socially excluded groups such as prisoners, refugees and people with learning disabilities.

CAUSES

The World Health Organization (1999) indicates that type 1 diabetes may be linked with both genetic and environmental causes and that type 2 diabetes may be caused by a number of contributory factors (see table 10.1)

SIGNS AND SYMPTOMS

In type 2 diabetes the symptoms are mild or even absent; they develop gradually and people are often unaware of the development of the disease, which can remain undiagnosed for many years. In type 1 diabetes the symptoms are more obvious and usually develop over a few weeks (see table 10.2).

Prevention of type 2 diabetes

There is strong evidence that both diet, physical activity and, where appropriate, drug therapy can prevent progression to diabetes and CVD (JBS, 2005). In people with impaired glucose regulation a physical activity programme of at least 150 minutes a week of moderate to vigorous activity is recommended, alongside a healthy diet (ADA, 2004).

Table 10.1	Causes/risk factors for diabetes
Type 1	**Type 2**
• Genetic link: however, even if a person has genes associated with type 1 diabetes they will not automatically develop diabetes. • Environmental trigger: the disease may develop after an encounter with a trigger, possibly linked to certain viruses and chemicals, which causes the body's immune system to attack the beta cells in the pancreas.	• Family history of type 2 diabetes • Increasing age • Obesity or central obesity • High blood pressure • Lack of physical activity • *Impaired glucose tolerance (IGT) • *Impaired fasting glycaemia (IFG).

*Impaired glucose tolerance (IGT) and impaired fasting glycaemia (IFG) indicate that the body is not processing glucose effectively. IGT is a stage of impaired glucose regulation and IFT is used to classify individuals who have fasting glucose levels above a normal range, but below those diagnostic of diabetes (Diabetes UK, 2000). Both IGT and IFG are associated with an increased risk of developing diabetes and CVD (JBS, 2005).

DIAGNOSIS

A GP will usually make a diagnosis based on symptoms, physical examination and the results of the following laboratory tests to measure blood glucose levels:

- fasting plasma glucose ≥6.0mmol/l, or
- 2-hour plasma glucose ≥11.1mmol/l following an oral glucose tolerance test (OGTT).
  (Adapted from Diabetes UK, 2000; Joint British Societies Guidelines, 2005)

If it is difficult to tell whether the person has type 1 or type 2 diabetes the GP will carry out a test which checks for the presence of antibodies that attack the body or a substance called C-peptide (NICE, 2004). The presence of antibodies or C-peptide indicates type 1 diabetes.

HbA1c

Another blood test for diabetes is called haemoglobin A1c (HbA1c). This test is not used as a diagnostic test; however, it is usually carried out on a 2–6-month basis and gives an idea of a client's overall average glucose control. HbA1c is formed when glucose in the blood 'sticks' to the haemoglobin in the red blood cells. The HbA1c measures the amount of glucose attached to the haemoglobin in the red blood cells. The Joint British Societies Guidelines (2005) recommend an HbA1c of ≤6.5 per cent.

Table 10.2	Signs and symptoms of diabetes
Excessive thirst (polydypsia)	
Excessive urination (polyuria)	
Blurred vision	
Unexpected weight loss (more evident in type 1)	
Recurrent infection such as thrush (evident in type 2)	
Tiredness	

Table 10.3	Signs and symptoms of hypoglycaemia and hyperglycaemia
Hypoglycaemia (low blood glucose level)	**Hyperglycaemia (raised blood sugar levels)**
Trembling	Restlessness and nervousness (initially)
Sweating	Increased thirst
Anxiety	Dry mouth
Blurred vision	Decreased appetite
Feeling faint	Fatigue
Feeling hungry	Nausea and vomiting (developing over time)
Paleness	Acetone breath
Mood change	
Confusion	
Elevated pulse	
Slurred speech	

Blood glucose levels

Ideally, blood glucose levels should be between 4 and 7mmol/l before meals and <9mmol/l two hours after meals (NICE 2004). The new Joint British Societies Guidelines recommend a slightly lower fasting or pre-prandial glucose value of 4.0–6.0mmol/l as an optimal target for glycaemic control. Not everyone is able to maintain such a tight control and realistic goals for blood glucose management will need to be negotiated and agreed between the client and their health professional. It is important to maintain blood sugar levels as near to normal as possible to reduce the risk of developing complications of diabetes and the development of CVD.

COMPLICATIONS

The aim of diabetes treatment is to maintain blood glucose levels within appropriate margins, so that they are not too high (hyperglycaemia) or too low (hypoglycaemia). There are a number of complications (short and long term) from poor management.

Hypoglycaemia

Hypoglycaemia is used to describe a low blood glucose level and is often called a 'hypo'. This refers to a blood glucose level below 4mmol/l. However, everyone is different and some people may experience hypoglycaemic symptoms (see table 10.3) at higher blood glucose levels or if there is a sudden drop in blood glucose levels. Hypoglycaemia occurs when there is too much insulin in the body, which may be caused by a number of factors including:

- a change in food intake, irregular or missed meals;
- the type and timing of medications such as insulin or insulin secretagogues;
- exercise;
- alcohol consumption.

It is important for the client and exercise professional to be aware of the signs and symptoms of hypoglycaemia (see table 10.3) and to know what to do in the event of a hypo.

Signs and symptoms can vary from person to person so ask the client to describe how hypoglycaemia affects her or him. Sometimes a carer or relative may be able to provide this information. A person on insulin therapy or insulin secretagogues such as sulphonylureas is at an increased risk of hypoglycaemia during or after exercise (see table 10.8).

Hyperglycaemia

Hyperglycaemia refers to a raised blood glucose level above 10mmols/l (Diabetes UK, 2003a). The signs and symptoms of hyperglycaemia

(see table 10.3) may include restlessness or nervousness initially, with more characteristic signs and symptoms such as thirst, fatigue and nausea developing over time. Factors that may lead to hyperglycaemia are listed in table 10.4. Long-term hyperglycaemia increases the risk of diabetes-related complications.

Diabetic ketoacidosis (DKA)

This is caused by an inadequate concentration of insulin in the blood, which prevents the cells of the body taking up glucose and using it as a source of energy. The cells begin to rely on the body's

Table 10.4	Causes of hyperglycaemia
Insulin/diabetes medication	A reduced dose or change in timing may cause blood glucose levels to rise (including missing medication or taking too little). If a client is taking medication appropriately and is experiencing hyperglycaemia, a change in treatment may be required. A client who is managing diabetes with healthy eating and physical activity may need to begin taking tablets if they frequently experience raised blood glucose levels.
Change in physical activity	A decrease in level of physical activity will result in a decreased use of glucose by the body and an increase in blood glucose levels. If a client is on insulin or insulin-like medication and their blood glucose levels are not well controlled, they are at an increased risk of hyperglycaemia during exercise.
Food intake	An increase in the amount of food and a change in type of food will cause an increase in blood glucose level e.g. more starchy foods eaten.
Stress/hormone change	Stress hormones such as cortisol and adrenaline can affect the action of insulin and lead to a rise in blood glucose levels. Women may find that glucose levels are affected by the menstrual cycle and during the menopause (Walker & Rodgers, 2004).
Illness	During illness glycogen in the liver is converted to glucose. Increased levels of stress hormones will also be released, reducing the effectiveness of insulin. Both these actions result in an increased blood glucose level, requiring frequent monitoring (around 4 times a day).

Adapted from NHS Choices (2012f); Diabetes UK (2009)

fat reserves as a source of energy and the levels of blood glucose begin to rise. The by-products of fat metabolism are called ketones, which cause the blood to become more acidic. This can lead to drowsiness and coma and is a potentially life-threatening condition. DKA is rare in people with type 2 diabetes and is only likely to occur when there is another illness or infection; when insulin management is insufficient; or with cocaine use (Diabetes UK, 2003a and 2009).

Hyperosmolar hyperglycaemic state (HHS), previously known as hyperosmolar non-ketotic acidosis (HONK)

This occurs in people with type 2 diabetes who may be experiencing high blood glucose levels, often over 40mmol/l. It develops over a few weeks and symptoms include frequent urination, increased thirst, nausea and, in later stages, drowsiness and gradual loss of consciousness. In people with type 2 diabetes who are still producing some insulin, the acidic by-products associated with DKA are less likely to be produced. Hospital treatment is required to replace lost fluids and bring blood glucose levels down (Diabetes UK, 2003, 2009a).

Long-term complications

If blood glucose levels remain elevated over a long period of time, the walls of the blood vessels become damaged. Microvascular damage affects the small arteries, veins and capillaries and can lead to additional complications.

People with diabetes, especially people with type 2 diabetes, are at an increased risk of macrovascular damage, which affects the walls of the larger blood vessels supplying the heart, brain and peripheries. This can lead to CVD including:

Table 10.5	Microvascular damage
Peripheral neuropathy	Damage to nerves supplying the lower limbs, which can lead to loss of sensation, ulceration and lower limb amputation.
Autonomic neuropathy	Damage to the nerves can affect the involuntary function of the body including the cardiac, gastrointestinal and genitourinary systems.
Retinopathy	Damage to the small arteries of the retina at the back of the eye leads to visual impairment and blindness.
Nephropathy	Damage to the kidneys can lead to progressive kidney failure.

Adapted from DoH (2001)

- coronary heart disease (angina and myocardial infarction);
- stroke and transient ischaemic attack (TIA);
- peripheral arterial disease, which can lead to pain on walking (claudication), leg and foot ulcers and limb amputation. (DoH, 2001c.)

The risk of dying from cardiovascular disease is doubled in men with diabetes and the risk of a heart attack is 50 per cent higher. For women with diabetes the risk of dying from cardiovascular disease is four times higher and the risk of a heart attack is 150 per cent higher (AACVPR, 2004).

In order to reduce the likelihood of long-term complications it is important to try to keep the blood sugar level as normal as possible and to address other cardiovascular risk factors (high blood pressure, cholesterol, smoking, inactivity, obesity etc.).

Metabolic syndrome

A clustering of the risk factors (see box) is often found in people with central obesity and is referred to as the metabolic syndrome. An individual with metabolic syndrome is at an increased risk of cardiovascular disease. Weight reduction can play an important role in improving elements of the metabolic syndrome (NICE, 2004b; JBS, 2005).

Metabolic syndrome

Risk factors include:
- blood pressure >135/80mmHg;
- waist measurement more than 90 cm in women, or 100cm in men; or 10cm less in men and women with a South Asian background;
- low levels of high-density lipoprotein (HDL), the protective cholesterol;
- elevated triglycerides (type of blood lipids);
- insulin resistance;
- impaired glucose regulation including diabetes.

MANAGEMENT OF DIABETES

According to the Joint British Societies Guidelines (2005), people with type 1 and type 2 diabetes are considered at high risk of CVD (≥20 per cent over 10 years) and of developing atherosclerotic disease. In order to manage diabetes effectively and lessen the increased risk of CVD, a combination of lifestyle measures and drug therapies is recommended. Empowering people with diabetes is central to the National Service Framework (NSF) for diabetes (DoH, 2001c). This is advocated through effective education, partnership with health professionals and shared decision making about health.

General goals for working with people with diabetes

- Maintain blood glucose levels within an appropriate range.
- Support lifestyle change to help control diabetes and reduce the long-term complications associated with diabetes.
- Provide individualised, culturally appropriate diabetes-specific advice about exercise and physical activity.
- Reduce the risk of cardiovascular disease.

People with long-term conditions such as diabetes are more likely to get anxious and depressed, which can have a detrimental effect on the management of their diabetes (NICE, 2004). Education can play an important role in managing diabetes, and help to improve knowledge, blood glucose control, weight and dietary management, physical activity and psychological well-being (DoH, 2001c). Education is particularly effective when it is tailored to the needs of the individual and addresses attitudes, skills and knowledge.

Lifestyle measures include:
- stopping smoking;
- eating more healthily;
- increasing levels of physical activity;
- achieving optimal weight and weight distribution.

Risk factor targets

Blood pressure In people with diabetes a BP target of <130mmHg systolic and <80mmHg diastolic is recommended. People with diabetes and elevated blood pressure will be offered antihypertensive medication (see medication tables in chapter 12, page 186).

Blood glucose control Tight control of glycaemia is recommended (JBS, 2005):

- fasting or preprandial glucose of 4–6.0mmol/l, and
- HbA1c <6.5 per cent.

Cholesterol The optimal target for total cholesterol is <4.0mmol/l *and* low-density lipo-protein (LDL) cholesterol <2.0mmol/l, or a 25 per cent reduction in total cholesterol *and* a 30 per cent reduction in LDL cholesterol, whichever achieves the lowest value (JBS, 2005). Cholesterol-lowering medication called statins will be recommended to improve cholesterol levels (JBS, 2005; NICE, 2004*b*). (See medications table in chapter 12.) Statins are recommended for all people with diabetes (type 1 and 2) over the age of 40 and for some younger people with diabetes who have diabetic complications or an increased risk of CVD.

Antithrombotic therapy Aspirin is recommended for some people with diabetes to reduce the risk of CVD (NICE 2004*b*). If aspirin is not appropriate, an alternative, clopidogrel, might be prescribed (refer to medications table in chapter 12).

EXERCISE RECOMMENDATIONS

The aim of an exercise programme is to maximise the benefits of physical activity and minimise the complications associated with diabetes. The American College of Sports Medicine (2005*a*) recommends that people with diabetes planning moderate- to high-intensity activity should undergo a graded exercise test if the following criteria apply:

- age ≥ 35;
- Type 2 diabetes >10 years duration;
- Type 1 diabetes >15 years duration;
- presence of any additional risk factor for cardiovascular disease;
- presence of any microvascular disease (retinopathy or nephropathy);
- peripheral vascular disease;
- autonomic neuropathy.

This would provide useful information; however, a graded exercise test is not standard practice in the UK. In the absence of a graded exercise test it is advisable for a client with diabetes to be assessed by their GP prior to increasing their levels of physical activity. This should include taking a medical history and a comprehensive physical examination, especially in relation to diabetic complications affecting the heart and circulatory system, eyes, kidneys, feet and nervous system. This will ensure that the diabetes is well controlled and will identify any conditions that require referral to a specialist and/or a specific exercise prescription.

Benefits of exercise

Exercise can benefit insulin sensitivity, hypertension, and blood lipid control. It has an important role in reducing the risk of cardiovascular disease and improving overall health and well-being. In many cases, type 2 diabetes can be effectively managed by lifestyle measures such as a healthy diet, weight loss and increasing levels of physical activity. Exercise has a role in improving self-efficacy, psychological well-being and stress management, which can contribute to better self-management and improved quality of life (Diabetes UK, 2003*b*).

Key considerations before starting an exercise programme

- Client is assessed by GP, is stable and exhibits no contraindications to exercise.
- Diabetes is well controlled.
- Client is taught about appropriate footwear and ongoing foot care.
- Client is aware of the effect of activity on blood glucose levels (hypoglycaemia and hyperglycaemia).
- Client knows the signs and symptoms of hypoglycaemia and knows what action to take.
- Client is able to self-monitor blood glucose levels.
- Client has discussed treatment changes such as adjusting insulin dosage and/or carbohydrate intake prior to exercise and for 24 hours afterwards.

Note: Refer also to chapter 4 for other contraindications to exercise, and chapter 6 for management of hypoglycaemia and hyperglycaemia in the exercise environment.

General guidelines for management of blood sugar levels before exercise

Monitoring blood glucose before exercise will ensure that it is safe to exercise and minimise the risk of worsening hyperglycaemia and hypoglycaemia in clients on insulin or oral hypoglycaemic agents. It important to take into account other factors including:

- intensity and duration of the activity;
- timing and dose of medication;
- time of the exercise session;
- type of insulin or oral medication;
- timing of last meal;
- individual response.

The general guidelines below are based on current UK (Diabetes UK), American College of Sports Medicine (2005) and American Diabetes Association (2004) recommendations. There are differences between these recommendations and it is important to work within guidelines that are developed locally between diabetes specialists and physical activity providers. Much of this advice

on glucose monitoring is specific to clients on insulin or insulin secretagogues (see medications table, chapter 12). It is important to remember that every individual has a different metabolic response to exercise. Appropriate monitoring and observation will help you learn more about your client's response to exercise, develop an individualised programme and enable the client to exercise more safely and effectively.

In America, milligrams per decilitre (mg/dl) are used to measure glucose levels, which can make it confusing when trying to compare with UK or European guidelines. To convert mmol/l of glucose to mg/dl, multiply by 18. To convert mg/dl of glucose to mmol/l, divide by 18 or multiply by 0.055 (see table 10.6).

Some of the recommendations below may be more appropriate to clinical settings, especially where ketone testing is advised.

Pre-activity screening If blood glucose level <5.5mmol/l (<100mg/dl) the client will need to eat some additional carbohydrate (ACSM, 2005).

Table 10.6	Conversion chart
Mg/dl	**Mmol/l**
80	4.4
100	5.5
240	13.2
250	13.75
300	16.5

The amount of carbohydrate needed will depend on the intensity and duration of the planned exercise. Check that blood glucose levels have increased before starting to exercise and that the client has no symptoms of hypoglycaemia. These recommendations are appropriate for individuals on insulin and/or insulin secretagogues. Hypoglycaemia is rare in individuals who are not on insulin or insulin secretagogues and supplementary carbohydrate is not generally necessary (ADA, 2004).

If blood glucose levels are >13mmol/l (Diabetes UK, 2004a), discuss possible reasons for blood glucose level and ask client to test for ketones in urine. Test strips are available from the GP. If ketone levels are elevated, refer client to GP.

Do not exercise if:
- Blood glucose level is >13mmol/l and ketone testing is inappropriate or not possible.
- Blood glucose level is >13mmol/l with ketones (Diabetes UK, 2004a).

The American Diabetes Association (2004) suggests that this may be over-cautious for a person with type 2 diabetes, especially if the person has recently eaten. If the person feels well and ketones are negative, it may not be necessary to postpone low to moderate exercise based simply on hyperglycaemia. However, it is important to encourage good glycaemic control and the aim is to exercise in the presence of optimal glycaemic control.

Exercise with caution if:
- Blood glucose level is >13mmol/l without ketones, as there may not be enough insulin to mobilise sufficient glucose for exercise (Diabetes UK, 2004).

Practical recommendations for community exercise setting

Blood glucose levels should be in the range of 5.5–13mmol/l (Diabetes UK, 2004a). Some people are more cautious and recommend postponing exercise for clients on insulin when glucose levels are >200mg/dl, which is approximately equivalent to 11mmol/l (Russell & Sherman, 1999).

If you have any concerns about a client exercising you can let him or her begin the session and ask them to monitor his or her blood glucose during exercise. If the blood glucose levels stay the same or begin to rise, you can ask the client to stop exercising and take appropriate action.

During exercise

If activity is vigorous or lasts more than an hour the client may need to check if blood glucose levels have fallen during activity and consume additional carbohydrate, e.g. a sugary drink or carbohydrate snack.

After exercise

Check blood glucose level after exercise to identify if food intake is necessary. If the client feels shaky, anxious, confused or has a low blood glucose level, encourage her or him to have a fast-acting snack, followed by a sandwich or piece of fruit. A client with type 2 diabetes who is not on insulin therapy or insulin secretagogues is unlikely to have a hypoglycaemic episode during exercise, but may need to have something to eat after exercise.

An individual who has a tendency towards hypoglycaemia may need to adjust her or his treatment by reducing the dose of insulin or insulin secretagogue or increasing carbohydrate intake before or during exercise. If you have any concerns about the client's diabetes control, refer her or him to the GP or specialist diabetes team.

GUIDELINES FOR EXERCISE

The guidelines for type 1 diabetes are very similar to those for apparently healthy adults; however, the guidelines for people with type 2 diabetes are more closely aligned to those for obesity, with a focus on increased caloric expenditure (ACSM, 2005). There are differences between the ACSM (2005) and the American Diabetes Association (2004) guidelines based on emerging research. These are highlighted below.

Table 10.7 summarises the current recommendations for exercise.

Cardiovascular

The main aim of cardiovascular exercise is to improve glycaemic control, reduce the risk of cardiovascular disease and help with weight loss or weight maintenance. Clients with type 2 diabetes can be encouraged to accumulate a minimum of 1000kcal a week of physical activity. If weight loss is a goal an additional caloric expenditure of ≥2000kcal per week may be required (ACSM, 2005). Daily exercise may be required to meet this

challenge. The American Diabetes Association (2004) recommends the following:

- moderate intensity activity (40–60 per cent VO_2max, 50–70 per cent HRmax) for at least 150 minutes per week; and/or
- vigorous intensity activity (>60 per cent of VO_2max or >70 per cent of HRmax) for at least 90 minutes per week;
- distribute physical activity over at least three days a week, with no more than two consecutive days without physical activity.

The duration and intensity of the activity will depend on the specific goals of the individual and co-morbidities. In the absence of exercise stress testing and in a community setting, it may be more appropriate to exercise at moderate levels of intensity.

Muscular strength

There is a growing body of evidence for the value of resistance training in type 2 diabetes (ADA, 2004). The ACSM (2005) recommend a low-resistance (40–60 per cent 1RM) strength programme for clients with diabetes. The American Diabetes Association (2004) previously endorsed a similar programme; however, in the light of new research they currently recommend a moderate intensity (60–80 per cent 1RM) strength-training programme. A conservative approach is suggested, beginning with one set of 10–15 repetitions 2–3 times a week at a moderate intensity, and progressing to three sets of 8–10 repetitions at a weight that cannot be lifted more than 8–10 times (8–10 1RM). Although one set is sufficient for building strength, three sets produce greater metabolic benefits for

Table 10.7	Exercise guidelines for diabetes	
Exercise modality (type)	**Exercise aims (goal outcome)**	**Frequency Intensity Time**
Aerobic/ cardiovascular Large muscle groups	Improve aerobic capacity Reduce cardiovascular risk factors Improve work capacity Improve BP Assist weight management Anaerobic/high intensity only for athletes with well managed diabetic control	4–7 days a week 20–60 minutes 50–80% peak HR Monitor RPE
Muscle strength Fixed resistance machines Dumbbells Body weight exercises Bands and tubing	Improve posture and strength of postural muscles Increase maximal number of repetitions Target areas of weakness	Low resistance and high repetitions 1 set, 10–15 reps, 40–60% 1RM (ACSM, 2005) Build to 3 sets of 8–10 1RM (ADA, 2004), i.e. a weight that cannot be lifted more than 8–10 times Higher resistance is okay for clients with well managed diabetes
Flexibility and neuromuscular Stretching Yoga	Increase/maintain ROM Improve gait Improve balance and coordination	2–3 times a week Static stretches
Functional	Increase or maintain ADL Increase confidence Specifically for clients at risk of falls (peripheral neuropathy)	Specific to individual

Adapted from Hornsby & Albright in Durstine & Moore (eds) (2009:188)

people with type 2 diabetes. It is important to consider co-morbidities when recommending higher-intensity resistance training, as it may be inappropriate or contraindicated for people with hypertension, retinopathy or joint problems.

Flexibility

There are no diabetes-specific guidelines for flexibility. The guidelines included reflect guidelines for the general population (see table 10.7).

EXERCISE LIMITATIONS AND CONSIDERATIONS

- *Encourage clients to measure their blood glucose levels before and after exercise. If the exercise lasts for more than one hour, monitor blood glucose levels during the session as well.
- *Clients should reduce their insulin dose for planned activity/exercise. This will involve some degree of experimenting, as everyone responds differently; it will also depend on the duration and intensity of the activity and the dose and timing of insulin. Advise clients to discuss this with their diabetes team or healthcare professional.
- Plan exercise 1–2 hours after meals. It is best to avoid exercising during the peak insulin action as this, combined with exercise, increases the risk of hypoglycaemia.
- *Use injection sites away from areas of the body predominantly used during exercise. The abdomen is the preferred site.
- *Clients should always carry fast-acting carbohydrate snacks or drinks when exercising.
- *Delayed hypoglycaemia can occur up to 36 hours after intense exercise as the muscles refuel. Make adjustments to the timing of exercise or encourage clients to eat a snack before going to bed. This is important if the client exercises in the evening, as there is an increased risk of nocturnal hypoglycaemia.
- Clients with type 2 diabetes who are not on insulin or suphonylureas are unlikely to have a hypo, however, they may need to eat soon after exercise.
- Certain medications can mask or increase the risk of hypoglycaemia, including beta-blockers, calcium channel blockers and diuretics.
- Clients should drink plenty of water before, during and after activity to avoid dehydration.
- Alcohol inhibits glucose production, causing a hypoglycaemic effect. This hypoglycaemic effect can last up to 24 hours.
- Encourage daily foot inspection and remind clients to inform you about any changes such as blisters or inflammation.

*Specific considerations for people on insulin or insulin secretagogues, who are more at risk of hypoglycaemia during exercise or after exercise.

(Adapted from ACSM, 2005; AACVPR, 2004; NICE, 2004)

See also table 10.8.

Nutritional guidance

Individuals with diabetes should always speak with their GP and be referred to a registered dietician for a tailored eating plan. Diabetes UK (2009) offer the following guidance:

- Eat regular meals (including breakfast) to maintain blood sugar levels.
- Make sure each meal contains foods from the starchy carbohydrate group with lower glycaemic index and fibre to prevent constipation (potatoes, wholemeal bread, wholemeal pasta, yams, oats, wholegrain cereals).
- Don't use diabetic foods or drinks. Apart from being expensive they contain just as much fat and calories of other foods and will still effect blood sugar levels.
- Reduce saturated fat (grill and bake instead of frying, choose low fat dairy options, skimmed or semi-skimmed milk, lean meat, less dairy products and creamy sauces).
- Eat more fruit and vegetables, at least five a day.
- Eat more beans and lentils (kidney beans,

Table 10.8	Recommendations and precautions for clients with diabetic complications
Complications	**Recommendations/precautions**
Retinopathy	Avoid contact sports. Avoid activities that raise blood pressure (high intensity resistance or CV). Avoid activities that lower the head (some yoga positions) or activities that jar the head or involve breath holding or straining. Have regular eye examinations to check progression of retinopathy. Low-intensity training.
Peripheral neuropathy	Avoid prolonged weight bearing (stepping, walking, high impact) and use non-weight-bearing alternatives – chair-based, cycling, rowing, exercise in water (unless ulcers present) or use a circuit training approach combining these approaches. Wear cushioned shoes. Loss of sensation can lead to problems with balance and increase risk of falls and other orthopaedic or musculoskeletal injuries. Include specific balance exercises.
Autonomic neuropathy	There is a risk of cardiac dysfunction, hypoglycaemia, silent ischaemia and dehydration. There may be an abnormal heart rate and blood pressure response at rest and in response to exercise. Avoid rapid changes in body position. Be aware of post exercise orthostatic hypotension. Ensure adequate hydration. Use RPE, alongside careful monitoring. May require a clinical exercise setting.
Nephropathy	Avoid activity that increases blood pressure (high intensity CV or resistance training). Perform low-intensity aerobic and resistance training. Ensure adequate hydration.

Adapted from ACSM (2005); AACVPR (2004)

chickpeas, lentils) as they have less effect on blood sugar levels and may help to manage cholesterol.

- Eat at least two portions of oily fish each week to boost omega 3 which helps to protect against heart disease.
- Reduce sugar.
- Reduce salt.
- Drink within safe guidelines and never drink on an empty stomach as alcohol may lower blood sugar levels.

Diabetes and Ramadan

Ramadan is a holy month in Islam, and all healthy adult Muslims are expected to fast. Ramadan lasts between 29 and 30 days and Muslims abstain from eating, drinking, smoking or using oral medications between dawn and sunset. The Koran exempts people with medical conditions, however, many people with diabetes decide to fast, often against the advice of the medical profession. Fasting can lead to complications such as hypoglycaemia, hyperglycaemia, diabetic ketoacidosis and dehydration. The level of risk will depend on the type of diabetes, level of control and ability to self-manage.

People with diabetes who decide to fast should have a pre-Ramadan assessment and educational counselling to reduce the risks (American Diabetes Association, 2005).

Normal levels of physical activity can be maintained, however, excessive physical activity or exercise may increase the risk of hypoglycaemia, especially in the hours before breaking the fast at sunset. People with poorly controlled type 1 diabetes may be at an increased risk of hyperglycaemia. The daily prayers after sunset (*tarawaih*) can be considered as part of the person's daily physical activity. If your client wants to continue his/her exercise programme during Ramadan, it is important to work closely with the client and the diabetes team to ensure that diabetes is well managed and the exercise programme adapted to minimise risk.

MEDICATION FOR TYPE 2 DIABETES

Some people with type 2 diabetes may be able to maintain target blood glucose levels by making lifestyle changes such as losing weight and increasing physical activity levels. If glucose levels remain high, medication is usually advised (see table 10.9) in addition to the recommended lifestyle changes. If, over time, blood glucose start to rise, additional medication may be prescribed. The main groups of medication are listed in table 10.9.

MEDICATION FOR TYPE 1 DIABETES

People with type 1 diabetes need to take insulin every day to manage their blood glucose. There are numerous types of insulin and it is important for people to find the type and pattern of insulin that suits their lifestyle and helps them to manage their glucose levels effectively.

Insulin

The goal of insulin treatment is to supply the body with the insulin it lacks and to mimic the normal pattern of insulin release throughout the day. There are a number of different types of insulin, including:

- **Rapid-acting insulin analogues** A synthetic form of insulin that aims to work like normal insulin to cope with a meal. The effects are short-lasting.
- **Short acting** Work more slowly, with the effect lasting up to eight hours.
- **Intermediate acting** Have an effect that can last through the night.
- **Long acting** Can last for a longer period, e.g. a whole day.
- **Biphasic insulin** A mixture of rapid- or short-acting and intermediate-acting insulin (NICE, 2004).

These work for different lengths of time in the body and are often prescribed in different combinations to control blood glucose levels adequately. The prescribed type and combination of insulin is called a regimen. Generally, an insulin regimen will provide a background level of insulin with additional boosts during the day. The insulin regimen may need to be adjusted to meet the needs of changes, such as increasing levels of physical activity, eating patterns or periods of feeling unwell. In the longer term, changes in health and lifestyle may necessitate a change in regimen.

As an exercise specialist it is appropriate to give your client general advice about physical activity and insulin treatment, however, it is important to ask your client to discuss any proposed change in physical activity and insulin regimen with his or her GP or specialist diabetes health professional. Insulin cannot be taken as a tablet because it would be digested by the body before getting into the blood supply, so it has to be injected (NICE, 2004).

Table 10.9	Medications for type 2 diabetes		
Drug name	**Purpose/action**	**Side effects**	**Exercise implications**
Biguanide	Usually prescribed for someone who is overweight and unable to control blood glucose adequately through lifestyle intervention alone.	Mild diarrhoea, sickness when first taken Not prescribed for persons with kidney problems	None known
Insulin secretagogues	Increases insulin secretion and include sulphonylureas and prandial glucose regulators (nateglinide and repaglinide).	Can cause weight gain, hypoglycaemia, nausea, mild diarrhoea or constipation	There is a risk of hypoglycaemia during and after exercise with these medications.
Thiazolidinediones (e.g. glitazones)	Increases the amount of glucose taken up from the blood and reduce blood glucose levels. Prescribed for people who can't take metformin and insulin secretagogues.	Weight gain, fluid retention (oedema), slight risk of liver damage, hypoglycaemia possible but uncommon	No risk of hypo unless given with other drugs
Alpha glucosidase inhibitor	Delays the absorption of carbohydrate, reducing the rise in glucose levels that occurs after eating. Prescribed for people who are unable to use other oral drugs.	Wind, bloating, diarrhoea	There is a risk of hypoglycaemia
Insulin	May be used for people with type 2 diabetes, to control blood glucose levels if other medications have not been effective.	As per secretagogues plus injection site irritation	There is a risk of hypoglycaemia
Orlistat	May be prescribed for people with type 2 diabetes who are overweight, as part of a plan to lose weight and maintain blood glucose levels.	Oily stools, flatulence, hypoglycaemia, anxiety, nausea, abdominal pain and headaches	There is a risk of hypoglycaemia

Adapted from Diabetes UK (2005, 2009); NHS Choices (2012)

RESPIRATORY DISORDERS

Respiratory disorders can be divided into restrictive and obstructive disease (see table 11.1). This chapter will focus on the obstructive conditions COPD and asthma, and the role of exercise within these conditions.

CHRONIC OBSTRUCTIVE PULMONARY DISEASE

Chronic obstructive pulmonary disease (COPD) is now the preferred term for conditions that were previously diagnosed as chronic bronchitis and emphysema (NICE, 2010*b*, Patient UK, 2012*b*). COPD is a chronic disabling condition in which the airways and sometimes the lungs themselves have become obstructed (by chronic bronchitis, emphysema, or both), causing persistent and progressive damage which can greatly impair the ability to lead a normal life. The disease is predominantly caused by smoking and nearly all sufferers are over 35 (NICE, 2004/2010).

CHRONIC BRONCHITIS

In chronic bronchitis the bronchi (airways) become irritated or inflamed, often in response to cigarette smoking. As a result of the inflammation mucous starts to build up in excessive amounts,

Table 11.1	Respiratory diseases
Restrictive disease	
Characterised by reduced lung volume as a result of a wide range of disorders that affect the thorax or the lung parenchyma (lung tissue), such as ankylosing spondylitis, kyphoscoliosis, spinal cord injury, and pulmonary fibrosis.	
Obstructive disease	
Characterised by increased airway obstruction and expiratory resistance. Airway obstruction is caused by conditions such as bronchitis, emphysema (collectively referred to as COPD) and asthma. Chronic obstructive pulmonary disease (COPD) can also include chronic asthma.	

causing a chronic productive cough. The bronchi become narrowed, obstructing the flow of air in and out of the lungs. These symptoms may lead to breathlessness (dyspnoea).

EMPHYSEMA

This is caused by permanent enlargement and damage of the alveoli or air sacs in the lungs. This makes them much less efficient in transferring the gases of respiration between the lungs and the bloodstream, often leading to lower oxygen levels in the blood. The damage to the walls of the alveoli reduces the elastic recoil of the lungs. This means that expiration becomes an active rather than a passive action. It becomes difficult to push air out of the lungs and air becomes trapped, causing hyperinflation of the lungs. The muscles surrounding the bronchi can also become tighter, which results in bronchospasm, or 'wheeze', as air is squeezed through the airways.

CAUSES

Smoking is the main risk factor for the development of COPD, however, according to the Global Initiative for Chronic Obstructive Lung Disease (GOLD), the American Thoracic Society (ATS) and European Respiratory Society (ERS) (2005) other genetic and environmental factors may also play a part in the development of the disease, such as:

- genetics;
- gender;
- occupation – where there is long-term exposure to certain types of dust or chemicals;
- environmental pollution (indoor air pollution in poorly ventilated living conditions and outdoor air pollution);
- socio-economic status;
- passive smoking also contributes to respiratory symptoms and COPD;
- respiratory infections in early childhood are associated with reduced lung function and respiratory conditions in adulthood.

PREVALENCE

COPD is one of the leading causes of morbidity and mortality worldwide and results in an economic and social burden that is both substantial and increasing (ATS & ERS, 2005).

It is estimated that around 3 million people in the UK have COPD, with around 900,000 people being diagnosed and a further 2 million remaining undiagnosed (NICE, 2010a, 2010b). COPD is accountable for around 30,000 deaths each year in the UK (most in the over 65 age group) and is the fifth leading cause of death in the UK (NICE, 2010b:24). 'Most patients are not diagnosed until they are in their fifties' and rates of COPD are higher in more deprived populations; while it is more common in men, there is evidence of increasing prevalence in women (NICE, 2010b:23).

It is also estimated that an average GP practice in the UK, caring for around 7,000 patients, will have around 200 patients with COPD (many undiagnosed) and it accounts for approximately 1.4 million GP consultations each year, around four times more than consultations for angina (NICE, 2010b:25).

SIGNS AND SYMPTOMS

COPD affects people in different ways. NICE (2010) suggests that any person over the age of 35 should be considered for diagnosis if they present with other symptoms. The main symptoms (NICE 2010, GOLD, 2005) are:

- a productive cough (coughing up sputum/ phlegm);
- a chronic cough (intermittent or every day);
- breathlessness that is:
  - worse over time;
  - present every day;
  - worse on exercise;
  - worse during respiratory infections;
- an increase in chestiness or wheezing during cold weather;
- peripheral muscle weakness;
- fatigue.

A cough is usually the first symptom. Initially the cough will come and go, but over time the cough becomes more persistent (chronic). As the airways become more damaged they produce more mucous, and phlegm may be coughed up every day. This occurs mainly with bronchitis, but not emphysema.

Breathlessness (dyspnoea) is one of the main symptoms of COPD and is the term used to describe subjective feelings of breathing discomfort. Dyspnoea may occur if the respiratory muscles have to work harder than expected to produce a given amount of ventilation (Ambrosino & Scano, 2004). Dyspnoea is one of the most debilitating and frightening symptoms of COPD and often leads to people avoiding any activities that might make them breathless. Many people with COPD can get stuck in a cycle of inactivity, which leads to a decrease in fitness and functional capacity. This in turn results in an increase in respiratory effort and breathlessness to carry out daily activities. Before a diagnosis of COPD has been made, many people experience breathlessness that limits activity involving heavy exertion. They often associate this with getting old and don't access health services until their condition deteriorates further. Activities of daily living and recreational activities become increasingly difficult and uncomfortable as the disease progresses. This cycle of inactivity can lead to isolation, anxiety and depression. Patients can benefit from learning techniques to relieve feelings of breathlessness.

Learning to manage breathlessness is an important part of a pulmonary rehabilitation programme as it can give people more control over their condition, and contributes to an improved quality of life.

DIAGNOSIS

A diagnosis will be based on a history of the patient's symptoms and the results of several tests:
- over 35 with a risk factor (generally smoking);
- history of chronic progressive symptoms (see symptoms, page 147) such as a cough, wheeze or breathlessness;
- airway obstruction confirmed through use of spirometry (discussed later in this chapter);
- no clinical features of asthma (with asthma, inflammation of the airways makes the muscles in the airways constrict and causes the airways themselves to constrict).

Symptoms vary in severity and may come and go. Treatment to reduce inflammation is usually effective. However, with COPD the damage is permanent. The narrowing of the airways is fixed and the symptoms are persistent. Treatment to open airways is of limited effect (Patient UK, 2012b). Asthma and COPD are different conditions; however, some people may have both conditions. Table 11.2 highlights the differences between COPD and asthma.

A full assessment by a GP should include: spirometry, breathlessness, weight loss and frequency of exacerbations (NICE, 2010b).

Spirometry

A common test to help diagnose COPD is spirometry, which estimates how much air can be blown out/expelled from the lungs in one breath. A device called a spirometer is used to measure how well the lungs are working and identify any reduction in expiratory flow. Two measurements are taken: the forced expiratory volume in one second (FEV1) and the forced vital capacity (FVC):

- FEV1 (forced expiratory volume in 1 second) measures the maximum amount of air that someone can force out of the lungs in one second.
- FVC (forced vital capacity) measures the total amount of air that someone can force out of his or her lungs after a maximal inspiration.
- The FEV1/FVC ratio is the FEV1 divided by the FVC.

A FEV1 (forced expiratory volume in 1 second) of less than 80 per cent predicted and a FEV1/FVC ratio of less than 70 per cent (0.7) indicates airway obstruction and the possibility of COPD (NICE, 2010). FEV1 is influenced by age, gender and ethnicity and is expressed as a percentage of a normal predicted value. There is a gradual decrease in both these measurements with age; however, smoking significantly accelerates this process and stopping smoking causes the decline in lung function to return to a 'normal' rate (GOLD, 2005).

Spirometry is required to make a diagnosis of COPD, and can be used to monitor the progression of the disease. Table 11.3 indicates FEV1 values and the severity of airflow obstruction.

Breathlessness (dyspnoea)

The level of dyspnoea does not necessarily relate to the severity of airway obstruction and it is possible for someone to have mild airway obstruction and severe dyspnoea. Dyspnoea is a subjective sensation of the severity of breathing discomfort experienced; however, it can be quantified using a scale. The effect of breathlessness on functional status or daily activities can be measured by using the Medical Research Council dyspnoea scale (see table 11.4).

Table 11.2	Differences between COPD and asthma (NICE, 2010b)	
	COPD	**Asthma**
Smoker or ex-smoker	Nearly all	Possibly
Symptoms under age of 35	Rare	Common
Chronic productive cough	Common	Uncommon
Breathlessness	Persistent and progressive	Variable
Night-waking with breathlessness and/or wheeze	Uncommon	Common
Significant diurnal or day-to-day variability of symptoms	Uncommon	Common

Table 11.3	Severity of air flow obstruction
Severity of airflow obstruction	**FEV1 % Predicted**
Mild (stage 1)	At least 80%
Moderate (stage 2)	50–79
Severe (stage 3)	30–49
Very severe (stage 4)	<30

Adapted from NICE (2010); Patient UK (2012b)

Table 11.4	Medical Research Council (MRC) dyspnoea scale
Grade	**Degree of breathlessness related to activities**
1	Not troubled by breathlessness except on strenuous exercise
2	Short of breath when hurrying or walking up a slight hill
3	Walks slower than contemporaries on the level because of breathlessness, or has to stop for breath when walking at own pace
4	Stops for breath after walking about 100m or after a few minutes on the level
5	Too breathless to leave the house, or breathless when dressing or undressing

Adapted from NICE (2010*b*)

Weight loss

Weight loss due to inadequate dietary intake, increased resting energy expenditure and muscle wasting may lead to a low body mass index (BMI) in patients with COPD. If a person's BMI is below the normal range of 20–24 they may need to supplement their diet to increase their calorie intake. This is especially relevant if the person is increasing their energy expenditure through increased physical activity.

Exacerbations

Managing exacerbations (flare-ups) is one of the key priorities of the NICE COPD guidelines (2004/2010). An exacerbation may occur from time to time, with a worsening of symptoms such as breathlessness, cough and volume of sputum. Symptoms may also include a cold or sore throat, reduced exercise tolerance, fluid retention and fatigue. An exacerbation can be infectious or non-infectious (ATS & ERS, 2005). It is important that patients are aware of the symptoms of an exacerbation and know how to respond promptly. Appropriate use of inhaled corticosteroids, bronchodilators and an annual influenza vaccination should reduce the frequency of exacerbations. An exacerbation will usually require a change in medications.

Additional tests used to diagnose COPD (NICE, 2004)

- Chest X-ray to rule out any other causes of the symptoms (lung cancer).
- Blood test to find out if symptoms are caused by anaemia.
- Breathing tests using a peak flow meter to check for asthma; this will be carried out at different times of the day, over several days.
- A blood test for alpha-1 antritrypsin, an enzyme that protects the lungs from harmful substances such as cigarette smoke; this test is more likely to be used if a person is under the age of 40 and has never smoked.
- A TLCO (transfer factor for carbon dioxide) test to assess the lungs' ability to transfer oxygen to the bloodstream; this will usually be carried out if the results of a spirometer test are especially low.
- A computed tomography (CT) scan for a more detailed assessment of the condition of the lungs.
- An (ECG) electrocardiogram and/or an echocardiogram to assess any damage to the heart caused by COPD.

- Pulse oximetry to measure the degree to which the arterial blood is saturated with oxygen.
- A sputum test to check for signs of infection.

ADDITIONAL COMPLICATIONS OF COPD

Cor pulmonale

Cor pulmonale is right-sided heart failure, which can develop as a result of pulmonary disease. Peripheral oedema is a common symptom. Cor pulmonale will usually require long-term oxygen therapy (LTOT) and medications such as diuretics to reduce fluid retention.

Anxiety or depression

It is important to be aware of the increased likelihood of anxiety or depression, which is more common in people with long-term illness. The current recommendations for treating anxiety and depression include the provision of support and medical therapy (NICE, 2004/2010b). People may also benefit from stress management, relaxation techniques and support groups such as Breathe Easy Groups. These local groups are part of the British Lung Foundation and provide support for everyone affected by lung disease, including friends and family.

TREATMENT AND MANAGEMENT

COPD cannot be cured, however, with effective treatments quality of life can be improved. The aim of treatment is to reduce risk factors, manage stable COPD, manage exacerbations, optimise function and improve quality of life. Treatment usually includes smoking cessation, inhaled and oral medications, supplementary oxygen and pulmonary rehabilitation.

Smoking cessation

One of the most important aspects of COPD management is to stop smoking. No other treatment may be needed if the condition is in an early stage and symptoms are mild (Patient UK, 2010b). Depending on the patient's readiness to change, he or she should be offered nicotine replacement therapy (unless contraindicated) and given access to support. Exercise professionals often see clients on a regular basis and are well placed to provide advice, support and encouragement. Positive encouragement towards smoking cessation should be offered at every available opportunity (Patient UK, 2012b & NICE, 2010b).

Pulmonary rehabilitation

Pulmonary rehabilitation is a multidisciplinary programme of care (see table 11.5), tailored to meet the needs of the individual. Comprehensive pulmonary rehabilitation usually consists of key components: exercise, education and psychosocial and behavioural interventions. The goals of pulmonary rehabilitation include:

- reduction in symptoms;
- increased participation in physical and social activities;
- improved overall quality of life.

NICE (2010b:53) suggest that: 'Pulmonary rehabilitation should be made available to all appropriate people with COPD including those who have had a recent hospitalization for an acute exacerbation.'

Medications

The use of oral and inhaled medications play an important role in the management of COPD and

Table 11.5	Multidisciplinary pulmonary rehabilitation care
Exercise professional	Monitor endurance, flexibility, strength, body composition and modify exercise prescription to meet individual needs and correct physical deconditioning
Respiratory therapists	Teach effective use of bronchodilator medications and oxygen therapy
Occupational therapist	Monitor ADLs and teach energy conservation and improved body mechanics to reduce oxygen requirements for specific activities Teach diaphragm breathing to slow respiratory rate
Counselling	To assist with management of anxiety and depression linked with breathlessness and other symptoms limitations

include drugs to control or reduce symptoms and improve exercise capacity (see table 11.9). The main role of medications in COPD is to relax and dilate the airways (bronchodilators), reduce inflammation (anti-inflammatory drugs such as steroids) and reduce the thickness of sputum, making it easier to cough (mucolytic medicines). Antibiotics will be prescribed for chest infections. Many patients will be on a combination of drugs to increase benefits (this may include medications to manage other co-morbidities). There are various methods for the delivery of inhaled medication including inhalers, spacers and nebulisers; the type used will depend on the preference and physical and cognitive skills of the individual and compatibility with other delivery systems used. In more severe cases, where oxygen levels in the blood are low, supplementary oxygen may be required.

Short-acting bronchodilator inhalers An inhaler with a bronchodilator medicine may be prescribed to relax and dilate the muscles in the airways (bronchi). These are often called relievers and include:

- Beta-agonist inhalers (e.g. salbutamol), usually (but not always) blue inhalers
- Antimuscarinic inhalers, e.g, ipratropium.

The inhalers work in different ways, some people need to use both.

People with stable COPD who remain breathless or have exacerbations, despite using short acting broncho-dilators are recommended to have the following prescribed for maintenance therapy:

- Long-acting beta2 agonosts (LABA) or long-acting muscarinic antagonist (LAMA) if FEV1 >50% predicted.
- Inhaled corticosteroids (ICS) in a combination inhaler, or LAMA if FEV1 <50% predicted.
- LAMA + LABA and ICS in patients who remain breathless or experience exacerbations despite taking LABA and ICS, regardless of FEV1 (NICE, 2010*b*:52).

Long-acting bronchodilator inhalers These are longer lasting and may be prescribed if short-acting bronchodilators are of limited effect. Example medications may include beta-agonist inhalers e.g. salmeterol, formoterol and antimuscarinic inhalers, e.g. tiotropium.

Steroid inhalers These are often prescribed in addition to a long-acting bronchodilator inhaler for individuals with more severe COPD or who experience regular flare-ups (exacerbations) to reduce inflammation. Examples include Beclometasone, Budesonide, Ciclesonide, Fluticasone, Mometasone (Patient UK, 2012*b*).

Combination inhalers These contain both a steroid medication and either a short-acting or long-acting beta-agonist. They are usually prescribed for those who have severe symptoms or who experience regular exacerbations. Examples include: Fostair® (formoterol and beclometasone); Seretide® (salmeterol and fluticasone).

Bronchodilator tablets Theophylline is sometimes prescribed to open the airways. It is used in stable COPD rather than in an acute exacerbation. The toxic (dangerous) dose for theophylline is only just above the dose that is needed for the medicine to work (Patient UK, 2012*b*).

Blood tests are done to measure the amount of theophylline in the blood, to check it is neither too high nor too low. Theophylline interacts with lots of other medicines too, so sometimes it cannot be prescribed, due to other medicines taken by the patient.

Mucolytic medicines These are usually prescribed for moderate to severe COPD with frequent flare-ups. They make the sputum less sticky and thick, and easier to cough up and may also reduce exacerbations. Examples include carbocisteine and mecysteine.

To check the currency of medications prescribed, readers should refer to other references (BNF National Formulary, NICE guidance etc.)

Oxygen

Oxygen may be prescribed if the lungs are not able to deliver sufficient oxygen to the body. Some of the signs and symptoms include:
- swelling in legs;
- skin has a bluish tinge;
- an increase in the number of red blood cells (polycythaemia) which indicates chronic hypoxia;
- raised pressure in jugular vein;
- oxygen level is below 92 per cent saturation.

A PaO_2 (partial pressure of oxygen in arterial blood) measurement will indicate the amount of oxygen being transferred from the lungs to the blood. Oxygen may be required in the short term or long term depending on oxygen levels. Oxygen may be used during an infection or exacerbation.

Lung surgery

Surgery may be appropriate for selected patients with COPD and procedures include:
- bullectomy, which involves removing a large bulla (pocket of air) from the lung;
- lung-volume reduction, which involves removing part of the damaged lung;
- lung transplant, which is usually carried out in the final stages of lung disease and involves replacing the diseased lung with a healthy one. The limited supply of donors means that many people are not able to benefit from this procedure.

EXERCISE RECOMMENDATIONS

People at all stages of the disease can benefit from exercise training. Exercise training improves the exercise tolerance and functional capacity of people with COPD, although it has little impact on lung function measurements or disease outcome (for example, survival rates). The main benefits of exercise are improvements in exercise tolerance and managing symptoms of dypsnoea and fatigue (GOLD, 2005 & Patient UK, 2012b).

Exercise improves quality of life and additional benefits include:

- reduction in fear and anxiety;
- reduction of depression;
- improvement in efficiency of skeletal muscles;
- ability to return to work or continue employment;
- improved ability to carry out everyday activities.

Exercise intolerance

People with COPD find it difficult to exercise due to dyspnoea and muscle fatigue and it is important to be aware of the factors affecting exercise intolerance. Exercise intolerance in people with COPD is mainly affected by ventilatory limitations, skeletal muscle dysfunction and cardiovascular and psychological factors.

Ventilatory limitation

In COPD the loss of elastic recoil and airway obstruction increase expiratory resistance and make it difficult to expire normally. This expiratory resistance can triple the normal cost of breathing at rest (McArdle et al, 1991). The effects of increased airway obstruction and the reduced expiratory drive increase the time needed for expiration, which makes it difficult to adequately empty the lungs. This results in an elevated end-expiratory lung volume (EELV) and hyperinflation of the lungs. The diaphragm becomes shortened and flattened and less able to generate the force required for effective breathing.

During exercise, hyperinflation of the lungs increases (dynamic hyperinflation) contributing to dyspnoea and a reduced exercise tolerance (Berry & Woodard, 2003; Cooper, 2009).

Skeletal muscle dysfunction

As well as lung damage, COPD also causes skeletal muscle dysfunction and deconditioning, characterised by a reduction in muscle mass and a change in muscle fibre type. These changes may be caused by a number of factors, including:

- a decrease in levels of physical activity;
- hypoxemia (reduction of oxygen concentration in the arterial blood);
- chronic hypercapnia (high concentration of carbon dioxide in the blood);
- poor nutritional status/malnutrition.

(Adapted from Berry & Woodward, 2003; Cooper, 2009)

The combination of lung damage and skeletal muscle dysfunction contributes to the decrease in exercise tolerance that is characteristic of COPD.

Psychological factors

Fear and anxiety play an important part in decreased exercise tolerance and the cycle of inactivity (described earlier in the chapter). The symptoms of COPD can be frightening, contributing to chronic anxiety, and the physical limitations may result in social isolation and helplessness, which contribute to depression (Cooper, 2009).

Cardiovascular limitations

Cardiovascular function is affected by an increased workload of the right ventricle caused by structural changes in the pulmonary circulation and dynamic hyperinflation (Sietsema, 2001). However, people with COPD are more likely to be limited by other factors such as ventilatory limitations and skeletal muscle dysfunction.

GUIDELINES FOR EXERCISE

There is no current consensus for the optimal exercise prescription for pulmonary patients, however, a comprehensive programme including cardiovascular and muscular strength and endurance training is generally recommended. Patient UK (2012*b*) suggest that any regular exercise or physical activity is beneficial and recommend the activity should make the individual a little out of breath, and be sustained for at least 20–30 minutes, a recommended 4–5 times a week. They suggest a daily brisk walk is a good starting point for those not used to exercise.

The American College of Sports Medicine *Guidelines* (2005*a*) provides a framework, which can be adapted to meet the specific needs of individuals with pulmonary disease.

Cardiovascular training

Many patients with COPD reduce their levels of physical activity to avoid the discomfort of breathlessness. This results in a loss of muscle mass and a decrease in exercise tolerance, which usually results in a reduction in the ability to walk and carry out activities of everyday living.

Pulmonary rehabilitation usually focuses on a combination of strengthening and aerobic activities, such as walking, stepping and stationary cycling. Stationary cycling is especially useful for people with COPD as the forward leaning position reduces the respiratory workload and the fixed arm position enables the accessory muscles to work more efficiently. This will enable clients to perform sufficient levels of cardiovascular training. Supported upper arm ergometry, such as arm cranking, can also be used within a cardiovascular programme, however, upper body cardiovascular exercise is less functional than leg exercise and at a given workload there is an increase in pulmonary ventilation, VO_2max and systolic blood pressure than at equivalent workload with leg exercise (ACSM, 2001).

Until recently it was thought that people with COPD were unable to exercise at sufficient levels of intensity to elicit beneficial physiological adaptations, due to ventilatory limitations. However, recent research has demonstrated that patients with COPD may be able to achieve the aerobic training levels required for physiological adaptations (ATS, 1999). Ideally, the intensity level of exercise will be based on the results of a sub-maximal exercise test such as a 6-minute walk test (6MWT) or incremental shuttle walk test (ISWT), which are commonly used in pulmonary rehabilitation programmes (ATS, 1999). If this information is not available, a conservative exercise prescription is advisable, using exertion or dyspnoea scales to monitor intensity. The traditional method of monitoring exercise intensity using heart rate is less effective in people with COPD and an alternative approach using dyspnoea rating is recommended (ACSM, 2005; Cooper, 2009*b*). A modified CR10 Borg scale is often used to rate dypsnoea during physical activity (see table 11.6). Patients are encouraged to exercise to a dyspnoea rating of 3–4 (moderate to somewhat severe). When determining exercise intensity, it is important to remember that high-intensity exercise may affect exercise compliance (Berry & Woodward, 2003).

The amount of time that the patient can sustain exercise will depend on the health

Table 11.6	Modified Borg dyspnoea scale	
0	Nothing at all	
0.5	Just noticeable – very, very slight	
1	Very slight	
2	Slight	
3	Moderate	Exercise training zone
4	Somewhat severe	
5	Severe	
6		
7	Very severe	
8		
9	Almost maximal – very, very severe	
10	Maximal	

Adapted from Australian Lung Foundation (2012)

Instructions:
1. This scale asks you to rate the difficulty of your breathing.
2. At 0 your breathing is causing no difficulty at all.
3. At 10 your breathing difficulty is maximal.
4. How much difficulty is your breathing causing right now?

status of the individual and his/her level of conditioning. Most people with COPD find it difficult to maintain a higher intensity of exercise for prolonged periods and an interval approach to training is more manageable. This consists of short bouts of higher-intensity exercise (2–3 minutes) alternating with short intervals of rest. After an initial period of training the duration of each bout of higher-intensity activity can be gradually increased (ACSM, 2005).

Muscle strength and endurance training

There has been limited research into the effectiveness of strength training in people with COPD. Peripheral muscle weakness contributes to exercise limitation and strength training is often used to supplement aerobic training within pulmonary rehabilitation.

Lower limb strengthening exercise Exercises, such as sit to stand, squats, lunges and leg extensions are often included to strengthen the lower limbs, with an emphasis on the quadriceps muscles (which are commonly weaker in patients with COPD), the hip extensors and gastrocnemius. These muscles are important for everyday activities such as walking, getting on and off a bus and climbing stairs.
- Squats
- Sit to stand
- Lunges
- Seated leg extensions
- Leg press

Upper limb strengthening exercise Current guidelines recommend that upper limb training is included in pulmonary rehabilitation, however, the research about upper limb training is less clear. Patients with COPD often develop compensatory mechanisms such as use of accessory muscles or fixing of the upper body to help with their breathing. They often have difficulty performing tasks that involve their arms as these compensatory mechanisms are removed. Activities that involve the upper limbs can provoke dyspnoea and fatigue. However, upper body muscular strength and endurance are required for activities of daily living, such as shaving, brushing hair, etc., so it seems appropriate to strengthen the muscles of the upper body. The Australian Lung Foundation (2012) suggests focusing on strengthening the accessory muscles of inspiration (pectoralis major and minor, serratus anterior, latissimus dorsi and trapezius), and biceps and triceps for functional tasks. Exercises using body weight, free weights, resistance machines and therapy bands can be used to train the upper body.

- Chest press
- Wall press-up
- Lat pull-down
- Lateral raises
- Bicep curls
- Tricep extensions
- Seated row

It is important to focus on maintaining optimal posture, good technique and appropriate breathing during resistance training.

Respiratory muscle training

Respiratory muscle weakness may be a contributory factor to breathlessness, exercise limitation and an increased level of carbon dioxide (hypercapnia) in some people with COPD. Much of the research is focused on inspiratory muscle trainers using small hand-held devices. Muscle training with adequate loads does improve the strength of respiratory muscles in people with COPD; however, the benefits are not well established and more research is needed (ATS, 1999).

Mobility and flexibility

Mobility exercise helps maintain the range of movement around joints. People with COPD often have a restricted range of movement in the spine, especially the thoracic spine. Mobility of the thoracic spine, including rotation, flexion and extension, is important for effective breathing.

Spinal mobility can be included as part of the warm-up and cool-down. The exercises can be performed seated or standing, although seated spinal mobility is particularly effective for encouraging good technique.

A combination of inactivity, ageing and breathlessness often leads to hunched posture and limited range of movement. Stretching helps to maintain range of movement and can be used to address poor posture and increase flexibility. Consider a whole body approach with an emphasis on muscles that become shortened due to postural changes, for example the pectorals. Use appropriate positions and props such as therapy bands to ensure stability and effective technique. See tables 11.7a and b for a summary of exercise recommendations for COPD from different sources. Exercise professionals should consider both sets of guidance and apply this in accordance with the specific needs of individual clients.

KEY CONSIDERATIONS

- Ensure appropriate screening to identify co-morbidities such as cardiovascular disease, osteoporosis and arthritis and to check risk stratification is within current competence.
- Use RPE and breathlessness scale to monitor intensity.
- Ensure medical management is optimised and client presents no exercise contraindications.
- Ensure ongoing assessment and modification of exercise programme in response to changes in health status.

Table 11.7a	Summary of exercise guidelines for COPD		
Training guidelines	**Cardiovascular**	**Muscle strength**	**Flexibility and neuromuscular**
Frequency	3–5 sessions per week. An individual with very limited functional capacity may require daily exercise	2–3 days per week (non-consecutive days)	3–7 days per week
Intensity	3–4 on Borg CR10 scale	Begin at 50–60% 1RM and progress to 80% 1RM	Lengthen muscle to point of tightness but not discomfort
Time	20–30 minutes (Interval training may be more appropriate for some individuals)	One to three sets of 8–10 repetitions	15–30 seconds; repeat stretches 2–4 times
Type	Walking, stepping, stationary cycling. Activities involving the upper body such as rowing may promote excessive dyspnoea in some individuals	8–10 exercises using major muscle groups. Whole body approach with an emphasis on quadriceps, gluteals, hamstrings and gastrocnemius, accessory muscles of inspiration (pectorals, latissimus dorsi, serratus anterior, trapezius), and biceps and triceps for functional tasks	Static stretch of all major muscle groups to improve joint range of movement and address postural changes, e.g. pectoral muscles
Functional	Include activities that reflect activities of daily living such as reaching, stair climbing, sit to stand. Core muscle training, balance and coordination exercises to address posture and balance		

Adapted from ACSM (2005); Australian Lung Foundation (2004/2012)

- Progress exercise programme gradually.
- Mid-late morning or early afternoon may be best time to exercise due to decreased dyspnoea.
- Avoid exercise in extremes of temperature and humidity (Cooper, 2003).
- Encourage people to plan their exercise and activities to avoid doing too much in one day.
- Provide opportunities for development of social networks.
- Emphasise optimal posture and good technique.
- Any significant change in condition will require reassessment of goals and risks of exercise (Cooper, 2009).

Table 11.7b	Updated exercise guidelines for COPD		
Training guidelines	Cardiovascular	Muscle strength	Flexibility and neuromuscular
Aims	Increase VO$_2$ peak Lactate threshold and ventilator threshold Improve ADL Reduce sensitivity to breathlessness Promote more efficient breathing	Increase lean body mass Increase maximal number of repetitions	Increase ROM Improve balance, breathing efficiency and gait
Frequency Intensity Duration	1–2 sessions on 3–5 days per week 30 minutes (shorter, accumulated targets initially) RPE 11-13 (on RPE 20 scale) Monitor breathlessness Emphasise progression of duration rather than intensity	Low resistance High repetitions 2–3 sessions per week	3 sessions per week

Adapted from Cooper, C. in Durstine et al (2009)

- If client experiences excessive breathlessness, remain calm and encourage client to adopt a comfortable position and use breathing techniques learned within pulmonary rehabilitation. Leaning forwards, either seated or standing with arms supported, reduces the respiratory effort and will help relax the upper chest while encouraging the use of the lower chest during breathing.
- Provide support and encouragement to promote adherence.
- Be sensitive to anxiety, fear and depression experienced due to breathlessness and disability.
- Living with a long-term condition such as COPD can be stressful. The relaxation component is an ideal time to practise relaxation techniques and effective breathing, emphasising the use of the diaphragmatic breathing (see chapter 14).
- Develop an effective working relationship with local respiratory physiotherapists. This will enhance client care and provide opportunities for continued professional learning and development.

ASTHMA

Asthma is a chronic inflammatory condition that affects the airways (bronchi) of the lungs. This causes narrowing (constriction) of the airway, which is usually reversible, either spontaneously or with medication, usually an inhaler (Prodigy 2005a/2012; Patient UK, 2011). However, in some people with chronic asthma, inflammation may lead to irreversible airflow obstruction (SIGN & BTS, 2005). In asthma the airways are hypersensitive and constrict in response to a trigger, which results in a range of symptoms including shortness of breath, coughing, chest tightness and wheezing. Asthma can start at any age, but it more usually starts in childhood. Adult-onset asthma is usually triggered by exposure to substances in the workplace (occupational asthma) (Prodigy 2005a/2011).

CAUSES

Asthma is caused by inflammation of the airways (Patient UK, 2011). The cause of the inflammation is not completely understood, however, it usually occurs when the person comes into contact with a trigger that irritates the airways and causes the symptoms of asthma to flare-up. Common triggers (some of which can be avoided) include:

- **Viral or bacterial infections** Infections such as colds, coughs and chest infections are common triggers. Some people with asthma may be advised to have a yearly flu injection; this will depend on their age and the severity of their asthma.
- **Exercise** For some people exercise is a trigger (exercise-induced asthma – EIA). However, exercise is beneficial for overall health so it is important for people with asthma to remain as active as possible. Asthma symptoms that worsen during or after exercise may indicate poorly controlled asthma, and may require a review of treatment. Exercise may help to control the frequency and severity of asthma attacks (Clark & Cochrane, 2009).
- **House dust mite** Some people are sensitive to house dust mites that live in soft furnishings, mattresses and carpets around the home.
- **Pollution** There is evidence that air pollution increases the likelihood of acute asthma attacks and aggravates chronic asthma (SIGN & BTS, 2005). On hot days when ozone levels are high it is better to avoid exercising outside.
- **Animals** Pets such as cats and dogs can be a common trigger; finding a new home for the pet or excluding the pet from certain areas of the house, such as the bedroom or living room, might help.
- **Emotion** Feeling down or under pressure or trying to cope with ongoing stressful situations can trigger symptoms of asthma. A prolonged episode of laughter can also be a trigger.
- **Certain drugs** Beta-blockers, which are taken for heart disease and glaucoma, and non-steroidal anti-inflammatory tablets such as aspirin, can trigger symptoms of asthma.
- **Pollens and moulds** Asthma is often worse during the hay fever season.
- **Cigarette smoke** Smoking or being in smoky environments can irritate the lungs, trigger asthma and cause permanent damage to the airways.
- **Occupations** Higher risk occupations include pastry making, metal work, chemical processing, baking, spray painting, farming etc.

(Adapted from Prodigy 2005a/2011; Patient UK, 2011; BTS/Sign, 2011)

Clients can reduce the severity of existing disease by avoiding known triggers. Sometimes a link is obvious, but sometimes there can be a delayed response to a trigger, making it more difficult to identify.

Some people may experience occupational asthma that is caused by exposure to specific substances at work, or they may already have asthma that is aggravated by substances or fumes in the workplace.

PREVALENCE

There are approximately 5.4 million people in the UK with asthma (Asthma UK, 2005). It can start at any age, but usually starts in childhood. Approximately one in ten children and one in twenty adults have asthma and it can run in families. About half the children who develop asthma grow out of it when they reach adulthood. It is estimated that three people die from asthma every day and many asthma-related hospital admissions (75 per cent) and deaths (90 per cent) are preventable (Prodigy 2005a; Patient UK, 2011; Asthma UK 2012).

Signs and symptoms can range from mild to severe and include:

- wheeze;
- shortness of breath;
- cough;
- chest tightness.

People may have some or all of the symptoms of asthma and the severity can vary at different times. The symptoms can sometimes last for just an hour and at other times may continue for a few days or even weeks if untreated. The symptoms of asthma are often worse at night and in the early morning and are often provoked by triggers such as pollen, cold air, exercise and some medications (aspirin or beta-blockers). Asthma does not always follow a predictable pattern and the severity and duration of symptoms may vary. During an exacerbation there will be wheeze and reduced lung function, which can be measured using a peak flow and spirometer (SIGN & BTS, 2005/2011).

DIAGNOSIS

A doctor usually diagnoses asthma based on typical signs and symptoms. Additional information will also contribute to a diagnosis of asthma:

- family history of asthma or atopic conditions such as eczema or allergic rhinitis;
- worsening of symptoms after using drugs such as aspirin, beta-blockers and non-steroidal anti-inflammatory medication;
- recognised triggers such as pollen, exercise, dust, or tobacco smoke.

Some of the symptoms of asthma are common to a range of diseases and conditions, which can make it difficult to diagnose. Asthma can also coexist with other conditions such as chronic obstructive pulmonary disease.

Objective measurements

Objective measurements such as peak expiratory flow (PEF) and forced expiratory volume in one second (FEV1) can be used in the diagnosis of asthma. In obstructive disease there will usually be a decrease in both these measurements, however, measurements may be normal if they are taken between episodes of bronchospasm. The following objective measurements demonstrate variability and reversibility of airway obstruction and can be used to confirm a diagnosis of asthma:

- more than 20 per cent daily variation on at least three days a week for two weeks, using a peak expiratory flow diary, is suggestive of asthma;
- more than 15 per cent (and 200ml) increase in FEV1 after taking short-acting beta2 agonists or steroid tablets or an increase in airflow limitation after six minutes of running;
- more than 15 per cent decrease in FEV1 after six minutes of running.

(Adapted from Prodigy, 2005)

Patients may be encouraged to monitor or home chart their peak flow readings as part of a personalised action plan. This can be used for the initial diagnosis and ongoing management of asthma (SIGN & BTS, 2005).

COMPLICATIONS

If people do not have optimal control of their asthma, they will often feel tired and either underperform at work or need time off. In the UK approximately 1500 people a year die from asthma (BTS, 1997). Some people experience psychological problems associated with the development of the role of a sick person (Prodigy, 2005a).

TREATMENT

General goals for working with people with asthma are:
- to maintain optimal control of asthma;
- to minimise symptoms during the day and the night;
- reduce the need for rescue medication;
- to avoid limitation of physical activity and work towards current recommendations for health;

- to maintain 'normal' lung function (FEV1 and/or PEF >80% predicted or best) (SIGN, 2010);
- to prevent exacerbations;
- to work in partnership with the client to encourage self-management of condition.

It is important to find a balance between optimal control and the inconvenience involved in taking medications and the side effects of medications (Prodigy, 2005a). The client's goals need to be individualised and s/he needs to be actively involved in decisions about the treatment of his or her asthma.

Self-management

Self-management plays an important part in the management of long-term conditions. The Scottish Intercollegiate Guidelines Network (SIGN, 2005) recommended the use of a set of educational resources produced by Asthma UK, 'Be in Control', which are designed to support self-management.

Avoidance of triggers

There is evidence that avoiding the exposure to a trigger or allergen may help to reduce the severity of existing asthma (SIGN & BTS, 2005/2010).

Smoking cessation

Smoking cessation is advisable not only for general health, but it may also help reduce the severity of asthma. It is important that adults are aware of the health implications for children of passive smoking, which include an increased likelihood of developing respiratory disease and an increase in the severity of asthma.

Weight management

Weight reduction is recommended for obese clients to improve asthma symptoms (SIGN & BTS, 2005/2010) and exercise can contribute to a weight loss programme.

Medications

Inhalers are the most common treatment to prevent the symptoms of asthma (for medications see table 11.9). Inhalers deliver the medication direct to the airways, minimising side effects. Inhalers are classified as 'relievers', 'preventers' and 'long-acting bronchodilators'. A stepwise approach is used to maintain optimal control of asthma. This involves stepping up treatment when required and stepping down treatment when the control of asthma is good (SIGN, 2011). Any change the client makes to her or his treatment needs to be negotiated with the GP and written in her or his personal action plan.

Relievers (blue inhaler) Relievers are used to relieve the mild to moderate symptoms of asthma by dilating the airways. They are *short-acting beta2-agonists* and include salbutamol and terbutaline. If a reliever is required more than three times a week to ease symptoms, a preventer inhaler is usually prescribed.

Preventers (brown or maroon inhaler) A preventer is usually taken twice daily, once in the morning and once in the evening, to prevent symptoms developing. It does not have an immediate effect so it cannot be used for instant relief of asthma. Steroids are the drugs commonly used in preventers. *Steroids (inhaled)* are very effective in the management of asthma as they reduce inflammation of the airways. This causes a reduction of oedema and secretion of mucus into the airways, and decreases the likelihood of the airways narrowing.

Long-acting bronchodilator Salmeterol and formoterol are inhaled *long-acting beta2-agonists*, which may be prescribed in addition to the inhaled steroids if further control is required.

Corticosteroids Steroid tablets, such as prednisolone, may be required if the symptoms of asthma are severe or prolonged. If clients are on long-term steroid use (e.g. longer than three months) there is likely to be a reduction in bone density. A long-acting bisophonate should be prescribed to reduce the effects of steroids on bone density.

EXERCISE RECOMMENDATIONS

People with asthma often have worsening symptoms when they exercise and this can be a barrier to increased levels of physical activity. This can lead to a cycle of inactivity with people avoiding activities that might make them breathless, resulting in decreased levels of activity and decreased fitness levels. Exercise contributes an increase in cardiopulmonary fitness and should be promoted as part of a general approach to improving lifestyle.

Many people with asthma report that they feel better and have fewer symptoms when fit.

Habitual physical activity increases physical fitness and reduces the likelihood of provoking exercise-induced asthma (EIA).

Exercise training may reduce the perception of breathlessness through a number of mech-anisms, including strengthening respiratory muscles (Ram et al, 2005).

Exercise-induced asthma (EIA)

Exercise can lead to an increase in airway resistance in people with asthma, leading to EIA. It is important to give clients advice about how to reduce or prevent EIA by pre-treatment with appropriate medication and appropriate exercise recommendations (Ram et al, 2005). Exercise-induced asthma usually begins during exercise and symptoms worsen about 15 minutes afterwards (Asthma, UK 2004). The mechanism behind EIA is not fully understood, but it may be connected to an increase in breathing rate, changes in airway temperature and airway drying.

Certain types of activity are likely to trigger exercise-induced asthma:

- exercising at higher levels (>75 per cent age-predicted maximum) of intensity is more likely to provoke asthma, although people with severe asthma may experience symptoms at lower levels of intensity;
- prolonged activity, such as long-distance running;
- exercise outside in cold, dry air;
- heavily chlorinated swimming pools.

(Adapted from Asthma UK, 2005)

Exercise-induced asthma is usually related to poorly controlled asthma. Once asthma is more effectively controlled, the symptoms of EIA usually stop. If a client is on preventative treatment for asthma but still experiences problems with EIA, s/he may need to have a review of medication and an assessment of inhaler technique. Using an inhaled short-acting beta2-agonist is recommended just before exercise, to prevent the symptoms of EIA. This may need to be repeated during prolonged exercise (SIGN & BTS, 2005/2010). Asthma UK (2004) recommends an extended warm-up and cool-down to decrease the likelihood of EIA.

Exercise recommendations for people with asthma are in line with general ACSM (2005) guidelines. All components of the exercise programme and the basic principles of frequency,

intensity, time and type will need to be tailored to meet the needs of the individual. See table 11.8 for a summary of exercise guidelines.

EXERCISE CONSIDERATIONS AND LIMITATIONS

- Check the asthma is well controlled and if not, refer the client back to their GP.
- Postpone exercise and advise client to visit GP to discuss asthma control if they answer YES to any of the following questions:
  - Is sleep affected by night-time cough or wheeze?
  - Has asthma interfered with everyday activities or exercise?
  - Are peak flow readings lower than normal?
  - Is client using a reliever more frequently than usual?
- Check that the client has regular check-ups with GP and has a written personal asthma plan.
- A dose of reliever just before exercise may help to prevent symptoms.
- Check client has appropriate medications such as reliever inhaler close to hand during exercise.
- Teach client to monitor exercise intensity using the RPE and breathlessness scale (table 11.6).
- A prolonged warm-up and cool-down will decrease the likelihood of EIA symptoms developing.
- Progress the programme gradually.
- Best time to exercise may be mid to late morning (Clark & Cochrane, 2009).
- Avoid exercising in extremes of temperature and humidity.
- Be aware of environmental triggers such as hot

Table 11.8	Summary of exercise guidelines for asthma		
Training guidelines	Cardiovascular	Muscle strength	Flexibility and neuromuscular
Aims	Improve breathing patterns Improve ADL Reduce sensitivity to breathlessness Increase VO_2max. Increase lactate and ventilator threshold	Increase maximal number of repetitions	Increase ROM (flexibility) Improve gait, balance and breathing efficiency (neuromuscular)
Frequency	3–5 days per week	2–3 days per week	Minimal 3 days per week Ideally 5–7 days per week Neuromuscular – daily
Intensity	55%/65%–75% HRmax 11–13 RPE (20 scale) Monitor breathlessness Emphasise progression of duration over intensity	Low resistance and higher repetitions Stop 2–3 reps before fatigue (e.g. RPE 15–16)	To position of mild tension, not pain or discomfort
Time	30 minutes (continuous or intermittent) activity)	1 set of 8–10/12–15 repetitions	Develop or maintain range of motion 15–30 seconds Repeat x 2–4
Type	Large muscle groups, dynamic activity	8–10 muscle groups that train major muscle groups Target specific areas of weakness Full range of movement	Static stretch (focus on muscles with a reduced range of movement)

Adapted from ACSM (2005); Asthma UK, Cooper & Cochrane (2009:147)

or humid days when ozone levels are high, or cold air. Use a scarf to cover the mouth and nose during cold weather.

- An interval approach to exercise, where periods of aerobic activity are interspersed with short breaks, is less likely to provoke EIA.
- Swimming is an ideal activity due to an environment of warm, humid air, and strengthening of the upper body.

- Make sure you know what to do in the event of an asthma attack (see chapter 6, page 76).
- Be sensitive to anxiety, depression and fear in response to breathlessness and disability.
- Consider side effects of any medications.
- Modify frequency, intensity, time and type of activity to suit individual needs and abilities and any co-morbidities.

Table 11.9	Medications for COPD and asthma		
Medication	Action	Side effects	Exercise considerations
Short-acting bronchodilators (relievers)			
Beta2-agonist inhalers (e.g. salbutamol)	Relax and open up (dilate) the muscles in the airways Quickly reduce airway obstruction and reduce symptoms of breathlessness and fatigue Rapid onset action and relieve symptoms for 4-6 hours	Common: Fine tremor in hands Nervous tension Headaches Restlessness Rare: Palpitations Tachycardia Muscle cramps	Tachycardia May improve exercise capacity in clients limited by bronchospasm
Antimuscarinic inhalers (e.g. ipratropium) Anti-cholinergic	As above	Common: Dry mouth Nausea/headache Rare: Palpitations Tachycardia Constipation Cough	As above
Long-acting bronchodilators			
Beta2-agonist inhalers (e.g. salmeterol)	Relax and open up (dilate) the muscles in the airways To control ongoing symptoms not relieved by short acting bronchodilators The duration of their action lasts up to 12 hours They reduce bronchospasm and reduce hyperinflation	Common: Tremor Rare: Palpitations Headaches Muscle cramps	Salmeterol may help prevent exercise induced asthma
Antimuscarinic inhalers (e.g. tiotropium) Anti-cholinergic	Relax and open up (dilate) the muscles in the airways	Common: Dry mouth Sore throat Rare: Nosebleeds Palpitations Tachycardia Blurred vision	Tachycardia

Medication	Action	Side effects	Exercise considerations
Steroid inhalers (preventers) May be prescribed in addition to a bronchodilator inhaler for more severe COPD or regular flare-ups (exacerbations)			
Beclometasone Budesonide Ciclesonide Fluticasone Mometasone	Prevent flare ups Reduce airway inflammation, oedema and secretions	Oral thrush Sore throat Hoarse voice Sore tongue Mouth infection (thrush) A prolonged high dose may lead to side effects for oral coticosteroids	Consider exercise recommendations and limitations for osteoporosis
Bronchodilator tablets			
Methylxanthines Theophylline Aminophylline	Open the airways	Potential for toxicity and drug interactions May cause tachycardia, arrhythmias, headache, malaise, palpitations Nausea/ headache Convulsions NB: Toxic (dangerous) dose for theophylline is only slightly above the dose that is needed for the medicine to work well	May increase exercise capacity Tachycardia and arrhythmias, palpitations
Oral corticosteroids			
Prednisone Metylprednislone	Similar to inhaled corticosteroids	Long term use associated with osteoporosis, weight gain, thin skin, bruising, altered diabetic control, mood swings	Also consider exercise recommendations and limitations for osteoporosis

Medication	Action	Side effects	Exercise considerations
Leukotriene receptor antagonists			
Montelukast Zaafirlukast	Blocks the effects of chemicals called leukotrienes that are produced in response of a trigger, in people with asthma	Common: Abdominal pain Headache Rare: Nausea Dizziness Weakness Worsening chest symptoms Productive cough Numbness	May be of benefit in exercise induced asthma

CARDIOVASCULAR DISEASE

12

Cardiovascular disease (CVD) is an umbrella term that refers to all conditions that affect the heart and circulatory system, including coronary heart disease (angina, myocardial infarction or heart attack, heart failure), hypertension (high blood pressure), stroke and peripheral vascular disease (PVD).

This section will explore the risk factors for CVD/CHD and will discuss lifestyle recommendations for managing these risk factors. It will also discuss the exercise implications and considerations for CHD related conditions including:

- angina (a brief introduction only, as this condition is outside the scope of practice for a Level 3 exercise referral instructor and would be managed by a Level 4 BACR instructor);
- hypertension.

Exercise as part of cardiac rehabilitation including post-myocardial infarction (MI), re-vascularisation procedures and cardiac surgery is covered in the Level 4 British Association for Cardiac Rehabilitation (BACR) course and would need to be managed by an instructor who had completed this training.

PREVALENCE

Cardiovascular disease is the leading cause of global death. It is responsible for around 200,000 deaths each year in the UK and it is estimated that over 3 million Britons suffer from CVD (BHF, 2008). In 2009, CVD was responsible for approximately one-third of all deaths in the UK, with around 82,000 deaths caused by coronary heart disease and 49,000 deaths from stroke (BHF, 2012).

CAUSES

The underlying cause of all CVD is atherosclerosis. Atherosclerosis is a complex process, which involves the build-up of fatty material (atheroma) and atherosclerotic plaques in the walls of the arteries, in response to irritation or injury to the inner lining of the wall of the arteries. These plaques lead to narrowing of the arteries, which restricts blood flow and the delivery of oxygen to the affected areas; they may also trigger a local thrombosis (blood clot), which completely blocks the flow of blood to the area (BHF, 2008). Atherosclerosis can affect:

- the **coronary arteries**, causing coronary heart disease (CHD). Reduced blood flow to the *heart* can result in angina (causing pain and discomfort in the chest). Alternatively, if a piece of atheroma breaks away, it may cause a clot which cuts off supply of blood to the heart, resulting in a heart attack.

- the **cerebrovascular arteries**, leading to stroke or transient ischaemic attacks (TIA), caused by a clot blocking the arteries to the *brain*.
- the **peripheral arteries**, causing peripheral arterial disease (PAD), which may affect one or both legs causing intermittent claudication (pain in the calf muscle) or ischaemic leg (BHF, 2008), caused by a blood clot restricting blood flow to the leg/s.

RISK FACTORS

A number of CVD (and CHD) risk factors have been identified and include various genetic, environmental and lifestyle factors (see table 12.1 and also table 4.2 in chapter 4, page 54). Risk factors are measurable factors that predict the development of the disease. The main risk factors that are routinely assessed in clinical practice are often classified as modifiable and non-modifiable (see table 12.1). Non-modifiable risk factors are fixed and cannot be changed, whereas modifiable risk factors can be changed.

Non-modifiable risk factors

Family history Family history is defined as CVD in a male first-degree relative, aged <55 years or in a female first-degree relative, aged <65.

Ethnicity Some groups within a country are at a higher risk of developing CVD than others because of genetic or racial factors (Smith et al, 2004). For example, South Asians (Indians, Bangladeshis, Pakistanis and Sri Lankans) living in the UK have a higher than average premature death rate from CHD.

Table 12.1	Risk factors for CVD/CHD
Non-modifiable or fixed risk factors	**Modifiable risk factors**
• Age • Gender • Family history of premature CVD • Ethnic origin	• Smoking • Physical inactivity • Obesity/overweight • Unhealthy diet • Excess alcohol • Stress (and how managed) • High cholesterol • Hypertension/high blood pressure • Diabetes or elevated blood glucose • Socio-economic (type of work and income)

Adapted from BHF (2008, 2012)

Age Age is a major risk factor. Prevalence increases with age, approximately doubling with each decade. CVD is common in over 60s but rare below age 30 (BHF, 2008). Although increasing age does not cause CVD, there is more time for the development of atherosclerosis, which can lead to CVD events.

Gender Women tend to present with CHD about 10 years later than men; onset in women may be linked to falling levels of oestrogen around the menopause, which causes an increase in cholesterol levels (BHF, 2003/2008). CHD is often considered a man's disease, but this is not the case. In 2001, 54,491 women died of CHD compared to 66,400 men. One in six women die from CHD, and after the age of 75 more women than men die of CHD (BHF, 2003*b*).

Modifiable risk factors

Smoking Smoking is one of the main modifiable risk factors for CHD. Smoking influences the formation of thrombus, plaque instability and arrhythmia. People who smoke are more likely to have ischaemic heart disease and have a higher risk of dying from it. The more cigarettes smoked, the greater the risk. South Asian men, who are already at a greater risk of CHD, continue to smoke more than the general population. Twenty-nine per cent of the general UK population smoke, compared to 42 per cent of Bangladeshi men (BHF, 2005d).

High blood pressure (hypertension) Persistently raised blood pressure is a key risk factor for CVD and people with high blood pressure run a higher risk of having a stroke or a heart attack. A person will be diagnosed as having hypertension if their systolic blood pressure is higher than 140mmHg or their diastolic blood pressure is higher than 90mmHg (NICE, 2004c).

High cholesterol Cholesterol is a fatty substance produced by the body. It plays a vital role in the functioning of cell walls. It is made up of high-density lipoproteins (HDLs) and low-density lipoproteins (LDLs), which are responsible for transporting cholesterol around the body. People with high levels of LDL are at a high risk of atherosclerosis, whereas high levels of HDL appear to have a protective effect. Other blood lipids such as triglycerides also have a role in the development of atherosclerosis: a high level of triglycerides increases the risk of CHD.

Familial hyperlipidaemia Approximately 1 in 500 people in the UK have an inherited condition called familial hyperlipidaemia or familial cholesterolaemia. Diagnosis requires:
- cholesterol >7.5 mmol/l, or

- low-density lipoproteins >4.9 mmol/l in adults, plus clinical signs of hyperlipidaemia such as tendon xanthomas. These appear as lumps on the tendons at the back of the ankles or on the tendons on the back of hands. People with familial hyperlipidaemia have an increased risk of CHD and aggressive treatment is recommended with lipid-lowering therapy and dietary advice (Patient UK, 2004).

Diabetes In people with diabetes, good glycaemic control is essential. This has a beneficial effect on cholesterol and decreases the risk of coronary heart disease. Men with type 2 diabetes have a two- to fourfold greater annual risk of CHD. Women with type 2 diabetes have a three- to fivefold annual risk of CHD (BHF, 2005c).

Psychosocial well-being The British Heart Foundation (2005c) identifies a number of psychosocial factors that are associated with an increased risk of CHD including:
- lack of social networks;
- stress related to employment;
- depression;
- personality (hostile).

Stress Stress can result in chemical changes in the body, which can increase heart rate, blood pressure and cholesterol levels. Psychosocial factors can also have an impact on health-related behaviours such as smoking, diet, physical activity and alcohol consumption.

Diet An atherogenic diet can contribute to CHD in many populations (Smith et al, 2004). In the UK fat intake, especially of saturated fats, is considered too high and daily salt intake is well above recommended levels. Consumption of fresh fruit and vegetables is low and in the UK only 13 per cent of men and 15 per cent of women eat the recommended five portions of fruit and vegetables a day. There are also marked socio-economic differences, with people on lower incomes eating fewer portions of fruit and vegetables than people on higher incomes (BHF, 2005).

Overweight and obesity Excess weight is associated with type 2 diabetes, raised blood pressure and raised cholesterol, which are all risk factors for CVD. Central obesity substantially increases these risks. See chapter 9 for further information.

Excess alcohol Alcohol needs to be considered within the context of dietary advice, in particular when an individual is overweight and needs to restrict calorie intake. However, a small amount of alcohol can be beneficial to the heart, possibly by increasing HDL. The pattern of drinking is important, with binge drinking associated with an increased risk of fatal myocardial infarction and stroke (Prodigy, 2003).

Sedentary lifestyle A physically active lifestyle decreases the risk of cardiovascular disease mortality, especially CHD mortality (DoH, 2001a). Only 37 per cent of men and 24 per cent of women currently achieve the current recommendations for health (BHF, 2005c).

Social inequality Social inequality is considered a risk factor for CHD. Premature death rate from CHD is 58 per cent higher for men who are manual workers than for non-manual workers (BHF, 2005). Factors such as psychosocial stress, behavioural factors and access to healthcare may contribute to an increased risk in people who are from lower socio-economic groups (Smith et al, 2004).

Multiple risk factors increase the possibility of an individual developing CVD/CHD (e.g. three risk factors place an individual at higher risk than two risk factors); however, even single risk factors such as long-standing and severe high blood pressure can lead to premature CVD. Some risk factors offer a much greater risk (smoking, hypertension) than other risk factors (overweight/obesity). Many risk factors are not modifiable, others are, and the aim should be to reduce modifiable risk factors (Patient UK, 2012). See table 12.2.

CARDIOVASCULAR RISK ASSESSMENT

Cardiovascular risk assessment is used in primary care as a tool to guide practice and to help health professionals and patients make decisions about appropriate interventions, for instance in the areas of lifestyle and drug therapy.

Cardiovascular risk assessment aims to estimate the probability (percentage chance) of an individual developing CVD over a defined period of time by calculating and accounting for all risk factors (see table 12.1). Risk factor assessment would include consideration of: ethnicity, smoking, family history of CVD, weight, waist circumference, age, blood pressure, total cholesterol and HDL cholesterol. The risk prediction charts can be downloaded from www.bnf.org.

Current guidance suggests that persons with a two in ten risk within the next ten years should be started on a treatment plan (Patient UK, 2012) which may include:

- medication to lower blood pressure;
- medication to lower cholesterol;
- aspirin (for persons with angina) to reduce the risk of clots;
- lifestyle interventions, activity, smoking cessation, dietary changes etc.

Table 12.2	Lifestyle recommendations for prevention of CVD and CHD
Smoking	All people who smoke should be encouraged to stop and be offered appropriate support, including access to smoking cessation specialists and nicotine replacement therapy (NRT)
Dietary management	Reduce saturated fats and trans fats and replace with unsaturated fats such as rape seed oil or olive oil Increase level of fruit and vegetables (a minimum of 5 portions of fruit and vegetables a day) Consumption of at least 2 portions of oily fish a week or other sources of omega fatty acids Reduce salt intake to <6g of sodium chloride or <2.4g/day sodium per day
Weight control	Encourage people to aim for a body mass index (BMI) of 20–25 If this is too difficult for people, encourage more realistic target of 5–10kg weight loss Avoid central obesity
Alcohol	Encourage people to limit alcohol consumption to 1–2 units of alcohol per day For men limit intake to <21 (no more than 4 units in one day) For women limit intake to <14 (no more than 3 units in one day)
Exercise	Encourage adults to do at least 150 minutes over the course of one week This could be 30 minutes moderate aerobic activity most days of the week or vigorous activity on fewer days (see chapter 1 for guidance) Note: Any exercise recommendations need to take account of specific conditions such as diabetes, *hyperlipidaemia or obesity (see relevant chapters)

*Adults with hyperlipidaemia are encouraged to exercise at least 5 times a week at a moderate intensity for up to 60 minutes. The aim is to increase calorie expenditure by exercising for 200–300 minutes per week, >2000 calories per week (ACSM, 2005).

Adapted from JBS (2005); Patient Plus UK (2005); NICE (2010c); DoH (2011)

CARDIOPROTECTIVE DRUG THERAPIES

All high-risk people will be prescribed an antiplatelet drug such as aspirin, and a statin to reduce cholesterol levels. People with established cardiovascular disease, such as CHD, may also be prescribed additional drugs including beta-blockers, ACE inhibitors and calcium channel blockers. See table 12.7 for medications.

CORONARY HEART DISEASE (CHD)

CHD refers to the narrowing of the coronary arteries supplying the heart muscle. Atherosclerotic plaques can develop over many years, causing narrowing of one or more arteries and the reduction of blood flow through the **coronary arteries**. The first indication of the disease may not be recognised until an individual presents with

Table 12.3	Risk factor targets for CVD prevention in high-risk people		
Risk factor	People with atherosclerotic cardiovascular disease	Asymptomatic people at a high risk (CVD risk ≥ 20% over 10 years)	People with diabetes
Body weight distribution	White caucasian: men <102 cm or 40 inches, women <88 cm or 35 inches		
	Asian: men <90 cm, women <80cm; Body mass index (BMI) <25		
Blood pressure	<130 mmHg systolic <80 mmHg diastolic	<140 mmHg systolic <85 mmHg diastolic	<130 mmHg systolic <80 mmHg diastolic
Cholesterol			
Total cholesterol	<4.0 mmo/l or a 25% reduction		
Low density lipoproteins (LDL)	<2.00 mmol/l or a 30% reduction		
Glucose (Fasting Plasma glucose)	≤6.0 mmol/l	≤6.0 mmol/l	≤6.0 mmol/l HbA1c <6.5%

(Taken from Joint British Societies Guidelines' 2005)

angina or experiences myocardial infarction (heart attack) or sudden cardiac death. People with other manifestations of atherosclerosis such as stroke or peripheral arterial disease are likely to have CHD.

STABLE ANGINA

Stable angina is caused by the temporary shortage of oxygen to the heart muscle, which is often the result of emotion or exertion. Angina is a **symptom**, not a disease, per se. Coronary heart disease (CHD) is the main cause of angina. Stable angina has an established pattern; it is characterised by symptoms at a predictable level of exertion and it is well controlled with medication.

SIGNS AND SYMPTOMS

Angina pectoralis describes the classic symptoms of chest pain, which is often described as a crushing pain, pressing or tightness. The most common symptom of angina is a pain across the front of the chest. This may feel like an ache or discomfort, which can radiate to the jaw, neck, arm, or abdomen and is often accompanied by shortness of breath. Some people describe it as feeling like a band of steel being tightened across the chest, or a crushing weight. Although the term 'pain' is often used to describe the symptoms of angina, it is not always perceived as pain and some people describe it as a troublesome ache. It is often related to exertion and is relieved by rest. It can also be triggered by other situations, including:

- vivid dreams;
- eating a heavy meal;
- being out in cold windy weather;
- emotional stress.

Many people find angina very distressing and get frightened. These feelings can cause other symptoms such as palpitations, sweating and feeling sick. Angina doesn't usually last longer than 10 minutes with rest, or is quickly relieved by taking glyceryl trinitrate (GTN). Some people find it difficult to tell the difference between the symptoms of angina and other chest pain such as:

- musculoskeletal pain;
- referred pain from the thoracic spine;
- oesophageal disorders;
- pulmonary disease.

Chest pain is more likely to be linked to coronary heart disease in someone with two or more CHD risk factors; however, someone with CHD may still experience non-cardiac chest pain (SIGN, 2001*b*).

UNSTABLE ANGINA

Unstable angina is a contraindication for exercise and it is important for the individual to seek immediate medical attention. Unstable angina is the term used to describe angina that has changed in some way and is less predictable than stable angina. One or more of the following defines unstable angina (BHF, 2005*b*):

- newly diagnosed angina;
- established angina that is getting worse, for example, angina that comes on with lower levels of exertion;
- frequent episodes of angina, not related to exertion;
- sudden onset of severe chest pain at rest.

Unstable angina is associated with atherosclerotic plaque instability and there is an increased risk of a myocardial infarction (see chapter 6, page 73).

DIAGNOSIS

The diagnosis of angina is based on history-taking to establish a clear description of the symptoms, including precipitating factors such as climbing stairs or emotions such as anger, anxiety or excitement. A physical examination and a number of both non-invasive and invasive investigations will be carried out by a health professional to confirm the diagnosis. Individuals diagnosed with angina are considered to be high-risk.

Investigations may include: blood test, resting electrocardiogram (ECG), exercise stress test, coronary angiography.

TREATMENT OF ANGINA

The aim of angina management is to alleviate the symptoms, to limit the development of atherosclerotic plaques and to reduce overall cardiac risk. Management of angina involves lifestyle modification and drug therapy. In poorly controlled angina or if patients are classified as higher risk, revascularisation procedures may be considered.

Lifestyle recommendations

Lifestyle measures focus on the modifiable risk factors of CHD such as smoking, poor diet, physical inactivity, stress and excess alcohol. See table 12.2 for lifestyle recommendations.

Goal-setting and pacing

Some people with angina find that they overdo things when they are feeling well, which can lead to an increase in angina or feelings of exhaustion, meaning they have to rest. Goal-setting and pacing can help people manage their angina more effectively and avoid overdoing things by planning their weekly activities. By gradually stepping up their levels of activity over time, it is often possible to return to activities that had previously been abandoned.

Relaxation

Sometimes the pain and worry of angina causes an increase in adrenaline, which can trigger a vicious cycle of more worry, causing a further increase in adrenaline, which increases heart rate and blood pressure, placing more workload on the heart, resulting in more angina. Some people find that simple diaphragmatic breathing exercises and relaxation techniques can help them remain relaxed and calm and more in control of their angina (see chapter 17).

Medication

A range of medications may be prescribed for the short-term and longer-term management of angina (see table 12.7, page 186), these include:
- Glyceryl trinitrate (GTN)
- Beta-blockers
- Calcium channel blockers
- Other medications to help reduce CHD risk factors, including:
  - Aspirin, which reduces the risk of a blood clot causing a heart attack. An alternative drug, clopidigrel, may also be prescribed in the event of an allergy to aspirin.
  - Statins may also be prescribed to lower the cholesterol level. If there is evidence of a previous MI and left-ventricular dysfunction (damage to left ventricle), ace inhibitors may also be prescribed.

Revascularisation

If a person is assessed as high-risk and has poorly controlled angina they may be considered for revascularisation treatment. This involves procedures to improve the blood supply to the heart muscle by widening the blocked arteries or replacing blocked arteries with grafts. The main revascularisation treatments include:
- percutaneous coronary intervention (PCI). This includes an angioplasty with or without a stent;
- coronary artery bypass graft (CABG).

EXERCISE RECOMMENDATIONS AND CONSIDERATIONS

Individuals who wish to work with clients with angina are recommended to attend the Level 4 BACR instructor training programme.

Exercise has an important role in the management of angina and as with other people with risk factors for CHD, they should be encouraged to increase their aerobic exercise within the limits set by their disease state (SIGN, 2001b). Exercise training improves the ability of the peripheral muscles to extract and utilise oxygen and increases the amount of work that can be carried out at a given rate pressure product (heart rate x systolic blood pressure). As a result, sub-maximal exercise and activities of daily living can be performed at a lower rate pressure product, reducing the oxygen consumption of the heart (MVO_2) and decreasing the symptoms of angina. The ACSM (2005a) recommends setting the upper heart rate (HR) for exercise at 10 beats below the ischaemic threshold. If you have the results of an exercise stress test (on medication) you can establish a safe training heart rate range. The ischaemic threshold may vary depending on the type of activity, for example, upper body activity is more likely to precipitate angina due to increased peripheral resistance. It is important to ensure

Revascularisation treatments explained

Angioplasty An angioplasty is carried out to widen a constricted or narrowed part of a coronary artery. A catheter or fine tube is inserted into a large artery in the groin or the arm and, under the control of X-ray, is guided to the lumen of the affected coronary vessel. A guide-wire is threaded through the catheter and down the coronary artery until it is accurately positioned. An angioplasty balloon is then threaded over the guide-wire and the balloon is inflated with sufficient pressure to widen the lumen. A tiny metal cage called a stent is usually inserted at the angioplasty site to help prevent restenosis (re-narrowing) of the artery.

Coronary artery bypass graft (CABG) This is a major operation that involves using healthy blood vessels, harvested from other parts of the body, to bypass the narrowed arteries and ensure blood flow to the heart muscle. There may be up to five grafts, depending on the site of the disease.

that clients understand the importance of working within an appropriate heart-rate range to prevent the onset of angina during exercise. Tools such as heart-rate monitoring and ratings of perceived exertion (RPE) can help clients to self-monitor.

If a client experiences angina during a supervised exercise session, document the exercise activity (mode, workload) and associated signs or symptoms, such as light-headedness or fall in blood pressure (AACVPR, 2004). Advise the client to stop exercising and follow the procedures for managing angina (see chapter 6, page 72).

The exercise programme should be tailored to the overall needs of the individual, taking into account age, co-morbidities, fitness level, current physical activity levels, skill level, confidence, preference, lifestyle and personal goals.

GUIDELINES FOR EXERCISE

It is important to be aware of any changes in the pattern of an individual's angina. There is an increased likelihood of an MI when stable angina becomes less stable. Unstable angina is a contraindication for exercise and it is important for the individual to seek immediate medical attention.

- Client should be risk-stratified in line with BACR guidelines.
- Exercise may not be appropriate for someone who experiences angina at low levels of exertion (i.e. below 3 METs).
- Exercising in cold weather and after a heavy meal is more likely to trigger angina.
- Ensure client is able to recognise symptoms of angina, and especially their own, individual symptoms of angina.
- Encourage client to identify activities that trigger angina and, if appropriate, modify activities.
- Check that your client carries a GTN spray and knows how to use it.
- Record any changes in angina symptoms and notify their GP.
- Some clients will benefit from taking pre-exercise GTN. Advise client to discuss this with their GP.

Table 12.4	Summary of exercise guidelines for CHD		
Training guidelines	**Cardiovascular**	**Muscle strength**	**Flexibility**
Aims	Reduce CHD risk factors Reduce blood pressure Improve functional capacity	Improve functional capacity	Improve ROM and reduce risk of injury
Frequency	3–7 times per week	2/3 times a week	Minimum of 2–3 days a week, ideally 5–7 days a week
Intensity	Training heart rate (THR) should be set at 10–15 beats below the threshold for angina. Rating of Perceived Exertion (RPE) will be a useful tool to use alongside THR	Light resistance 40–50% of 1RM	Stretch to a position of mild tension without discomfort
Time	30 minutes. An intermittent approach may be more appropriate for this client group. This can be achieved by exercising more frequently for shorter periods of time such as bouts of 5–10 minutes performed two or more times a day	15–20 minute session 1 set x 8–12 repetitions 8–10 muscle groups	Hold stretches for 15–30 seconds 2–4 repetitions of each stretch.
Type	Aerobic-type activities such as walking and cycling using large muscles of the lower body Note: Upper body exercise is more likely to precipitate angina than lower body activities	8–10 exercises including major muscle groups Circuit training approach Dynamic resistance exercises	Static stretches with a focus on muscle groups which have a reduced range of movement

Adapted from ACSM (2005); Gitkin et al (2003); Friedman & Roberts in Durstine et al (2009)

- Include a prolonged warm-up and cool-down to reduce the likelihood of angina.
- Advise client to remain seated for a few moments after using GTN as there is a risk of hypotension. The client can resume exercise if the symptoms ease, but you need to encourage the client to do some gentle pulse-raising activity as a warm-up.
- Ischaemia can occur without symptoms of angina (silent ischaemia) and is more common in people with diabetes.
- Level 4 instructors who are specifically trained to work with CHD clients should supervise clients in line with *Exercise Protocols for the Management of CHD Patients* (BACR, 2005).

HYPERTENSION

Blood pressure is the pressure the blood exerts on the artery walls. The pressure increases when the heart contracts and decreases as the heart relaxes. Systolic blood pressure (SBP) is the pressure exerted during the contraction of the heart and diastolic blood pressure (DBP) is the pressure exerted when the heart relaxes. This pressure is recorded as systolic blood pressure over diastolic blood pressure and is measured in millimetres of mercury (mmHg), for example 120/70mmHg. Cardiac output and total peripheral resistance are the main determinants of blood pressure. Cardiac output is the total amount of blood ejected from the left ventricle in a minute and total peripheral resistance (TPR) is the resistance to blood flow offered by the peripheral vessels. This is influenced by the tension in the walls of the peripheral blood vessels and degree of vasodilation (increase in diameter) or vasoconstriction (decrease in the diameter).

Blood pressure is expressed by the equation:
Blood pressure = cardiac output × TPR

A diagnosis of hypertension will be made if blood pressure is consistently >140/90mmHg (see table 12.5).

When there is no clear cause of hypertension it is called essential hypertension. Essential hypertension is the most common type of hypertension and may be linked to genetics and a number of lifestyle factors such as obesity or smoking. If hypertension is the result of an underlying definite cause, such as kidney disorders or thyroid problems, it is called secondary hypertension. This section will focus on the management of essential hypertension.

PREVALENCE

There is a concern that hypertension remains undiagnosed, untreated and poorly managed in most people (BHS, 2004). Prevalence of hypertension (<140/90mmHg) is estimated as affecting 32 per cent of men and 27 per cent of women over the age of 35 (Patient UK, 2012); and an estimated 16 million people in the UK are diagnosed. A further 5 million people in the UK are believed to have undiagnosed high blood pressure (BHF, 2012). It is also estimated that around 78 per cent of men and 66 per cent of women with raised blood pressures are not receiving treatment in the UK and in 2005, nearly 60 per cent of people being treated for hypertension were still hypertensive (BHF, 2005c).

Hypertension is more common in the following groups:

- Older people, affecting 50 per cent of people aged over 65 and one in four people of middle age with *at least* one in twenty adults having blood pressure of 160/100mmHg or above (NHS Choices, 2011).
- People of African-Caribbean origin have a higher risk of high blood pressure than the rest of the UK population, which increases their risk of stroke.
- South Asian people living in the UK are at a higher risk from diabetes and CHD, so blood pressure needs to be carefully monitored.
- People with a family history of hypertension.
- People with diabetes, with around three in ten individuals with type 1 diabetes and 50 per cent of individuals with type 2 diabetes developing hypertension.
- Individuals who are overweight, eat a lot of salt, are inactive, drink a lot of caffeine and/ or alcohol and who don't eat much fruit or vegetables.

Table 12.5	Classification of blood pressure levels	
Category	**Systolic blood pressure (mmHg)**	**Diastolic blood pressure (mmHg)**
Normal/optimal (Gordon in Durstine & Moore, 2009)	<120	<80
Normal (NHS Choices)	<130	<80
Pre-hypertension (Gordon in Durstine & Moore, 2009)	120–139	80–89
Stage 1 hypertension (mild)		
Clinic (NICE, 2011; Gordon in Durstine & Moore, 2009)	140–159	90–99
and subsequent ambulatory blood pressure monitoring (ABPM) day time average or home blood pressure monitoring (HBPM) (NICE., 2011)	135	85
Stage 2 hypertension (moderate)		
Clinic (NICE, 2011; Gordon in Durstine & Moore, 2009)	160–179	100–109
and subsequent ABPM day time average or HBPM (NICE, 2011)	150	95
Stage 3 Hypertension (severe)		
Clinic (NICE, 2011; Gordon in Durstine & Moore, 2009)	≥180	≥110
Isolated systolic hypertension (**British Hypertension Society, 2004**) Note: If diastolic and systolic measurements fall into different categories, the higher value is used to classify blood pressure (BHS, 2004)		
Grade 1	140–159	<90
Grade 2	≥160	<90

Adapted from NICE (2011); NHS Choices (2010); Gordon in Durstine & Moore (2009)

CAUSES

The exact cause of essential hypertension is unclear; however, it is likely that genetic factors predispose an individual to high blood pressure, especially when combined with environmental and lifestyle factors. The factors that contribute to hypertension overlap with the risk factors for coronary heart disease (see table 12.1).

SIGNS AND SYMPTOMS

Hypertension is sometimes referred to as the 'silent killer' (NHS Choices, 2010). Most people with hypertension feel well and are symptom-free (asymptomatic). If someone has really high blood pressure they may get headaches, but this is unusual. Other possible symptoms include sight problems, nosebleeds and shortness of breath (BHF, 2005).

DIAGNOSIS

A diagnosis of hypertension is made when an individual has a sustained blood pressure of >140mmHg/90mmHg (NICE 2004c/2011). The Joint British Societies Guidelines (2005) recommend that all adults over the age of 40 should have their blood pressure measured within primary care as part of opportunistic risk assessment for CVD, and Patient UK (2012) suggest that all adults have their blood pressure checked at least every five years up to the age of 80 and every year after age 80 (Patient UK, 2012).

Blood pressure can be affected by a number of factors including time of day, caffeine consumption and stress levels, so it important for it to be monitored on two or more occasions over a few months before a diagnosis is made. This process depends on the individual circumstances, and someone with very high blood pressure may be reviewed more frequently or referred to a specialist if there are additional signs and symptoms.

Blood pressure used to be measured using a mercury sphygmomanometer, which was considered the gold standard, but due to health and safety concerns over mercury in the environment, other automated or semi-automated devices have been introduced. Updated guidance recommends that a diagnosis of primary hypertension should be confirmed using 24 hour ambulatory blood pressure (ABPM) as the gold standard rather than basing diagnosis solely on measurements taken in the clinic. Home blood pressure monitoring (HBPM) is also suggested within the current guidance (NICE, 2011; BHS, 2011). All equipment used should be validated, well maintained and recalibrated on a regular basis (NICE, 2004c). Health professionals must be adequately trained and competent in order to take accurate blood pressure measurements. For full details about blood pressure monitoring methods see BHS and NICE guidance.

Some people become very anxious when having their blood pressure measured by a health professional, and experience 'white coat' hypertension. Hypertension increases the risk of cardiovascular disease, so a health professional will assess a hypertensive individual's overall CVD risk and treat the hypertension within that context. If there is no established cardiovascular disease, a cardiovascular risk assessment tool can be used. A number of routine tests can help identify or rule out the prevalence of other conditions, such as diabetes, or evidence of any target organ damage, including the heart and kidneys. These tests will also identify any secondary causes of hypertension such as kidney disease. The tests include:

- a urine test to check for protein or blood in the urine;
- a blood sample to assess plasma glucose, electrolytes, creatinine and cholesterol levels;
- an ECG (12-lead) to identify any ventricular hypertrophy (enlarged heart, affecting the left ventricle) or evidence of myocardial ischaemia (shortage of oxygen to the heart).

COMPLICATIONS

Hypertension affects the structure and function of the blood vessels and, if it is not managed effectively over a period of time, it can lead to organ damage including:

- kidney failure;
- retinopathy (damage to eyes);
- left-ventricular hypertrophy, heart failure;
- myocardial infarction, angina;
- stroke, transient ischaemic attacks;
- peripheral arterial disease;
- an accelerated rate of decline in cognitive function (JBS, 2005).

The likelihood of complications is increased by a combination of factors (NICE, 2004c), including:

- co-morbidities such as diabetes and obesity;
- lifestyle factors such as a high salt diet and lack of exercise;
- fixed risk factors such as family history, gender and ethnicity.

TREATMENT AND MANAGEMENT

The aim of treatment is to work in partnership with patients to:

- reduce overall cardiovascular risk;
- manage hypertension effectively through appropriate drug therapy and/or lifestyle modification.

Lifestyle recommendations

It is estimated that making dietary and activity changes can lower blood pressure by at least 10mmHg in around one in four people (Patient UK, 2012).

People often feel well and are symptom-free when they have hypertension. This can make it difficult for them to make the appropriate lifestyle changes. It is important for patients to be well informed about the risks of hypertension and the treatment options so they can take an active role in decision making about their health. Health promotion resources such as leaflets and audiovisual materials can be used to support one-to-one work with clients, and some clients may benefit from joining patient organisations or local groups that provide the opportunity to share information and experience and gain support. Some individuals who make lifestyle changes that lower blood pressure and reduce overall cardiovascular risk may reduce the need for long-term drug therapy (NICE, 2004c/2011).

The following lifestyle measures are recommended (NICE, 2004c/2011) in addition to those outlined in table 12.2:

- cut down on caffeine-rich drinks such as cola, coffee and tea (less than five cups of coffee per day);
- relaxation therapies such as stress management, or yoga and cognitive therapy, can reduce blood pressure. These treatments are not normally available on the NHS.

Dietary guidance (Patient UK, 2012) includes:

- ideally seven to nine (at least five) portions of fruit and vegetables per day;
- reduced fatty foods (fatty meats, cheese, full cream milk, fried food etc.);

- two to three portions of fish per week, at least one oily fish (salmon, pilchards, sardines etc.);
- eat lean meat;
- limit salt (use herbs and spices to flavour foods);
- use vegetable oil to fry (olive or sunflower oil);
- bulk of most meals should be starch-based (pasta, rice, bread, cereal, ideally wholegrain);
- alcohol in moderation (see chapter 3 for guidance on alcohol units).

Medication (see table 12.7)

Medication has an important role in reducing high blood pressure and the risk of cardiovascular disease. Medication is usually started as part of the treatment for:

- individuals' who have blood pressure of 160/100mmHg or above after making lifestyle changes;
- individuals' who have blood pressure of 140/90mmHg or above after making lifestyle changes AND have either:
  - diabetes
  - existing CVD
  - a 2 in 10 risk of developing CVD in the next 10 years.

There are several types of hypertensive drugs, including ace inhibitors or angiotensin II receptor blockers (ARB), calcium channel blockers (CCB), thiazide-like diuretics, beta-blockers and alpha-blockers (NICE, 2011). Generally a combination of medications will be offered depending on a number of factors, including age, ethnicity, presence of other co-morbidities and response to treatment. Ongoing review is important to monitor blood pressure and provide appropriate lifestyle support. If an individual has a low cardiovascular risk and her or his blood pressure is under control, it may be possible to reduce or stop medication; however, s/he needs to discuss any changes with the GP (NICE, 2004c).

Other medications such as aspirin and statins may also be prescribed as part of the primary and secondary prevention of CHD.

EXERCISE RECOMMENDATIONS AND CONSIDERATIONS
Role of exercise

Regular physical activity is an important lifestyle factor in the prevention and management of hypertension. Regular aerobic activity has been shown to reduce blood pressure, but the exact processes are not entirely understood. Exercise has an effect on the mechanisms that control and regulate blood pressure and immediately afterwards people experience post-exercise hypotension, which can last for two hours in healthy people and up to 12 hours in people with hypertension. In the longer term, the role of physical activity in preventing obesity, reducing insulin resistance and increasing the capillary density of muscle may contribute to a reduction in blood pressure (DoH, 2004a).

Blood pressure response to exercise

During cardiovascular exercise, such as walking, swimming and cycling, there is a linear increase in systolic BP with increasing exercise intensity. This is linked to the increase in cardiac output during exercise. The increase in systolic blood pressure will depend on the intensity of the exercise and the individual's resting blood pressure. Diastolic blood pressure does not normally rise in response to exercise, which is due to the blood vessels in the active muscles dilating, enhancing blood flow and reducing total peripheral resistance (McArdle et al, 2001). A decrease in SBP is an abnormal response to exercise that might indicate an underlying condition and is considered a contraindication to exercise.

During activity involving the upper body there is a different blood pressure response to exercise. Upper body exercise results in a higher systolic and diastolic blood pressure response than the lower limbs at a given VO$_2$max. This is because arms have a smaller muscle mass than legs, resulting in less vasodilation, greater resistance to blood flow and less reduction in total peripheral resistance.

GUIDELINES FOR EXERCISE

Although the optimal training prescription to lower blood pressure is unclear, the ACSM (2005) guidelines for cardiovascular, strength and flexibility training for the general population can be adapted. Table 12.6 outlines the most recent guidance.

Moderate-intensity cardiovascular training is recommended as the primary form of exercise training for people with high blood pressure. A resistance component of moderate intensity, using higher repetitions and lower resistance, contributes to a balanced exercise programme, but is not recommended in isolation, the exception being if using a circuit weight training approach (Gordon, 2009). The exercise programme should be tailored to the overall needs of the individual, taking into account age, co-morbidities, fitness level, current physical activity levels, skill level, confidence, preference, lifestyle and personal goals.

SPECIAL CONSIDERATIONS

- If a client has high blood pressure, ensure that s/he sees the GP and is on appropriate medication before beginning an exercise programme.
- Consider other co-morbidities (e.g. diabetes and obesity, see guidance in respective chapters).
- Contraindication: Do not exercise if:
  - resting blood pressure is >180/100mmHg;
  - a significant drop in blood pressure during exercise is a contraindication to exercise. If an individual feels light-headed or dizzy during exercise advise him or her to stop exercise and refer to GP (see chapter 6, table 6.3, page 72).
- Promote moderate intensity activity
- Discourage high-intensity aerobic activity.
- Clients taking medications such as beta-blockers and diuretics may have an impaired ability to regulate body temperature and need to be aware of the implications of exercising in hot and humid conditions.
- Clients taking medication such as alpha-blockers, calcium channel blockers or vasodilators will require an extended cool-down to avoid hypotension after exercise.
- Encourage appropriate breathing technique during resistance training to avoid the valsalva manoeuvre (forceful expiration against a closed glottis).
- Discourage isometric activity, such as over-gripping of equipment, to avoid the possibility of an excessive increase in blood pressure.
- Avoid heavy resistance training, as this increases blood pressure.
- Avoid high-intensity or sustained upper body exercise due to increased myocardial workload (ACSM, 2005).
- Avoid excessive overhead arm movements.

Table 12.6	Summary of exercise guidelines for hypertension		
Training guidelines	**Cardiovascular**	**Muscle strength**	**Flexibility**
Aims	Control BP at rest and during exercise Reduce CHD risk factors Increase calorie expenditure Weight management	Improve strength and endurance	Maintain and improve ROM As per general populations
Frequency	4–7 days a week. Daily exercise may provide optimal benefits due to the acute reduction in BP that follows a bout of exercise	2–3 times per week	Minimum of 2–3 days a week, ideally 5–7 days a week
Intensity	Moderate level 40–60% HRR (55–69% HRmax) Rating of perceived exertion (RPE) 12–13 (Borg 6-20)	Low resistance/high repetitions 60–80% of 1RM Circuit weight training approach	Stretch to a position of mild tension without discomfort
Time	30–60 minute session OR Continuous or intermittent activity of ≥30 minutes Intermittent bouts (minimum of 10 minutes) accumulated throughout the day recommended	1 set 8–12 reps	Hold stretches for 5–30 seconds, 2–4 repetitions of each stretch
Type	Using large muscle groups such as walking, cycling, dancing	8–10 exercises including major muscle groups Dynamic resistance exercises Maintain normal breathing pattern	Static stretch Whole-body approach with emphasis on muscles with a reduced range of movement

Adapted from Gordon in Durstine et al (2009)

Table 12.7	Medications for cardiovascular disease		
Drug	**Purpose/Action/ Treatment for**	**Side effects**	**Exercise implications**
Nitrates Glycerol Trinitrate (GTN) (tablets or spray) Isosorbide mononitrate	Relax and dilate the coronary arteries, increasing blood flow to myocardium Can be taken for immediate relief of angina or prior to undertaking activities likely to precipitate angina Prevent angina in the long term however become less effective with prolonged use Heart failure	Can cause a headache, flushing or dizziness Postural hypotension Nausea	Postural hypotension Care with transitions e.g. floor based work to standing and will need longer cool down If client uses GTN spray and wants to continue exercising, be aware of possible drop in blood pressure Can increase exercise tolerance by preventing angina and increasing ischaemic threshold
Betablockers • Atenolol • Meotoprolol • Acebutolol • Propranolol • Bisoprolol* • Carvedilol* • Sotalol** • Esmolol**	Beta-blockers block the action of the hormone adrenaline Reduces workload on the heart, reducing the incidence of angina Reduce recurrence rate of myocardial infarction Hypertension Stable heart failure* Betablockers** can also act as anti-arrhythmic drugs	Common: Lethargy and fatigue, cold extremeties (hands and feet) Rare: Fainting, palpitations May slightly raise blood glucose levels in someone with diabetes Sleep disturbances and nightmares Can precipitate bronchospasm in people with asthma or chronic obstructive pulmonary disease	Symptoms of hypoglycaemia may be altered/blunted Heart rate response suppressed Risk of postural hypotension with floor based work Use RPE alongside adjusted target heart rate Improved exercise tolerance
Calcium channel blockers • Amlodipine • Felodipine • Isradipin • Nifedipine • Verapamil • Diltiazem	Reduce contractility of the heart muscle Angina Hypertension Arrhythmia	Common: Dizziness, fatigue, headache, nausea, abdominal pain, facial flushing, ankle oedema (swelling), postural hypotension Rare: Skin rash, breathing difficulties, constipation (Verapamil)	Verapamil and Diltiazem can cause bradycardia

Drug	Purpose/Action/ Treatment for	Side effects	Exercise implications
Antiplatelets	These drugs decrease the clotting ability of platelets and may inhibit the formation of a thrombus or clot		None known
Aspirin	Aspirin is used in both primary and secondary prevention. It reduces the risk of MI, stroke or vascular deaths by 30% Aspirin is also used in atrial fibrillation, stable angina and intermittent claudication	Aspirin: (common) Indigestion Aspirin: (rare) Nausea, vomiting, rash, ringing in ears, breathlessness/ wheezing. Can bring on an asthma attack. Gastric bleeding (blood in vomit/ black faeces)	
Clopidogrel	Clopidogrel is used for the prevention of ischaemic events. It is often used if aspirin is contraindicated, or there are side effects	Clopidogrel (common) Diarrhoea, abdominal pain Bruising, nosebleeds Clopidogrel (rare) Sore throat/fever, rash/itching, headache/dizziness, constipation	
Alpha blockers Doxazosin Indoramin Prazosin	Hypertension not lowered by other drugs	Common: Nausea, weakness Rare: Runny nose, sleep disturbances, palpitations, chest pain, postural hypotension (dizziness, fainting) Urinary incontinence (women)	Postural hypotension Care with floor based work
Anti arrythmias Digoxin	To control arrhythmias Supra-ventricular tachycardia Atrial fibrillation Heart failure (limited use)	Headache, fatigue, dizziness, slow pulse, photosensitivity, metallic taste, nightmares, dizziness, visual disturbances	Possible reduced heart rate response Possible reduced exercise capacity
Amiodarone	Atrial fibrillation or flutter		
Flecainide	Ventricular tachycardia		

Drug	Purpose/Action/ Treatment for	Side effects	Exercise implications
Anticoagulants *Warfarin*	Use in atrial fibrillation for those at risk of blood clots Mechanical prosthetic valves	Need regular blood tests May cause, or make bleeding worse Rare: Nausea, vomiting, abdominal pain, diarrhoea, fever, hair loss, jaundice	Check environment to reduce likelihood of trips or knocking into equipment
Angiotensin II receptor antagonists • Candesartan • Losartan • Valsartan	Vasodilator drugs Blocks the receptor site of angiotension II (a powerful vasoconstrictor). Relaxes blood vessel walls, reducing blood pressure	Common: Dizziness Rare: Fatigue, diarrhoea, cough, hypotension, taste disturbance, skin rash	Dizziness, muscle or joint pain
Ace inhibitors • Captopril • Cilazapril • Enalapril • Ramipril • Lisinopril	Hypertension Post MI for LV function	Common: Dry cough rash, loss of taste Rare: Renal impairment, angio-oedema (swelling) of lips and tongue, dizziness, breathing difficulty, sore throat, mouth ulcers	There may be an increase in exercise capacity due to treatment of heart failure
Diuretics Group 1 • Thiazide diuretics • Bendroflumethiazide • Chlorothiazide Cyclopenthiazide Group 2 Potassium sparing diuretics • Furosemide • Bumetanide • Sprironolactone* Group 3 Loop diuretics	Hypertension Heart failure*	Rare: Diabetes, gout, hyperlipidaemia, Impotence, hypokalaemia (loss of potassium), leg cramps, dizziness	Aching legs Dehydration – encourage adequate fluid intake

Drug	Purpose/Action/ Treatment for	Side effects	Exercise implications
Lipid-regulating drugs	Reduce the progression of coronary atherosclerosis by decreasing concentration of low density lipoproteins and increasing the high density lipoproteins		Aching legs otherwise no exercise considerations
Statins • Pravastatin • Simvastatin	Statins are used in both primary and secondary prevention of CHD. Statins reduce coronary events, all cardiovascular events, and total mortality. They are used in primary prevention with patients who are at an increased risk of CHD. Statins are also used in secondary prevention of CHD, peripheral artery disease or a history of stroke	Common: Gastrointestinal upset Rare: Muscle weakness, Jaundice Generally well tolerated	
Fibrates • Bezafibrate • Clofibrate • Fenofibrate • Gemfibrozil	Reduce triglycerides and LDL cholesterol Increase HDL cholesterol	Common: Gastrointestinal upset Rare: Dizziness, gallstones, rash, headache, acute pain in calf or thigh muscle if kidney function impaired,	
Cholestyramine • (Questran)	Reduce LDL cholesterol	Gastro-intestinal problems, raised triglycerides	

Adapted from BACR 2000 and BMA (2011)

Note: To check the currency of medications prescribed, readers should refer to other references (BNF National Formulary, NICE guidance, etc.)

NEUROLOGICAL // DISEASE

13

This chapter introduces the following diseases:
- Multiple sclerosis (MS)
- Stroke
- Parkinson's disease.

NB: These conditions are outside the scope of practice for a level 3 instructor.

MULTIPLE SCLEROSIS (MS)

Multiple sclerosis is a condition affecting the central nervous system (CNS). It is an autoimmune disease, which means that the immune system mistakenly attacks the body's own tissue. Nerve cells (neurons) carry messages around the CNS. A sheath of fatty tissue called myelin surrounds the axon, which is a specialised part of the neuron. The myelin protects and insulates the neuron and facilitates the smooth transmission of messages between the CNS and the organs of the body. In MS the immune system attacks the myelin tissue causing damage and inflammation (demyelination). This causes scar tissue (sclerosis) to develop over the affected areas, forming plaques or lesions. These lesions interrupt and distort the messages travelling along the nerve fibres. There is also evidence of damage to the axons, resulting in axon loss. These axons cannot regenerate and their impairment causes the progressive disability characteristic of MS. These lesions can occur in multiple parts of the brain and spinal cord, causing a number of neurological symptoms. MS affects people in different ways, depending on the parts of the brain and spinal cord affected (MS Trust, 2005).

CAUSES

The cause of MS is unknown. Current theories suggest an interaction between genetic and environmental factors. MS is not directly inherited, however, a combination of genes may make a person more susceptible to MS. The incidence of MS is greater as one moves further away from the equator (MS Trust, 2005).

PREVALENCE

In the UK approximately 85,000 people have MS. The disease predominantly affects young adults, with most people being diagnosed between the ages of 20 and 30. Women are twice as likely than men to develop MS (MS Trust, 2004).

SIGNS AND SYMPTOMS

The signs and symptoms of MS are varied and are not specific to MS. The disease affects people in unpredictable ways; some people experience very few symptoms, some people experience different symptoms at different times.

Common symptoms include the following:

- Fatigue due to changes in the central nervous system can make physical and mental activity difficult. Depression, pain and disturbed sleep are experienced. Poor diet, lack of physical activity and loss of fitness may contribute to feelings of overwhelming fatigue.
- Problems with balance and co-ordination; vertigo.
- Visual problems such as double vision (diplopia). The eyes might move from side to side or up and down. This is called nystagmus.
- Sensory problems such as numbness or tingling in the hands and feet.
- Muscle stiffness or rigidity (spasticity) and uncontrollable jerk (spasm). MS affects the control and regulation of normal muscle activity and maintenance of posture; this leads to uncoordinated movement, which can affect activities of daily living such as walking, getting washed and dressed, and leisure activities.
- Joint contracture due to tissues around the joint permanently tightening or contracting can occur if people have ongoing muscular problems, such as weakness or spasticity, that limit normal range of movement around a joint. In some cases this can lead to pain.
- Pain, which can be neuropathic, caused by damage to the nerves in the brain or the spinal cord, or musculoskeletal pain (nociceptive). Nociceptive pain is often caused by lack of mobility and poor posture, or as a result of spasm and spasticity.
- Muscle weakness, due to damaged nerves, mainly in the spinal cord, which affect the transmission of messages, causing muscle weakness. If these weak muscles are not used they atrophy, leading to secondary weakness.
- Shaking (tremor) and uncoordinated, clumsy movements (ataxia) can be very disabling, making it difficult for people to carry out activities of daily living, work and leisure.
- Anxiety, depression and mood swings.
- Cognitive problems affecting memory, concentration, speed of information processing, reasoning and judgment.
- Speech problems such as dysarthria, where weakness or lack of coordination in the muscles leads to slurred or slow speech and difficulty controlling intonation. People may also find it difficult to find words or form sentences (dysphasia).
- Swallowing problems (dysphagia) can happen when the nerves that control swallowing are affected.
- Bladder problems can involve difficulties with frequency, urgency, hesitancy and incontinence. This can be very disabling, making it more difficult for people to go out. Bladder problems are often combined with mobility problems, making it even more difficult to get to a toilet quickly.
- Bowel problems, including urgent need to empty bowels, constipation or pain.
- Changes to emotional state such as laughing or crying for no obvious reason.
- Sexual problems, which are caused by a number of factors including neurological, psychosexual and relational.
- Mobility (the ability to move freely). A wide range of factors can affect mobility including fatigue, visual disturbance, posture, pain, depression, muscle weakness and spasticity. Inflammation around the spinal cord (transverse myelitis) can lead to leg weakness or paralysis.

Adapted from NICE (2003); MS Trust (2005)

The most common presenting symptoms at the onset of disease include:

- A sudden reduction or loss of vision in one eye. This is called optic neuritis and is caused by inflammation of the optic nerve.
- Sensory problems such as pins and needles in the hands and feet.

MS is characterised by periods of remission followed by relapses (sudden episodes of symptoms). A relapse is thought to occur when a part of the central nervous system (CNS) becomes inflamed or damaged. The symptoms will depend on the part of the CNS affected. New or worsening symptoms may not necessarily be caused by a new episode of MS, but may be aggravated by a number of triggers such as infection, heat and humidity (MS Trust, 2005).

DIAGNOSIS

MS is a complex disease that is not easy to diagnose and there is no single test to confirm MS. The symptoms are not specific to MS and might be caused by other conditions. A neurologist will carry out a number of investigations to try to identify any changes in movement, reflexes and sensation that indicate damage to the nerve pathways. A number of tests may also be carried out to exclude an alternative diagnosis or to support the potential diagnosis (NICE, 2003):

- A magnetic resonance imaging (MRI) scan of the brain and/or spinal cord can identify the site and severity of myelin damage.
- A visually evoked potential test monitors how the brain responds to patterns on a screen. The slower the response, the greater the myelin damage.

- A lumbar puncture obtains a sample of cerebrospinal fluid. This is analysed to check for the presence of antibodies, showing that the immune system has attacked the CNS.

Different types of MS are classified according to the patterns of progression:

Benign MS

In benign MS there are only a few relapses and little or no disability. If this pattern continues over a 15-year period the MS is classified as benign. See figure 13.1.

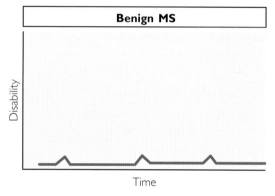

Figure 13.1 Benign MS

Relapsing/remitting MS

Relapsing/remitting MS is the most common type, affecting approximately two-thirds of people diagnosed with MS. At the onset many people have symptoms that come and go, with sudden relapses and remissions. A relapse typically occurs once or twice every two years and may last from 24 hours to a few months. During remission symptoms may disappear, but there may be some residual damage. See figure 13.2.

Secondary progressive MS

Approximately 50 per cent of people with relapsing/remitting MS gradually develop secondary progressive MS. This usually develops during the initial 10 years of the disease. There may be more or worsening symptoms and fewer remissions. See figure 13.3.

Primary progressive MS

Approximately 10 per cent of those diagnosed have primary progressive MS. From the onset of MS the symptoms steadily develop and worsen, without relapses or remissions. See figure 13.4.

TREATMENT

MS is an unpredictable disease, which can change from day to day or from one time of day to another. It is a lifelong disease that cannot be cured. However, it can be managed though a range of interventions. These include:

- access to a specialist multidisciplinary neuro-logical team including physiotherapists, continence advisers, psychologists, speech therapists and occupational therapists;
- drug therapy;
- advice on maintaining a healthy lifestyle.

The National Service Framework (NSF) for long-term conditions recommends a person-centred approach with an emphasis on:

- provision of appropriate information and education;
- the opportunity for people to make decisions about their health;
- involvement in the development of a care plan.

(Adapted from DoH, 2005c)

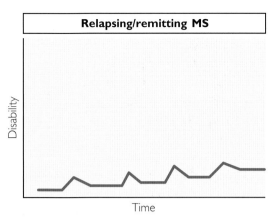

Figure 13.2 Relapsing/remitting MS

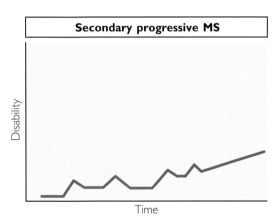

Figure 13.3 Secondary progressive MS

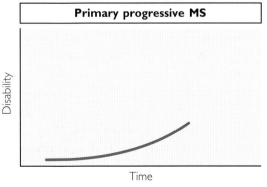

Figure 13.4 Primary progressive MS

MEDICATIONS

Drugs cannot cure MS, but they can be used to manage relapses, modify the disease and help manage symptoms.

Relapse management

Steroids are used to treat relapses. They help speed up the recovery from a relapse, but they cannot change the course of the disease. Steroids appear partly to suppress the immune system and reduce inflammation at the site of nerve damage. The NICE (2003) guidelines recommend the use of methyprednisolone in the short term (less than three weeks) and limiting the use to three times a year to avoid the long-term side effects of steroid treatment. The long-term side effects of steroids include bone cell degeneration, which can lead to osteoporosis.

Disease modification

Beta interferon 1a, beta interferon 1b and glatiramar acetate are called disease-modifying drugs. In the UK these drugs are licensed for the treatment of relapsing/remitting MS and secondary progressive MS, where relapses are a major feature (MS Trust, 2005).

Other drugs used in MS

Some immunoregulators have proved effective in the treatment of other autoimmune diseases such as rheumatoid arthritis. This has led to the use of immunoregulators such as azathioprine, mitoxantrone, intravenous immunoglobulins (IVIg) and methotrexate to treat MS. Some studies show a reduction in relapse and a reduction in the progression of disability. However, these drugs are only used in specific circumstances (MS Trust, 2005).

Medication to manage symptoms

Drug therapies are currently used to manage some of the symptoms of MS including bladder difficulties, depression, pain and spasticity, in conjunction with the support of a specialist neurological rehabilitation team.

- **Spasticity** Medications for spasticity generally act on the CNS and include baclofen, gabapentin, tizanidine and diazepam. These medications can cause drowsiness, muscle weakness, fatigue and dizziness and may have implications for exercise. Dantrolene is the only antispasmodic that works directly on the muscles, but is often not well tolerated. Cannabis is documented as improving spasticity and pain in people with MS, but it is not currently prescribed.
- **Bladder difficulties** Medications such as anticholinergics and vasopressin may be prescribed to help with urinary problems.
- **Depression** Depression will usually be treated with a combination of drug therapy and psychotherapy. Medications such as selective serotonin re-uptake inhibitors (e.g. Prozac) can be beneficial for depression. Imipramine and amitriptyline may also be prescribed. These act on a variety of chemical neurotransmitters in the brain associated with mood regulation. Many of the medications prescribed for other symptoms of MS such as corticosteroids have depressed mood as a side effect (MS Trust, 2005). Medication used for depression can cause an increase in postural instability.

OTHER THERAPIES
Healthy eating

A healthy diet is important for general health and well-being. Linoleic acid may help maintain a healthy nervous system and is recommended for people with MS (MS Trust, 2005). These essential fatty acids can be found in oils such as sunflower, soya and safflower and may help to slow the disabling effects of MS (NICE, 2003).

Environment

People with MS are more sensitive to heat and humidity (thermo-sensitivity). An increase in body temperature may trigger a transient increase in symptoms (Karpatkin, 2005).

Counselling

Counselling may help people develop coping strategies to deal with the change and uncertainty that is involved in living with MS.

Complementary therapies

There is limited evidence that some complementary therapies such as Tai Chi, reflexology, massage and neural therapy may benefit people with MS (NICE, 2003).

EXERCISE RECOMMENDATIONS

Appropriate exercise can help maximise muscular strength and endurance, flexibility and aerobic capacity. It can also help to:
- improve overall health and well-being;
- optimise and maintain function;
- reduce the disabling impact of relapses;
- reduce muscle wasting;
- reduce spasticity and avoid the development of contractures;
- improve posture.

(Adapted from NICE, 2003; MS Trust, 2003)

The exercise programme needs to take into account the client's health status, functional capacity, confidence, skills, preference and personal goals. A flexible, responsive approach is important to ensure the programme continues to meet the client's needs and reflects changing symptoms and energy levels. Exercise can contribute to fatigue, so it is important to plan exercise sessions to ensure an appropriate balance of rest and activity. Too much exercise may leave an individual feeling overtired and lacking the energy to carry out activities of daily living (ADL) and leisure pursuits. It is beneficial for the exercise professional to develop an effective relationship with the client's physiotherapist or healthcare team. This will facilitate communication and enable the exercise professional to respond appropriately to any changes in the client's health status and complement the work of the specialist healthcare team. See table 13.1 for a summary of exercise guidelines.

Cardiovascular

The type of activity will depend on the abilities and preferences of the client. Appropriate activities include cardiovascular machines such as stationary cycling and elliptical trainers, walking and water-based activity. Water-based exercise can help provide support for people with impaired balance and appropriate water temperature may help thermo-sensitivity (Karpatkin, 2005). Intensity and duration may need to be adjusted on a daily basis according to symptoms and energy levels. The current recommendation of 30 minutes of moderate physical activity on at least five days a week may not be realistic for people with MS and will depend on the degree of physical impairment. The ACSM (2005) recommends a more realistic and achievable goal of 30 minutes of moderate physical activity on three days a week. This can be

Table 13.1	Summary of exercise guidelines for multiple sclerosis		
Training guidelines	Cardiovascular	Muscle Strength	Flexibility
Aims	To maintain CV fitness	To increase functional strength and performance	To increase ROM and manage spasticity
Frequency	Structured exercise 3 days a week. ADL and leisure activities can be carried out on non-exercise days	2–3 non-consecutive days a week	5–7 days a week Ideally twice a day
Intensity	60–75 per cent HRmax Use RPE to monitor intensity. Lower levels may be more appropriate for older or more severely impaired clients, until their fitness level increases	40–80 per cent 1RM Allow adequate rest between exercises	To the point of mild tension but not pain
Time	Build up to 30 min (continuous or intermittent). This can be broken down into shorter sessions e.g. 3 ×10 min	1–2 sets 8–15 reps 50–70% maximum volume by contraction (MVC)	30–60 sec. More prolonged stretching may be appropriate for people with contractures. Repeat each stretch 2–5 times
Type	Low-impact, cycling, walking, treadmill, water-aerobics or chair-based aerobics	8–10 exercises Focus on major muscle groups Dynamic resistance Relate to ADL Modifications may be required to accommodate differences between limbs (strength and ROM)	Static stretching Use props such as therapy bands or assistance by partner Focus on muscle groups prone to contractures including hamstrings, gastrocnemius, iliopsoas and pectoralis major and minor

Functional

Include activities such as small squats, sit to stand, stair climbing.

Include balance exercises to address postural instability.

ACSM (2005*b*); Lambert (2003). Jackson and Mulcare in Larry Durstine et al (2009) broken down into shorter sessions of 10 minutes and may be more appropriate for people with low levels of fitness, while ensuring sufficient energy and time to carry out ADL and leisure pursuits. A training heart rate of 60–75 per cent HRmax is generally recommended, but some individuals (older or more severely impaired) may need to begin exercising at lower levels of intensity (ACSM, 2005).

Muscular strength and endurance

Muscle weakness is a common symptom of MS and everyday activities such as walking, climbing stairs and getting out of a chair become increasingly difficult. Strength training cannot alter the progression of the disease, but it can help maintain muscle mass and functional capacity. Lambert (2003) recommends training muscles unilaterally to accommodate differences in strength and range of movement between limbs. Fixed resistance machines provide more support and stability for controlled movement and may be more appropriate for people with balance and coordination problems. It is important to include activities such as small squats, step-ups and sit to stand, which can help an individual carry out activities of daily living and contribute to functional independence. It may be advisable for people with MS to perform strengthening and cardiovascular exercise on different days to avoid excessive fatigue. However, if an individual's condition is stable and their symptoms are mild, they may be able to tolerate aerobic training and strength training within the same exercise session. The ACSM (2005b) advise against strengthening work during an exacerbation, and suggest a focus on gentle ROM and stretching exercises if appropriate. Lambert (2003) recommends an exercise prescription for muscular strength and endurance for people with MS (see table 13.1), but there is no consensus on the optimal prescription for resistance training. There are limited studies in this area and the variable nature of MS may make it difficult to develop protocols for strength training (Karpatkin, 2005).

Flexibility

The muscle groups prone to tightness and contractures in MS are the hamstrings, gastrocnemius, iliopsoas and pectoralis major and minor (ACSM, 2005b). Over time tightness in these muscles affects posture, balance and gait, and can have an impact on ability to perform activities of daily living. People with more severe MS may have contractures and they will need to be assessed for more specific treatments, which may involve long periods of stretching in plaster casts or removable splints (NICE, 2003). For people with general tightness the ACSM (2005b) recommend performing stretching exercises once or twice a day, holding stretches for 30–60 seconds. Stretching programmes need to be tailored to meet the needs of the individual, taking into account ROM, balance and coordination.

Posture

Posture is important for efficient movement patterns, balance and respiratory function. In MS a number of factors such as muscle weakness, instability, fatigue and changes to eyesight can affect posture. Posture can also affect how an individual feels about her- or himself and how others perceive them. An exercise session is an ideal time to focus on standing and seated posture, with specific postural exercises and/or reinforcement of optimal posture throughout the programme. Betts (2004) recommends specific postural exercise for people with MS, with an emphasis on the position and the alignment of the pelvis.

Breathing

Breathing can become less efficient with changes in posture and a less active lifestyle. Breathing exercises such as diaphramatic breathing can play a role in improving posture, by exercising the diaphragm and abdominal muscles (Betts, 2004).

Balance

Balance exercises are important for people with MS and can be incorporated within an exercise programme. Ensure a safe environment for people performing balance activities, with stable support such as a wall bar. If balance is a particular problem, a qualified Postural Stability Instructor (Falls Prevention) may be able to provide a more tailored exercise programme and appropriate level of support.

EXERCISE LIMITATIONS AND CONSIDERATIONS

- **Fatigue** Be sensitive to daily variations in symptoms such as fatigue. This may be influenced by a number of factors such as medication, sleep patterns or temperature. Encourage exercise at times when energy levels are likely to be higher, usually in the morning.
- **Spasticity and spasm** Select a mode of exercise that is most appropriate for your client, for example, some people experience ankle clonus (jumping feet), which makes foot stability during cycling difficult. Many people with MS have problems with one or all limbs going into spasms at different times. Betts

(2004) describes a range of physical techniques involving posture and positioning that people can use to reduce the symptoms of spasm.

- **Relapse** Avoid exercising during a relapse. Gentle ROM and stretching exercises may be appropriate, depending on the severity of the symptoms. Exercise can be resumed when the person is in remission and the symptoms have either diminished or disappeared. The exercise programme may need to be reviewed following a relapse.
- **Balance, vertigo and dizziness** Use equipment such as stationary cycling as opposed to treadmill walking if balance is a problem. Ensure support is available for free-standing activities such as circuit training.
- **Muscle weakness** Muscle weakness can contribute to increased fatigue. It is important to exercise muscles to prevent atrophy. Gradually build up endurance and strength to avoid excessive fatigue.
- **Lack of coordination** Using fixed resistance machines can help provide support and stability and enable more controlled movement.
- **Sensory changes such as numbness** This may affect proprioception and balance during activities such as treadmill walking.
- **Thermo-sensitivity (heat intolerance)** Ensure the exercise environment is air-conditioned and a comfortable temperature. Encourage client to drink plenty of water before, during and after exercise to ensure adequate hydration. Some people may restrict their water intake to avoid problems with bladder urgency and incontinence. Dehydration might also contribute to fatigue. There is some evidence to suggest that cooling before or during exercise can enable a client to exercise for longer periods

of time. Cooling methods include cold showers, ice packs and cold drinks.

- **Ataxia** Encourage use of handrail support in treadmill walking.
- **Cognitive loss, memory, attention, concentration** Provide step-by-step instructions and use visual and verbal cues to reinforce information.
- **Depression** Depression may affect adherence to programme. Consider a range of support strategies.
- **Visual disturbances** You may need to modify activity or use alternative equipment such as the handrail on a treadmill, or changing to a stationary bike.
- **Bladder and bowel problems** Ensure accessible toilet facilities.
- **Autonomic nervous system dysfunction** There may be an abnormal cardiovascular response to exercise in some people with MS. This has been observed in response to isometric exercise and incremental dynamic exercise.
- **Medications** Medications for MS may cause weakness, drowsiness, dizziness, postural instability and impact on cognition.

(Adapted from ACSM, 2005*b*; Lambert, 2003; MS Trust, 2005)

STROKE

A stroke or brain attack occurs as a result of disruption of blood flow to the brain. A stroke is also called a cerebrovascular accident (CVA). This is commonly caused by an occlusion, which leads to a lack of oxygen reaching the brain cells, or a haemorrhage (bleed) in and around the brain. Brain cells are damaged or die, affecting the function of the central nervous system (CNS). The brain cells around the damaged areas may recover as the swelling caused by the stroke goes down.

A transient ischaemic attack (TIA) is similar to a stroke and is often called a 'mini-stroke'. It is caused by a temporary lack of oxygen to the brain and can last from a few minutes up to 24 hours. The symptoms are the same as a stroke and indicate that part of the brain is not receiving enough blood. Unlike a stroke, the symptoms soon go. It is important not to ignore a TIA, as people who have a TIA are at an increased risk of having a stroke. The greatest risk of a stroke is within the first 72 hours after a TIA (Royal College of Physicians, 2004).

PREVALENCE

In the UK, 150,000 people have a stroke each year (for 120,000 this is their first stroke and for the rest it is a recurrent stroke). This equates to about one person every 5 minutes. Approximately one-third of people die within 10 days of having a stroke, approximately one-third make a recovery and the remaining third are left disabled.

- 1 million people live with the effects from a stroke and half of these are dependent on others for support and care..
- Nearly 60,000 people die from a stroke every year.
- Stroke has a greater disability impact than any other disease.

(Adapted from Stroke Association, 2005*a*)

CAUSES

There are two types of strokes, ischaemic and haemorrhagic stroke.

Ischaemic stroke

Ischaemic stroke accounts for two-thirds of

strokes. An ischaemic stroke is caused when the blood flow to the brain is reduced or blocked. The main cause of ischaemia is atherosclerosis, which leads to the narrowing of the arteries leading to the brain. This narrowing increases the likelihood of a blood clot blocking the blood supply to the brain. Within a few minutes of being deprived of oxygen the brain cells of the affected area become damaged or die.

There are different types of ischaemic strokes:
- A **cerebral thrombosis** occurs when a blood clot develops in the major arteries (carotid or vertebrobasilar) that supply the brain with blood.
- A **cerebral embolism** occurs when a clot develops in another part of the body (embolus) and travels to the brain.
- **Lacunar strokes** occur when there is occlusion in the small branches of the major intracranial arteries deep in the brain.

Haemorrhagic

Bleeding from a ruptured blood vessel causes a haemorrhagic stroke. This may be due to weakness in the wall of a blood vessel (an aneurysm) that ruptures. This can occur either in the brain (intra-cerebral) or in the arachnoid space between the skull and the brain (subarachnoid haemorrhagic).

RISK FACTORS

The risk factors of ischaemic stroke overlap with the risk factors for coronary heart disease, and are often classified as modifiable and non-modifiable risk factors (see table 13.2).

The combined contraception pill (oestrogen and progesterone) and hormone replacement therapy (HRT) can increase the risk of stroke

Table 13.2	Modifiable and non-modifiable risk factors
Modifiable risk factors	**Non-modifiable risk factors**
• Hypertension • Smoking • Diet (high in salt, low in fruit and vegetables, low in potassium) • Excess alcohol • Overweight and obesity • Low levels of physical activity • High cholesterol • Diabetes	• Increasing age • Male gender • Asian, African, African-Caribbean • Positive family history of stroke

Stroke Association (2006), GP Notebook (2005a).

and the risks and benefits of hormone treatment should be discussed with a GP (Stroke Association, 2006).

PRIMARY PREVENTION OF STROKE

Primary prevention of stroke involves addressing the modifiable risk factors for stroke (see table 13.2) and managing existing medical conditions such as blood pressure, diabetes, atrial fibrillation (irregular heart rate) and high cholesterol. Stress and depression can contribute to long-term health problems and people should be advised to get help from a GP or health professional if this is a concern (Stroke Association, 2006). Primary care plays an important role in identifying people who have multiple risk factors and a high risk of CVD. Risk factor prediction charts can be used to calculate the likelihood of a person having cardiovascular disease (including a stroke) within a 10-year period (BHS, 2004). An asymptomatic individual with a CVD risk of ≥20 per cent over 10 years is considered high risk and should be offered the same advice on lifestyle and risk factor management as people who have already had a stroke or TIA (secondary prevention). See tables 12.2 and 12.3 in CVD section.

SIGNS AND SYMPTOMS

The common initial symptoms of a stroke include:

- weakness;
- paralysis or numbness in one side of the body;
- drooping face or dribbling mouth;
- slurred speech, difficulty speaking or understanding speech;
- loss of vision in one or both eyes;
- confusion;
- headache;
- sudden problems with balance and co-ordination.

The most common symptom of a subarachnoid haemorrhage is a sudden, severe headache, which is often followed by loss of consciousness. Some people feel sick and have a stiff neck. These symptoms can be confused with a migraine or meningitis.

DIAGNOSIS

The Stroke Association UK has expressed concern about the lack of awareness of the symptoms of a stroke in the general public and misdiagnosis of stroke by health professionals. It is important to recognise the symptoms of a stroke and act as quickly as possible to avoid delaying diagnosis and treatment. A stroke is a medical emergency and delay in diagnosis and treatment can lead to unnecessary disability and death. A tool called FAST has been developed to help people with accurate identification and is currently being used as part of a campaign called 'Stroke is a Medical Emergency' (Stroke Association, 2005b) to encourage people, including paramedics, to recognise the signs of a stroke and act promptly (see box below).

> ### How to recognise the signs of a stroke (FAST)
>
> - **F**acial weakness
>   Can the person smile?
>   Has their mouth or eye dropped?
> - **A**rm weakness
>   Can the person raise both arms?
> - **S**peech problems/disturbance
>   Can the person speak clearly and understand what you say?
> - **T**est all three symptoms
>
> (Adapted from Stroke Association, 2005b)

Diagnosis is based on the signs and symptoms of a stroke and the results of a brain scan to confirm the diagnosis. The Stroke Association (2005b) recommends that someone with a suspected stroke undergoes a brain scan and is given a diagnosis within three hours. A number of tests are commonly carried out to confirm the diagnosis and exclude other conditions:

- CT scan (computed tomography) to confirm the diagnosis of a stroke and exclude the possibility of a bleed or other diseases;
- MRI scan (magnetic resonance imaging), which gives more detailed information than a CT scan, but is less effective at excluding other conditions;

- blood tests to check for diabetes, cholesterol and blood-clotting factors that may have contributed to the stroke;
- blood pressure measurements to identify hypertension;
- chest X-ray to identify any underlying conditions such as heart disease;
- ECG to identify abnormal heart rhythms;
- echocardiogram to check for underlying heart conditions;
- a Doppler or duplex ultrasound to check for narrowing of the carotid arteries.

Effects of a stroke

The effects of a stroke will depend on the age and health of the individual, the severity of the stroke and the area of the brain affected. A severe stroke can cause death, while a mild stroke can cause minor problems that might resolve over time. The left side of the brain is responsible for language and the right side of the brain is responsible for perceptual skills, such as making sense of what you see, hear and touch, and spatial skills, such as judging depth, size, distance or position in space (Stroke Association, 2001). In most people the left side of the brain controls the right side of the body and vice versa. If the damage caused by a stroke affects the left side of the brain, there is likely to be paralysis on the right side of the body and problems with language.

COMMON PROBLEMS
Cognitive problems

Mental processes involved in remembering, communication, attention, learning and perception (making sense of what you see and hear):

Memory Most people will have some problems with memory after a stroke. Some people have problems with verbal memory, which involves remembering language-related information such as names, while other people have problems with visual memory, which is non-language related and involves remembering faces and shapes. Losing prospective memory involves forgetting to carry out activities such as taking tablets. Total amnesia affects only a small number of people.

Attention Problems with attention include:
- failure to concentrate on relevant or important information and filtering out less important information;
- difficulty focusing on important things such as the person talking to you or the traffic;
- being easily distracted.

(Adapted from Moore, 2001)

Communication Communication is one of the most common cognitive problems affecting people after a stroke. Language is usually affected when the left side of the brain is damaged, however, if the stroke has damaged the right side of the brain it can affect control of the muscles used in speech and affect concentration and the ability to organise language. The most common problems include:
- difficulty with language (dysphasia), which includes understanding what is being said (receptive dysphasia), making yourself understood (expressive dysphasia) and problems with reading and writing. Sometimes people feel that they are talking normally yet cannot be understood because they are missing out words or using words with related meanings;
- motor speech problems (dysarthria), which result from weakness or loss of control of the muscles used to make the sounds needed to speak. Some people have problems controlling their breath, using the voice to produce sounds

and controlling the speed and intonation of speech. This can lead to slurred or jerky speech;

- difficulty in performing complex tasks (dyspraxia) such as the control and coordination of movements required for speech, can affect the person's ability to speak clearly and understand conversations.

(Adapted from McLaughlin, 2000)

Perception Perception involves making sense of what is seen (visual perception), touched (tactile perception) and heard (auditory perception). A stroke can affect how people make sense of the world around them. Problems can include:

- inability to recognise objects and colour;
- difficulty judging space, distance or depth;
- difficulty understanding what is seen when it is looked at from an unusual angle;
- unilateral neglect, which means that people neglect one side of the body or the space around one side of the body. This may result in people bumping into things on one side of their body or forgetting to brush their hair on one side of their head.

Emotional and psychological problems

The type of problems experienced will depend on the site and severity of the stroke, for example damage to the right side of the brain may lead to impulsive behaviour, whereas damage to the left side of the brain is associated with anger and crying. Some of the emotional and psychological changes are related to physical damage to the brain and others may be related to the psychological effects of having to live with the consequences of a stroke. Common problems include:

- **Depression** Approximately 50 per cent of people who survive a stroke develop depression within the first year. Depression may be due to the disruption of electrical activity in the brain responsible for emotions, perceptions and thoughts, however, it is also linked to the effect of having a stroke and the impact of living with the changes.
- **Apathy** is common in people who have had a stroke. This may be linked to depression or be a result of damage to the area of the brain responsible for motivation and enthusiasm.
- **Emotionalism** refers to difficulty in controlling emotions, with exaggerated emotional responses and mood swings. Crying is a common problem after a stroke.

(Adapted from Stroke Association, 2005e)

Sensory impairment and pain

Pain and sensory impairment can be caused by a number of factors including:

- immobility and existing conditions such as arthritis: musculoskeletal pain should be appropriately assessed and managed through exercise, improved seating, passive movement or analgesics (Patient UK, 2005);
- shoulder pain in the affected arm, which occurs in approximately 30 per cent of people following a stroke;
- central post-stroke pain (CPSP), which can cause large areas of pain in the leg and/or arm on the affected side of the body. CPSP may be caused by the brain's attempt to compensate for damage to the pain pathways and results in a loss of control over the mechanisms that regulate intensity of feeling. CSPS can be made worse by stress and emotional upset and some people find that relaxation, meditation, visualisation and gentle yoga help (Stroke Association, 2005).

- CPSP may also respond to anticonvulsant medication or antidepressants (Patient UK, 2005).

Paralysis, weakness and spasticity

Weakness on one side of the body (hemiparesis) and paralysis on one side of the body (hemiplegia) is a common problem. This is often accompanied by spasticity and muscle stiffness. After a stroke it is common for muscles to be floppy (flaccid) and weak. If the strength does not return, the muscle will begin to get stiff. It is important to encourage movement to avoid contractures (tightening of muscles, which makes it difficult to move the joint).

TREATMENT
Rehabilitation

The aim of stroke rehabilitation is to help people adapt to their impairments and enable them to participate as fully as possible in life. A range of assistance is available, including physiotherapy, speech and language therapy, psychologists, occupational therapy and specialist nurses and doctors. After a less severe stroke the undamaged area of the brain may take over and compensate for the loss of brain cells in the affected part of the brain. Recovery is fastest in the first three months following a stroke, but recovery may continue even after a year (Patient UK, 2005).

Secondary prevention of stroke and TIA

People who have suffered a stroke are at an increased risk of a further stroke (30–40 per cent risk within five years). They are also at an increased risk of myocardial infarction or other vascular events. The risk of developing a stroke after a TIA can be as high as 20 per cent in the first month, with the greatest risk being within the first few days (Royal College of Physicians, 2004). The Royal College of Physicians (2004) recommend that all patients should be given appropriate information on lifestyle factors including: smoking cessation, physical activity, diet and weight management, reducing salt intake and avoiding excess alcohol (see table 12.2, page 173). Haemorrhagic stroke is not usually caused by atherosclerosis; however, hypertension is a modifiable risk factor for haemorrhagic stroke so it benefits from medical treatment (Smith et al, 2004).

Medications

Drug therapy plays an important part in the secondary prevention of cardiovascular disease and includes medication for blood pressure, cholesterol and anti-thrombotic treatment (see table 12.7).

Blood pressure High blood pressure is a risk factor for stroke and it is important to manage it effectively. A target systolic blood pressure of <130mmHG and a diastolic blood pressure of <80mmHG is recommended by the British Hypertension Society (2004). Drugs commonly used to treat hypertension include diuretics, beta-blockers, calcium channel blockers, ACE inhibitors and angiotensin11 receptor antagonists.

High cholesterol Treatment with a statin (unless contraindicated) is recommended for patients with ischaemic stroke or TIA to achieve optimal targets (see table 12.7).

Anti-thrombotic treatment The Royal College of Physicians (2004) recommends that all patients with ischaemic stroke or TIA should be on antiplatelet drugs such as aspirin or clopidogrel or a combination of dipyridamole modified release and aspirin.

Anticoagulants such as warfarin should be started in patients with atrial fibrillation unless contraindicated (e.g. in haemorrhage stroke).

Some medications such as baclofen, dantrolene and tizandine may also be prescribed for spasticity. The side effects of these drugs can include drowsiness, dizziness and fatigue.

Surgery

A procedure called a carotid endarterectomy can be carried out to remove the fatty deposits from the carotid arteries to reduce the risk of a blood clot. Recent research indicates that carotid endarterectomy may halve the risk of a stroke in some people (Stroke Association, 2005*g*).

After a subarachnoid haemorrage (SAH) surgery is carried out to seal off the aneurysm to prevent further bleeding (Stroke Association, 2005*c*).

EXERCISE RECOMMENDATIONS AND CONSIDERATIONS

After a stroke many people are deconditioned and are more predisposed to a sedentary lifestyle, which increases the likelihood of a further stroke or cardiovascular event. Physical deconditioning can limit functional capacity, affect the ability of individuals to carry out everyday activities and increase the risk of falls (Gordon et al, 2004). Exercise is beneficial for stroke survivors, but there are many barriers to physical activity (see box below), including physical impairments such as hemiplegia, spasticity and dysphasia, which are the primary neurological disorders caused by the stroke, and other factors such as intrinsic motivation, adaptability, coping skills, access to rehabilitation and appropriate exercise opportunities (Gordon et al, 2004).

These factors can make it increasingly difficult for people to remain active, and can lead to a downward spiral of activity leading to a decreased exercise tolerance, further deconditioning, muscle atrophy, osteoporosis and impaired circulation in the lower limbs (Gordon et al, 2004). Social withdrawal and social isolation is a major problem after a stroke and this can exacerbate depression, making it even more difficult for people to stay motivated and engaged in activity. Access to appropriate leisure facilities may help to address some of the external barriers to community-based exercise.

Barriers to physical activity

- Degree of impairment e.g. hemiplegia and spasticity
- Access to appropriate rehabilitation (i.e. as to amount and type)
- Motivation and mood
- Depression
- Communication
- Cognition and learning ability
- Adaptibility and coping skills
- Co-morbidities, e.g. cardiac disease
- Increased energy demands of physical activity leading to fatigue
- Impaired mobility and balance
- Perceived social stigma associated with physical and cognitive deficits
- Level of support
- Access to appropriate leisure facilities

(Adapted from Gordon et al. 2004)

EXERCISE GOALS

- To improve overall health and well-being.
- To reduce the risk of recurrent stroke and cardiovascular events.

- To improve fitness levels, functional capacity and ability to carry out activities of daily living.
- To provide opportunities for the development of social networks.
- To encourage long-term behaviour change.
- To involve family and carers in the process.

It is important for the client to undergo a comprehensive pre-exercise assessment to identify neurological complications and medical conditions that require special considerations and an appropriate level of supervision. Many clients will have co-morbidities such as cardiac disease and it is recommended that stroke patients undergo an exercise stress test before starting an exercise programme (Gordon et al, 2004). This is not always realistic or practical and a lower-intensity exercise programme may be required to minimise the risks associated with exercise.

Cardiovascular

Although there is limited evidence about the role of cardiovascular training in stroke clients, a number of studies suggest that stroke subjects can improve their aerobic capacity and fitness levels following training (Brownlee & Durward, 2005). Aerobic training may include leg, arm or combined leg and arm ergometry. In the absence of an exercise stress test it is important to have a conservative approach to exercise intensity and begin at very low levels of intensity, i.e. 50–60 per cent HRmax. A deconditioned client may need to exercise intermittently, gradually building up to a continuous aerobic bout of >20 minutes. Treadmill training is a functional activity important for everyday living and within the hospital setting treadmill walking is used for individuals with minimal motor impairments. An 'unweighting' device or harness can be used to lift the patients and decrease the amount of weight-bearing involved in walking. This increases safety and enables people who find it difficult to walk to get the training benefits associated with walking. These facilities are unlikely to be available in a community setting and treadmill walking may be inappropriate for clients with postural instability. Inclusive gym equipment can provide a more accessible and appropriate environment and enable clients with varying needs to exercise safely. Examples include the following:

- Straps on pedals or handgrips to help secure an affected lower limb: if straps are used to help secure an affected hand or foot, extra supervision may be required in the event of a fall as the client will not be able to extend an arm or leg to prevent a fall.
- Backrests and seat belts can be fitted to equipment to help with impaired sitting balance.
- Seated steppers are appropriate for people with poor balance and/or coordination. Some seated steppers have reciprocating levers that enable arm exercise.
- A stool or step can help people get on and off equipment such as an exercise bike. Encourage people to step up onto the step with the unaffected leg and step down with the affected leg.

(Adapted from Palmer-McLean & Harbst, 2003)

Strength

It is now accepted that strength exercises should be included in an exercise programme for clinically stable stroke clients. Strength training may contribute to an increased functional capacity and ability to carry out everyday activities and reduce postural instability. There are no current guidelines for how or when to initiate a resistance programme after an ischaemic or haemorrhagic stroke. The following guidelines are similar to those recommended for post-myocardial infarction:

- Low intensity and high reps (12–15)
- 2–3 times a week
- Minimum of one set of exercises targeting the major muscle groups.

(Adapted from Gordon et al, 2004)

Postural stability may be impaired and seated positions might need to be considered, or standing exercises using one hand to hold on to a stable support while exercises are done with the free arm.

Flexibility and neuromuscular

Flexibility training is important to increase range of movement of the affected side and prevent contractures. Many older people may already have orthopaedic conditions such as arthritis that may limit their ROM. Balance and coordination activities will be important to address postural instability and improve ability to carry out activities of daily living.

Table 13.3 summarises the exercise recommendations for stroke. The exercise programme should be individualised, taking into account the age, abilities, preferences, individual goals, skills and confidence of the client. It is important to be aware of any barriers to physical activity (see box on page 205) and find ways to provide a safe, effective and accessible exercise programme which meets the needs of the client.

EXERCISE LIMITATIONS AND CONSIDERATIONS

- Behavioural factors may influence the selection of an appropriate exercise environment. For some people a busy, noisy gym might be too distracting, and encouraging the client to attend during quieter periods might help. A client who struggles with motivation and initiative might benefit from participating in a group circuit class, whereas someone who is prone to exaggerated emotional responses could benefit from one-to-one attention.
- Group exercise sessions with a high level of support may help address the issue of social isolation that people often experience after a stroke.
- People with perceptual problems might experience unilateral neglect. They may bump into equipment on one side of the body or forget to carry out exercises on both sides of the body.
- People might have difficulty in learning and remembering. Allow more time for teaching and reinforcing exercises. Try to encourage a simple exercise routine. Provide written instructions and label exercise machines clearly.
- Allow more time for communication. Make instructions short and clear. Sometimes it helps if the client repeats what you have told them in their own words. Some people might find it easier to understand the written word.
- Involve family members or carers in the exercise programme. They will be able to provide additional support, encourage home-based exercise and enhance exercise compliance.
- Be aware of the side effects of medications for spasticity such as drowsiness, dizziness and fatigue.
- Clients with altered body structure and function, such as hemiplegia, use much more energy walking than an able-bodied person walking at the same speed.

Table 13.3	Summary of exercise recommendations for stroke		
Training guidelines	**Cardiovascular**	**Muscle strength**	**Flexibility**
Aims	To increase safety during ADLs Increase walking speed Decrease risk of CVD	Increase independence and performance of ADLs	Improve ROM Decrease contractures
Frequency	3–5 days per week	2–3 days per week	2–3 days per week
Intensity	50–80 per cent of HRmax RPE 11–14 (6–20 scale)*	No consensus on optimal intensity. Low intensity, high reps	Stretch to the point of tension, without pain
Time	20–60 mins (continuous or intermittent, multiple 10-min bouts)	1–3 sets of 8–12 reps	Hold each stretch for 10–30 sec, 2–4 reps
Type	Large muscle group activities such as walking, cycling, combined arm-leg ergometry	8–10 exercises including major muscle groups. Dynamic resistance exercises	Static stretching. Aim to increase ROM on affected side and prevent contractures

Neuromuscular
Co-ordination and balance activities 2–3 days per week (consider performing on the same day as strength activities)

*In the absence of an exercise stress test it is more appropriate to exercise at low to moderate levels of intensity (55–69 per cent HRmax). Compensate for lower levels of intensity by increasing the frequency and/or duration. Palmer-McLean and Harbst (2003 and 2009); Gordon et al. (2004)

- After a TIA or stroke, ensure the client has been under the care of a medical specialist, is on aspirin or equivalent (unless stroke was caused by a cerebral bleed) and is clinically stable. Liaise with GP and physiotherapist to ensure appropriate transition or return to community-based exercise programme.
- Many stroke patients will have co-morbidities such as cardiac disease, therefore it is important to focus on safety with appropriate screening, exercise programming, monitoring and client education.
- Monitor client's response to exercise and ensure clients are aware of warning signs and symptoms and what action to take, e.g. to stop exercise and inform instructor.
- Only work within your own levels of competence and confidence. Liaise with GP and physiotherapist and seek advice if needed.
- Where possible use inclusive equipment in line with Inclusive Fitness Initiative (2004).

(Adapted from Palmer-McLean & Harbst (2003); Gordon et al (2004))

PARKINSON'S DISEASE

Parkinson's disease (PD) is a chronic, progressive, degenerative neurological disease that results from a reduction in the neurotransmitter (chemical messenger) dopamine. The reduction in dopamine occurs as a result of the death of dopamine-producing cells within a component of the basal ganglia (part of the brain) called the substantia nigra. The basal ganglia have an important role in the output of voluntary movement and postural adjustments (ACSM, 2005). Over time more cells become damaged and levels of dopamine decrease, affecting movement, cognitive function, emotion and autonomic function. The symptoms of Parkinson's disease are also the main symptoms of a number of different conditions, which are grouped together under the umbrella term 'Parkinsonism'. Eighty-five per cent of all people with Parkinsonism have Parkinson's disease. It is sometimes called idiopathic Parkinson's disease (IDP), which means that the cause of the disease is unknown. The remaining 15 per cent have specific conditions that cause Parkinsonism, such as Alzheimer's disease or motor neurone disease or secondary causes such as viral infections, toxicity and head injury (Prodigy, 2005g).

CAUSES

The causes have not yet been identified but are believed to be a combination of factors including:

- genetic susceptibility
- environmental factors such as toxins, e.g. pesticides.

PREVALENCE

In the UK approximately 120,000 individuals have PD. It is more common in people over the age of 50, and is more likely to affect men than women. PD can also occur in younger people, and is known as young-onset Parkinson's disease (Prodigy, 2005g).

SIGNS AND SYMPTOMS

Some of the main features of PD relate to movement, and include slowness, stiffness, difficulty in initiating movement and tremor. The symptoms of PD do not appear until there is less than 80 per cent of dopamine left in the brain, and these levels of dopamine continue to decrease over time. People are usually affected on one side of the body at the onset of the disease, but over time both sides of the body are affected. PD affects people in different ways and they may experience different combinations of the symptoms described.

Tremor usually begins on one side of the body, affecting the hands and arms. Over time it can spread to all four limbs. When the affected part of the body is supported and rested, the tremor will be more apparent. When the affected limb is moving, tremor is reduced. Tremor can worsen as a result of stress, anxiety or tiredness.

Bradykinesia (slowness of movement), **hypokinesia** (reduction in the amplitude or size of movement) and **akinesia** (difficulty in initiating movement) are the main features of PD. Common symptoms include feeling tired, difficulty in performing more than one motor task at a time or doing activities that involve fine motor skills such as writing or doing up buttons, and reduced speed and size of repeated movements such as walking.

Rigidity (muscular stiffness) is caused by an increase in muscle tone and resistance to passive stretch in both the agonist and the antagonist muscles around joints (ACSM, 2005). This usually begins in one limb and over time spreads to the other limbs and other parts of the body. Sometimes the stiffness has a jerky quality and this is called *cogwheel rigidity*, and sometimes the rigidity has a slow, sustained quality and is called *lead-pipe rigidity*. When the trunk is affected, spinal rotation and extension become limited and postural reflexes are affected. It becomes increasingly difficult to perform functional activities that involve coordinating the trunk and extremities and limited trunk rotation makes everyday activities, such as turning over in bed, looking behind or getting out of a car, difficult.

Postural instability The impairment of postural reflexes affects postural stability, and when balance is challenged there is a delayed response and people are less able to right themselves and more likely to fall, often backwards. Over time their posture changes to a rounded upper back (kyphosis), a forward head position, and flexion at the hip and knee joints. People with PD may also find it difficult to shift their centre of gravity forward, and are at an increased risk of falling backwards when moving from sitting to standing.

Gait changes People may develop a characteristic gait with short, slow, shuffling steps, involuntary hurrying (festinating) and difficulty initiating movement. Gait is affected by the flexed posture, reduced trunk rotation and arm swing. Turning becomes more difficult and postural instability increases when turning.

Cognitive dysfunction Dementia, depression and hallucinations may also affect people with PD. Dementia and hallucinations may be part of the disease process, but they may be caused or aggravated by the medications taken for PD.

Autonomic dysfunction refers to the part of the peripheral nervous system that is responsible for the control of involuntary muscles. Features of autonomic dysfunction include:

- constipation and bladder problems;
- sweating;
- impotence;
- problems regulating temperature (thermo-regulation);
- problems with swallowing (dysphagia);
- in the later stages postural hypotension is common, although this may be aggravated by medications for PD.

Pulmonary Some people with PD may experience respiratory problems (obstructive and restrictive), which may be linked to changes in functioning of the respiratory muscles, loss of flexibility in the trunk and postural changes (ACSM, 2005).

Other features of Parkinson's disease include:
- sleep disturbances;
- altered sense of smell;
- changes in speech;
- lack of facial expression.

The symptoms will generally get worse over time, however, the rate of progression will vary from person to person.

DIAGNOSIS

Parkinson's disease is difficult to diagnose as many of the signs and symptoms may be due to other disorders or secondary causes such as:
- Alzheimer's disease;
- motor neurone disease;
- antipsychotic drugs;
- cerebrovascular disease;
- head injuries (e.g. in boxers);
- toxicity (e.g. carbon monoxide).

Patients with suspected PD should be referred to a neurologist or physician with a special interest in the disease for a diagnosis to be confirmed.

TREATMENT

There are no treatments to cure PD, or to prevent the progression of the disease. Current treatments aim to ease the symptoms. If someone has mild symptoms they will often decide to postpone drug therapy and focus on improving their lifestyle through healthy eating, exercise and relaxation. As the disease progresses and symptoms worsen, drug therapy will be introduced. Drug therapy and a healthy lifestyle (nutritious diet, relaxation and exercises) are essential components in the management of PD. Therapies such as physio-, occupational and speech therapy play an important part in the ongoing management of the disease.

Healthy eating

The current guidelines for healthy eating promoted by the British Nutrition Foundation (2005) are recommended for people with PD. Specific advice includes:

- Increasing intake of fluid and high-fibre foods and increasing physical activity levels are recommended for constipation.
- Timing of medications may need to be discussed with GP as protein in foods can interfere with the absorption of some medication such as Levodopa (Parkinson's Disease Society, 2003b).
- People with chewing and swallowing problems may need specialist advice from a speech and language specialist.

Relaxation

When a person has PD a lot of concentration and mental energy is used to carry out relatively simple activities of daily living. Relaxation can have a positive impact on well-being and can be used in isolation or within an exercise programme. Complementary therapies such as massage therapy and reflexology and relaxation techniques may also help relieve symptoms and help people with stress and low moods (Parkinson's Disease Society, 2005a).

Medication (see table 13.4)

The main aim of drug treatment is to control symptoms and improve quality of life. The medication can control symptoms by:

- increasing the levels of dopamine in the brain;
- stimulating the parts of the brain where dopamine works;
- blocking the action of chemicals such as acetylcholine that affect dopamine;
- blocking the action of other enzymes that affect dopamine.

(Adapted from Parkinson's Disease Society, 2005b)

There are complications associated with the long-term use of PD drug therapy, caused by an interaction between the disease and the drugs. People can experience 'early wearing off', where the effect of the medication does not last as long as necessary and loses its effect before the next dose. 'On/off syndrome' can also occur, where symptoms such as dyskinesia (involuntary movements) start and stop unexpectedly (Parkinson's Disease Society, 2004b). People with PD usually have postural instability and the drugs used to treat the symptoms can cause dizziness and postural hypotension. Depression is more common in people with PD and some

Table 13.4	Medication for Parkinson's disease		
Name of medication	**Action/purpose**	**Side effects**	**Implication for exercises**
Dopaminergics Levodopa Madopar Sinemet **Dopamime agonists** Bromocriptine Cabergoline Pergolide Ropinirole Apomorphine	Levodopa is a chemical that the brain converts into dopamine. It can dramatically improve symptoms of PD. Dopamine agonists stimulate the part of the brain where dopamine works. They are often used in addition to levodopa.	Nausea and vomiting. Orthostatic hypotension. Cardiac arrhythmias. Excessive drowsiness, sudden onset of sleep. Motor complications over time such as dyskinesia (involuntary movements), freezing and motor fluctuations. Nausea and vomiting. Confusion or hallucinations, drowsiness.	Orthostatic (postural hypotension). Timing of exercise. Motor complications. Cardiac arrhythmias. Improvement in stiffness and slowness of movement. Longer term motor fluctuations.
Anticholergics Trihexyphenidyl Benztropine Orphenadrine Procyclidine	Blocks the action of the chemical messenger acetylcholine. Useful for younger people with mild symptoms. More effective at improving tremor than slowness and stiffness. Reduces production of saliva when drooling is problematic, and reduces bladder contractions (urge incontinence).	Cardiac irregularities, mood changes, memory loss, confusion, blurred vision, dry mouth, nausea and vomiting. Not used in the elderly due to the side effects, which might be mental confusion and heightened glaucoma.	Be aware of possible cardiac irregularities. Improvement in tremor more than slowness or stiffness.
Monoamine oxidase type B inhibitor Selegiline	Blocks the enzyme MAO-B that breaks down dopamine in the brain.	Insomnia, headaches, sweating.	
COMT inhibitor Entacapone Tolcapone	Prolongs the action of levodopa by blocking the action of an enzyme that breaks it down. Reduces symptoms.	Nausea, vomiting and diarrhea. Can exacerbate involuntary movement (dyskinesia).	Possible exacerbation of involuntary movement (dyskinesia).

Parkinson's Disease Society (2005).

people may be on antidepressants, which can have a sedative effect and cause sleepiness, which in turn has implications for exercise.

EXERCISE LIMITATIONS AND CONSIDERATIONS

There is very limited research about the benefits of exercise in people with PD, but regular physical activity can influence survival rate by preventing the deconditioning and decline associated with inactivity (Northumbria University, 2005). There is no current evidence to suggest that exercise can affect the progression of the disease; however, it can help:

- improve quality of life;
- increase fitness levels;
- improve balance, posture, mobility and gait;
- alleviate some of the symptoms of the disease, including stiffness and slowness of movement;
- promote independence.

For people with mild to moderate PD a general fitness programme following ACSM guidelines is probably appropriate (ACSM, 2005b). The programme should be individualised and take into account the limitations of the client, including age and co-morbidities such as heart disease. It is important for the exercise professional to be in partnership with other health professionals working with the client, such as a physiotherapist who has more specialised skills, knowledge and experience of working with people with PD. This partnership becomes increasingly vital as the disease progresses and a more specialised programme addressing gait and balance is required. Orofacial and breathing techniques may also be included within a specialist programme. The progression of the disease will determine the level of supervision required and the exercise environment, which may need to change to meet the specific needs of the client. See table 13.5 for a summary of exercise guidelines.

Cardiovascular training

The evidence for cardiovascular exercise in people with PD is limited, but it may be appropriate to maintain aerobic capacity in people with mild or moderate levels. People with PD often have little physical activity, leading to low levels of cardio-respiratory fitness. Cardiovascular training is important for overall health and well-being as well as cardiovascular health. Where possible, functional activities, such as walking, are recommended. Treadmill walking may not be a safe option, although this will depend on the individual's symptoms. If postural instability is a concern a stationary bike or upper body ergometer may be more appropriate. Equipment such as cross trainers, which involve the upper and lower body, are a good option as they encourage a good ROM and encourage trunk rotation.

Muscular strength and endurance

The ACSM (2005b) acknowledge the lack of research in this client group. They suggest using the ACSM guidelines for the general population, provided the programme takes into account age, co-morbidities, individual limitations and impairments.

Further considerations for this component include:

- Ensure client performs an adequate warm-up that includes low-level aerobic activity, joint mobility exercise and stretches before beginning a resistance programme.
- Reinforce good posture during muscle strength and endurance activities.
- Emphasise extensor muscles such as lower and

middle trapezius, rhomboids, erector spinae, gluteus maximus and quadriceps.

- Include exercises such as standing squats, prone squeezes, leg extensions, calf raises, back extensions and toe lifts.
- Where possible use functional positions, e.g. standing squats.
- Use sound and visual cues such as clapping, body language or a metronome to help with movement and timing.

(Adapted from ACSM, 2005)

Flexibility

Low levels of physical activity and poor posture can lead to reduced ROM around joints and tight muscles. This can eventually lead to the development of contractures in certain muscle groups and a reduced ROM in hip and knee extension, dorsi-flexion, shoulder flexion, external shoulder rotation, trunk extension and axial rotation (ACSM, 2005). There is limited research on the effectiveness of flexibility training for people with PD. A general stretching programme is appropriate for people with mild muscle tightness, but people with severe muscle tightness or muscle contractures will require a more specialised stretching programme delivered by a physiotherapist. Refer to Norris (2004) for comprehensive information on the principles and practice of stretching.

Further considerations for this component include the following:

- Tailor the stretch programme, taking into account individual ROM and stability.
- Consider appropriate positions, including floor, standing, seated and using a couch for people who find it difficult to get down onto the floor.

- Reinforce optimal posture.
- Use a range of tools such as therapy bands, exercise balls and foam rollers and touch to encourage ROM and enhance stretching.
- Include a range of stretches with an emphasis on gastrocnemius, soleus, hamstring, hip flexor and pectoral stretch. Spinal extension, lateral flexion and rotation are particularly important to increase ROM in the spine.
- Include stretching exercises for the hands.
- Encourage a daily stretching programme.

Posture

It is important to reinforce optimal posture throughout the exercise programme. Poor posture not only affects walking and postural stability, but also breathing, swallowing and speaking loudly and clearly. A stooped posture can also affect the way people feel about themselves and the way other people perceive them. The Parkinson Society for Canada (2003) emphasises the importance of checking seated and standing posture throughout the day and recommends a number of specific exercises to practise daily including:

- Lie on the floor with legs outstretched. Provide support under head to ensure spinal alignment. Allow gravity to gently stretch out and lengthen tightened muscles.
- Back extension from a prone lying position to strengthen the back extensors.
- Shoulder squeezes (seated or lying prone) to strengthen the shoulder retractors (rhomboid major, rhomboid minor and trapezius).
- Chin tuck (seated or lying) to lengthen the cervical spine and reinforce optimal posture.

In 2003 the Parkinson's Disease Society developed an exercise programme called 'Keeping

Moving'. The programme was developed as a group exercise, but a booklet and video are available to enable people to exercise independently (Parkinson's Disease Society, 2004c). The programme aims to minimise musculoskeletal limitation and postural deformities and promote independence through the maintenance of functional capacity. The programme involves relaxation and an emphasis on slow, controlled movements synchronised with breathing, and elements of strengthening, balance, coordination and flexibility. Pilates and/or core stability trained exercise professionals will be familiar with the type of exercises within the programme. Examples of some of the exercises and the reasons for them include the following:

- Encourage backward chaining to get on and off the floor. This is a technique used by physiotherapists and postural stability exercise professionals to teach people how to get on and off the floor. It involves breaking the sequence into small component parts, teaching each part separately and arranging the parts sequentially.
- Pelvic tilt mobilises the pelvis and lumbar region, and encourages smooth, controlled movement. This is important for activities such as sit to stand and walking.
- Knee opening/knee drops develop trunk stability against limb loading and practise isolation and control of movement.
- Heel slides develop trunk stabilisation against limb loading and practise control and isolation of movement.
- Heel slide plus single arm pullover increases the complexity, controlling movements of opposing limbs.

Seated exercises:
- Sitting pelvic tilt to progress the lying pelvic tilt and practise it in a more functional position.
- Trunk rotations to increase range of movement and improve balance and coordination.

Standing exercises:
- Weight transference in standing position with both feet in contact with the floor. Encourage forward and backward sway that is gradually reduced until weight is appropriately balanced and steady. This can help with the weight transference needed for activities such as sit to stand and can help improve postural control and balance.
- Standing rotation to progress the seated version by maintaining upright standing posture.

(Adapted from Ramaswany & Webber, 2003)

Postural instability Not everyone with PD will fall, but as the condition progresses, the risk of a fall increases. There are several factors that contribute to falls, including the physical problems related to PD, ageing, the effects of medication and the environment. People often develop a kyphotic standing posture, with rigidity in the neck and shoulders spreading to the trunk and extremities. This stooping position and change in muscle tone places the individual at an increased risk of falling. Rigidity or contraction of the calf muscle can make it difficult to dorsiflex the foot, hindering a normal heel-toe walking action. This results in a shuffling type of gait with short steps. Rigidity around the ankle joint can eventually lead to walking on the balls of the feet, reducing the ability of the feet to absorb shock adequately and exacerbating balance problems. A client with postural instability may benefit from a targeted programme with specific fall-management strategies such as gait, dynamic posture, balance and functional floor activities to improve confidence and coping skills. Other approaches such as Alexander technique and Tai Chi may also contribute to improved balance and gait (Parkinson's Disease Society, 2005*a*).

Strategies to prevent falls

- Encourage client to focus on one activity and move slowly, to compensate for the body's inability to respond automatically.
- Avoid turning too quickly; don't turn on the spot; walk in a half circle; take more steps.
- Be aware of activities that increase the risk of falling such as stepping backwards or reaching for something while walking.
- Try to swing arms and lengthen stride when walking.
- Encourage upright posture and looking ahead.
- Practice striking the ground heel first.
- Encourage client to avoid doing too many things at once such as walking and talking and/or carrying objects.
- Encourage client to take time to perform activities that involve changing positions, e.g. to sit on the side of the bed for a while before getting out of bed. This is particularly important if client feels light-headed.
- Only perform floor-based exercises if clients can get themselves up off the floor.
- Check that any walking aid used has been recommended by a physiotherapist, as some walking aids may not be appropriate for people with PD and actually increase the risk of tripping or falling.
- Use a solid support such as a wall for standing exercises, especially for activities like calf raises that require balance.

- Ensure close supervision for balance exercises and gait training.
- Footwear with rubber soles tend to grip the floor and may cause a trip.
- Ensure a safe, clutter-free exercise environment to minimise the risk of trips and falls.

(Adapted from Parkinson's Disease Society, 2003)

Freezing

People with PD can also have problems with 'freezing'. When this happens people feel as though their feet are stuck to the ground, even though their upper body wants to move forward. This causes them to stop suddenly. Freezing often occurs when people are approaching doorways and narrow spaces. It is also more likely to occur when people are feeling anxious or are in crowded places or unfamiliar situations. Changes in the surface such as moving to an uneven surface or a different pattern on a carpet can also cause a freeze. It can also happen when trying to initiate other movements, such as getting out of bed, lifting a cup to drink or stepping off after getting up from a sitting position. This is sometimes referred to as 'start hesitation' (Parkinson's Disease Society, 2003*a*). The problems involved with initiating movement and freezing may leave people feeling unsteady on their feet and at an increased risk of falls.

Practical ways of helping with freezing There are a variety of methods that people find help them overcome 'freezing' and different methods will work for different people. If you are working with a client with PD, find out what works for them and if there is anything you can do to assist. Try not to distract the person when they are walking, as this will affect their concentration. The following cues can be used to help initiate and maintain movement and can be helpful for people experiencing freezing:

- **Proprioceptive cues, e.g. weight shift method** Instead of trying to move forward, focus on shifting the weight from one leg to the other as this can sometimes make it easier to step forward. Taking a step back before walking forward may also help. However, these methods may not be appropriate if balance is a problem.
- **Visual cues** Some people find it helps to identify a definite target and walk towards it. Stepping over a mark on the floor can help, or dropping a piece of paper and stepping over it. Other people find that trying to step over an imaginary obstacle can help initiate movement.
- **Auditory cues** Decide which leg to move first and then say '1, 2, 3, step' or 'ready, steady, go'. The client or the person with the client can say this. Counting from one to ten while walking or using a marching rhythm or a small metronome are methods that work for different people.
- **Cognitive cues** Some people find it helpful to memorise parts of a movement sequence, mentally rehearsing a movement or visualising the length of a step.

Communication

An inability to use facial expressions and changes in speech such as rhythm, rate and intonation can have a big impact on communication for people with PD. Communication problems can lead to withdrawal and isolation so it is important for the exercise professional to be aware of these difficulties. Try to avoid making assumptions about how a person is feeling or their ability to understand based on body language, gesture and facial expression. Allow more time, and try to find ways to enhance communication (Parkinson's Disease Society, 2003*b*).

GUIDELINES FOR EXERCISE

- Timing of an exercise will be influenced by a number of factors. People who are on medication will know when it is working well, and whether they feel well enough to exercise.
- It is not appropriate to exercise if the client is feeling tired, if there has been a change in medication or if there has been a worsening of symptoms.
- Don't make assumptions about what a person can or cannot do.
- Teach transitions carefully, taking into account postural hypotension.
- Break down complex movement sequences into smaller components.
- Encourage people to practise exercises at a conscious level. This approach is used in exercises such as Pilates, where the mind-body connection is a key principle.
- Use a range of visual, auditory or proprioceptive cues to help people initiate and maintain movement, and to facilitate learning.
- Take into account co-morbidities such as heart disease.
- Only work within your own levels of competence and confidence. Seek advice where appropriate.
- Be sensitive to possible increased levels of frustration and depression that people with PD may experience.
- Provide appropriate support to help clients continue with the programme, such as telephone calls, an inclusive environment and social support (family and friends).

NEUROLOGICAL DISEASE

Table 13.5	Summary of exercise guidelines for Parkinson's disease		
Training guidelines/ Aims	Cardiovascular/ Endurance to improve CV capacity	Muscle strength to improve capacity	Flexibility to improve ROM
Frequency	Structured exercise 3 times a week minimum ADL and leisure activities can be carried out on non-exercise days.	2–3 non-consecutive days a week.	5–7 days a week. 1–3 times a week.
Intensity	No consensus on optimal intensity. Moderate intensity may be appropriate 55–70 per cent of HRmax. Some people may need to initiate a programme at lower levels of intensity.	No consensus on optimal intensity. Initiate programme at low levels of intensity using light resistance.	To the point of mild tension but not to pain or discomfort.
Time	30 min. This can be broken down into smaller bouts e.g. 3 ×10 min. ≤60 min.	1 set of 8–12 reps.	Hold stretch for 20–30 sec. Repeat each stretch 2–5 times.
Type	Arm or leg ergometry, walking, rowing, water-based. Short walking sessions.	8–10 exercises including major muscle groups. Fixed equipment may provide more support. Emphasis on erector spinae, rhomboids, middle and lower trapezius, gastrocnemius and quadriceps. Include functional activities such as sit to stand, squats and step-ups. Closed kinetic chain.	Static stretching is appropriate for people with mild muscle tightness. General stretching programme with an emphasis on increasing ROM in muscles which promote extension of the spine, hips and knees, and rotation of the spine.

Neuromuscular
Postural and balance exercise to improve the mind-body connection and encourage smooth, controlled movement (Ramaswany & Webber 2003). As the disease progresses, a more specialised programme with an emphasis on transfers, balance and gait will be necessary.

(2005b); Protas and Stanley (2003).

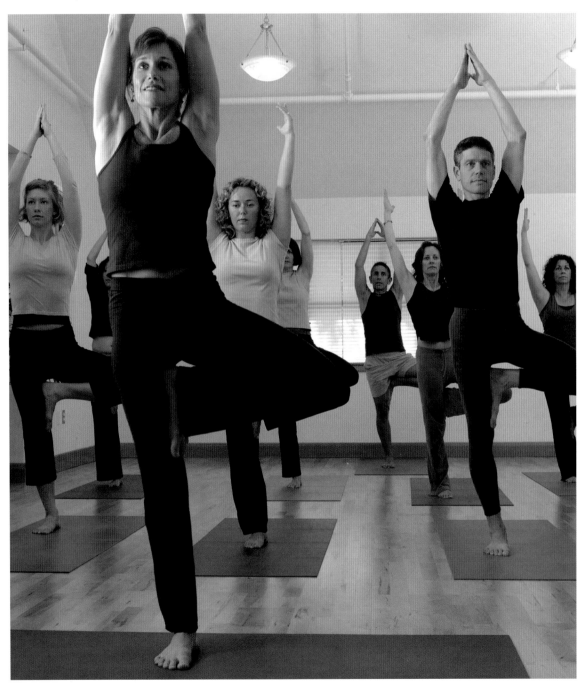

Yoga, is one of many holistic approaches to activity, that if suitably modified and adapted, can provide a wonderful alternative activity approach for referred populations

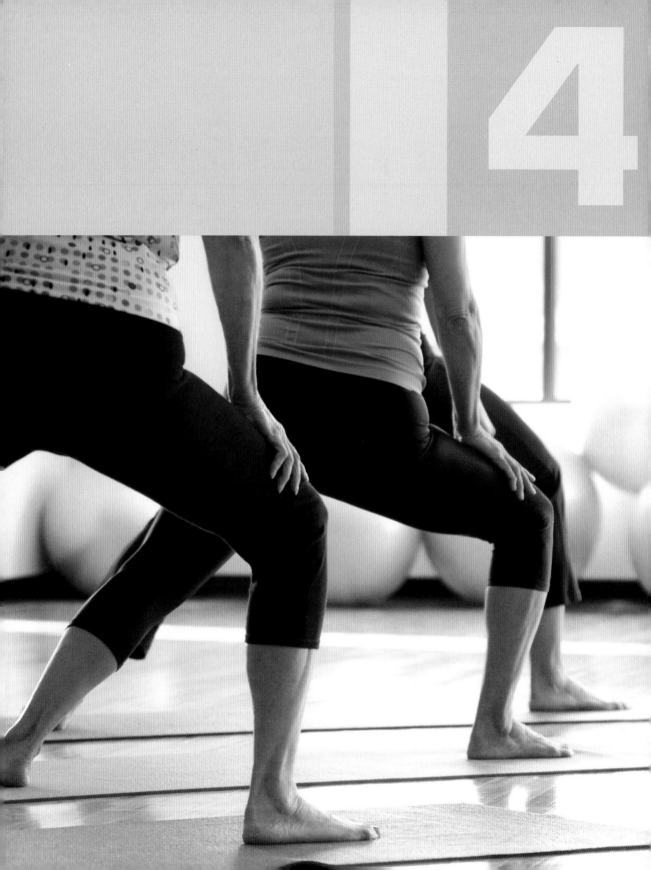

4

PART **FOUR**

SUPPORTING AND WORKING WITH CLIENTS

This section of the book describes a way of working with referred clients to assist with the process of change. It discusses how to create a helping relationship, focusing on how to work in a client-centred way using an empathetic, non-judgmental and relational style. It also explores one model of behaviour change, which can be used to increase the instructor's awareness of the stages people move through when undertaking change, and discusses some of the processes and strategies for assisting with the management of behaviour, thoughts and feelings in relation to the change process.

CREATING A HELPING RELATIONSHIP

14

THE ROLE OF THE EXERCISE PROFESSIONAL

The role of the exercise professional is to work directly with clients and make them the central focus to the work (client-centred); enabling and empowering them to make their own decisions about the life changes that will most enhance their health and well-being and which meet their needs.

The role includes:
• initial assessment and information gathering, negotiating a working contract, establishing a working alliance and building rapport and relationship (specific information and tools are discussed in chapter 4 and 5);
• planning an appropriate programme (session structure and health and safety are discussed in chapter 5 and 6);
• delivering the programme developed, with consideration to the needs of specific conditions (discussed throughout part 3);
• assessing and monitoring clients (progress checks etc.) and evaluating the impact of the programme (with consideration to all factors listed throughout parts 2 and 3 of the book);
• action planning, which may include making changes to the programme (progression,

regression) or teaching style, seeking additional training (Level 4 qualifications) or CPD etc.

BUILDING RAPPORT AND RELATIONSHIP

The rapport and relationship that is established between the client and the exercise professional is arguably one of the most important tools for helping the person to make changes, and is certainly a key factor in motivation and possibly adherence.

Similarities between client and exercise professional may have a bearing on the effectiveness of specific interventions, for example, matching of age, gender, ethnicity and social class may all impact the relationship and the effectiveness of specific interventions. For example, a male client may work better with a male trainer, an Asian client may work better with an Asian trainer, an older client may work better with an older trainer. These elements of difference are often ignored, but they can potentially make a significant difference to the rapport and relationship.

Early meetings with the client need to focus on making contact and connecting with them and gathering information (initial assessment, screening and risk stratification, discussed in chapter 4). However, it is also essential to get to know the person. For example: How open are they? How aware are they about their condition and the changes they need to make? How ready do they feel to make these changes? Do they have any fears or concerns? Do they believe they can make the changes (self-efficacy)? How motivated and committed are they?

The exercise professional will need to listen to the client to find out some of this information and may also need to read between the lines of the information the client gives. For example, a client may indicate they don't want to change something, when really they just feel scared and lack the belief in themselves to make the changes. In these instances, the exercise professional can use motivation interviewing techniques (change and sustain talk, discussed later) to work with the client (if they are trained to use these techniques). Alternatively, they can make a recommendation for the client to speak with a counsellor to help them work through the fears of making changes.

The relationship and rapport between client and exercise professional often develops over time and it is important that the relationship stays professional and that boundaries are maintained. See table 14.1.

THE WORKING CONTRACT

Most schemes offer short-term working contracts with clients (10–16 weeks) that are funded and supported by local commissioning services (GP consortiums etc.) or through funding received through specific grants etc. Some schemes have exit routes or strategies, where the client's continued progress and adherence can be monitored, and where the client can still have some access to their original point of contract with the scheme (even if this is just a simple 'Hello, how are you doing?').

Table 14.1	Responsibilities, roles and boundaries	
Action/responsibility	**Role**	**Boundary**
Provide information	Teacher	Without crossing the boundaries and providing information that is outside of scope of practice
Being friendly	Friend	Without crossing the boundary into becoming a friend, as this may create a conflict
Offer different strategies and interventions	Strategic planner	Without forcing strategies upon the client that may not really suit their needs or lifestyle
Help to establish goals	Goal setter	Without forcing goals upon the client
Actively listen	Counsellor	Without moving into the role of being a counsellor or sounding board for every problem the client has
Motivate and support	Nurturer and supporter	Without creating dependency or acting like a surrogate parent
Challenge clients and test/check their perception and beliefs that may influence change	Liberator	Without moving into the role of being the expert on what is best for the person. The person is always the best expert on themselves!

Personal trainers who work with private clients, may have the luxury of longer-term working contracts, because in most instances, the client funds their own training.

Short-term contracts

The disadvantage of short-term contracts is that they demand a more directive way of working and this does not suit all people. For example, a programme is written and this is what needs to be adhered to; or the inclusion of specific cognitive and behavioural techniques and strategies may be integrated to promote self-management and self-help. Directive approaches are effective and work for some people, and are probably most appropriate for making short-term interventions. However, they do not suit all people. Some people need to find their own way and try different things out and see what works and doesn't work, and this experimenting usually takes longer than a few weeks.

Longer-term contracts

An advantage of longer-term contracts is that the trainer can develop a deeper working alliance with the client and operate in a more exploratory and experimental way. The process of helping a client to make changes can include:

- identifying and exploring blocks to success as they present (for example, discussing relapses and helping to overcome these);
- encouraging an exploratory and creative attitude to confronting and managing these blocks and learning about the self;
- supporting the client as they work through these blocks and towards their goals.

A longer-term contract can offer more support to the person as they struggle to implement the changes they desire and work towards long-term behaviour change. They also provide the exercise professional with the opportunity to develop a greater understanding of the person they are working with. Longer-term working may help the client to access and sustain the level of motivation they need to maintain the changes more permanently.

In reality, a lifetime of choosing unhealthy behaviours and habits and the beliefs and attitudes the person holds that support these habits are unlikely to change overnight. For most clients referred to exercise, ongoing support and guidance will need to be provided.

The working alliance and reflective practice

To build and sustain an effective working alliance, the exercise professional needs to be able to reflect on their work and on their relationship with the client(s). They need to *reflect on action* (look back at the effectiveness of the relationship and interventions made after working with the client at each session and at the end of the work), and also *reflect in action* (being aware of the effectiveness of the relationship and communication during their work with the client and responding appropriately) (Boud et al, 1985).

The exercise professional will need to be able to adapt his or her working style to suit different client needs. Some clients may need a more directive approach at times (being guided towards what to do); others will need a more exploratory approach, where they can experiment with different changes and decide which changes suit them and their lifestyle. Some clients need lots of support and encouragement and may be more dependent on specific support interventions, while others will be more inclined towards self-management and will only need occasional reassessments to discuss their progress and are happier being left to get on with things. It is essential that the trainer is reflective and creative so that s/he can adapt his or her way of working to accommodate different needs. The approach taken may depend on the client's locus of control.

Locus of control

Locus of control is the extent to which an individual *believes* they have the power to influence their life through their own actions. Locus can be either *internal* or *external*.

- Clients with an **internal locus of control** believe that they have the power to make changes and have a level of control over their lives. They are more self-motivated and will keep going to achieve a goal; they need less external rewards and encouragement. Once their mind is made up, they are determined and less likely to succumb to peer pressure (e.g. resisting pressure to have another drink or eat a dessert).
- Clients with an **external locus of control** are 'fatalistic', and believe that life is more a matter of chance/luck, that is controlled by other factors, external to themselves. If they perceive any risk of failure, they are less likely to commit to engaging or making a change (learned helplessness). If they do engage, they may lose belief quickly and consequently, will change/modify their goal (or sometimes give up) to something more achievable.

A person with an external locus of control will most likely need a more directive approach:

- more direction (a step-by-step guide to how they can achieve their goal and make changes);
- more advice and guidance (what to do and when to do it);
- clear SMART (see page 238) goals (to help them achieve and make small steps and assist motivation and adherence);
- more ongoing support (supervised exercise);
- more encouragement (positive reminders of everything they are doing well and more praise for what they do, e.g. attending).

Individuals with an internal locus of control will need this support, but once they have made their commitment, they are more likely to stick with it (adherence) through self-determination and motivation.

Another factor which may influence the change process and the support needed may be cognitive dissonance.

Cognitive dissonance

When considering change most people will experience some inner conflicts. Cognitive dissonance is the state of inner conflict and discomfort that occurs when an individual holds two or more conflicting beliefs, which are contradictory to each other (Leith, 1994:13; Gross 1996:448.

For example, an individual who smokes, but also knows that smoking causes chronic diseases (CHD, COPD, cancer etc.) will have two conflicting cognitions: (1) 'I smoke' and (2) 'Smoking causes health problems' (Gross, 1996:448). Their behaviour is incongruent with their belief.

To resolve the dissonance, the individual needs to either change the *behaviour* or change their *attitude* and beliefs towards the behaviour and there are many ways of doing this. The healthiest option is to give up smoking (*change the behaviour*). The unhealthy option (and usually the road chosen) is to *change their attitude* about the behaviour, for example, dismissing the evidence base that links smoking with chronic conditions (not all smokers get cancer), or smoking low tar cigarettes (in an attempt to reduce the risk); convincing themselves that smoking brings pleasure and reduces uncomfortable stress or helps to prevent them gaining weight; or associating with others who smoke (e.g. I have seen nurses smoke, so it cannot be dangerous); flaunting the danger and continuing to smoke anyway (Gross, 1996:448).

One intervention could be to raise awareness of the very real fear that smoking is a high contributory factor to CHD, however, this can sometimes trigger more fear and may encourage an anxious person to smoke even more, particularly if it is deeper feelings of fear that trigger the person to smoke.

Another intervention could be to explore the fear that surrounds both polarities (change talk and sustain talk – see 'Motivational interviewing techniques', page 228) in thinking. Again this would require the skilled interventions of a counsellor, as these issues need to be dealt with sensitively and empathetically, as they are very real to the client's experience.

Any decision or choice to make changes ultimately lies with the client. It is not the role of the exercise professional to enforce specific changes, for even if the person complies with these changes in the short term, he or she is unlikely to do so in the long term. Attempting to coerce people to make the changes they are resisting is assuming they are not able to make effective choices for themselves. The issue here is that some of the choices people make are not the most effective for their health. However, the decision to change lies with the person. Chapters 16 and 17 introduce some processes for helping people to make changes.

Cognitive dissonance will apply to other lifestyle behaviours – use of alcohol, activity and exercise, eating behaviours, sexual behaviours etc.

PERSON-/CLIENT-CENTRED WORKING

Client-centred working evolves from the work of Carl Rogers (Rogers & Stevens, 1967). A patient-centred approach to working emphasises compassion and appropriate use of communication skills, relational skills and intimacy for helping individuals. As outlined in chapter 9, a person-centred way of working is for the exercise professional to be:

- empathic, as opposed to unconcerned, about the person's struggles in relation to their condition;
- unbiased, as opposed to judgmental, about the person. This includes being aware of any pre-judgments, self-righteousness and blame regarding the person's contribution to and responsibility for their condition from their behaviour choices (inactivity, smoking, alcohol, poor eating habits, etc.);
- supportive, as opposed to dismissive;
- accepting, as opposed to finding fault and blaming;
- optimistic, as opposed to skeptical, highlighting the positive changes that can be made by simple and achievable adjustments and the positive impact that each small change can make.

The core conditions

A key feature of client-centred working is that the person is the best expert on themselves; they intrinsically know what is right for them, but have along the way lost connection to the aspect of self (the organismic self) that knows this, and are instead living out of balance and connection (Rogers & Stevens, 1967:90). Rogers believed that in the presence of the core conditions (and being allowed to be their own self-expert) each person is capable of working out the solutions to his or her problems. The three primary core conditions are:

1. Congruency
2. Empathy
3. Unconditional positive regard.

Congruency This is being totally honest and genuine and living life by one's own standards and values. Incongruence is living to the expectations of others to gain approval and wearing a mask or façade.

Most people are able to sense incongruence, when someone is putting on a front to perform a role. People can also recognise when someone is not communicating genuine thoughts or feelings, and consequently will often hold back from revealing themselves at any deeper level. It is worth noting that 55 per cent of our communication comes from body language, 38 per cent from voice tone and 7 per cent from the words we use (see figure 14.1). Clearly, any discrepancy between what we say and how we feel will be communicated at some level. The response we get may actually tell us more about what we are communicating than what we say or how we say it.

Similarly, with a person who is unafraid to be who s/he is, others are more likely to develop trust and consequently reveal more of themselves.

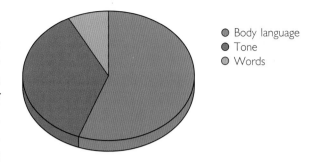

- Body language
- Tone
- Words

Figure 14.1 Communication model

However, it is essential not to just 'blurt out impulsively every feeling and accusation under the comfortable impression that one is being genuine' (Rogers & Stevens, 1967:91) as this is not helpful! The key is to be aware and recognise one's own inner responses and to process them in a way that is sensitive to the helping relationship.

Empathy This is the ability to see things from the other person's perspective, to put yourself into his or her position and understand his or her world as if it were your own, without losing the 'as if quality (Rogers & Stevens, 1967:93). In order to do this we need to be aware of any prejudices, self-righteousness and closed-mindedness within us and put these issues to one side. We also need to be able to sideline any need to analyse and evaluate, which only helps us see the other people's worlds from our perspective, not theirs! Removing these barriers to intimacy will help to minimise projection of our own issues into the client's world.

Rogers (Rogers & Stevens, 1967:93) quotes: 'If I am truly open to the way life is experienced by another person – if I can take his world into mine – then I run the risk of seeing life in his way, of being changed myself, and we all resist change. So we tend to view this other person's world only in our terms, not in his. We analyse and evaluate it. We do not understand it. But when someone understands how it feels and seems to be me, without wanting to analyse me or judge me, then I can blossom and grow in that climate.'

Unconditional positive regard This is about showing respect and warmth for the people with whom you are working. It is about prizing them as individuals in their own right, with their own unique way of being and valuing who they are without making judgments or decisions that they should be any other way.

An example: working with a client who frequently relapses from the activity plan. To deny or ignore any feeling of frustration, disappointment or intolerance you may be feeling inside may be missing an opportunity to gather some key information about what the client may actually be feeling about her- or himself. Awareness of one's own internal processes can often enable more effective inquiry about the client's experience. One's feelings can be communicated and worked with respectfully by asking: 'How do you feel about your relapse?' This may open the client to discussion of a series of events that proved to be a block to their activity programme, which may offer reasons for their relapse that can be worked with. The inquiry may also reveal that the client felt frustration and disappointment with him- or herself. Enabling this level of openness can provide the helper with an opportunity to show that these feelings are a natural response. The helper could then make an intervention that enables the person to recognise the *inner judge*, the aspect of oneself that likes to criticise and focus on the negative, and the *inner nurturer*, the aspect of oneself that is able to see the positive steps and focus on these, so validating oneself (Stewart & Joines,

1987). Raising awareness of these aspects of the self can be used to help balance any inner conflicts and move the client towards becoming his or her own best friend.

From an exercise professional's perspective, we need to recognise that while we have certain pieces of knowledge that the client needs, it is the client who knows his or her lifestyle and what changes will work for him or her in life. Resistance to any 'useful' suggestions offered should be acknowledged as an indicator that somehow this advice is not right for this client. A more effective approach than giving specific advice (Do this! Do that!) is to explore the client's world and his or her way of operating and identify a range of potential ways that s/he can work with to move towards making the desired changes. Asking them what they think is the best way forward for them. Relapse can be viewed as acknowledgement that the approach selected was not the 'best fit' for the client, and allows other ways of making changes to be explored. The key is to be creative and work with the client, helping her or him to choose approaches to change that work personally rather than imposing specific programmes. This way of working does not necessarily provide the quick fix, if indeed there is such a thing, but it is a way of working that enables effective change in the longer term.

MOTIVATIONAL INTERVIEWING TECHNIQUES

Motivational interviewing is a client-centred method of gathering information to explore a client's readiness to change. It can be used to elicit information about the client's concerns about specific areas of his or her life that s/he would like to change. This information can then be used to discuss with the person the advantages and disadvantages of making the changes proposed. The information collected can also indicate where the client is in relation to the 'cycle of change' model (contemplating, preparing, action) and can identify his or her personal levels of motivation, any support systems in place and any resistance or ambivalence to making changes. It can also help the exercise professional recognise the appropriate support and interventions that will help the client make a positive decision for her- or himself and negotiate goals and strategies to work towards with the client.

When contemplating change, clients often have mixed feelings. Part of them may really want to make the changes and part of them may not (resistant). Allowing the client to speak and hearing their *change talk* (reason for making the change) and *sustain talk* (reasons for not making the change) gives space for the client to hear themselves (sometimes for the first time). In motivational interviewing, the aim is to encourage the client to speak from their change talk position; facilitating them to motivate themselves towards making the change. Using the examples listed in table 14.2, the helper can ask more open questions (discussed later) such as: How do you think you will feel if you start exercising? How do you know this? What would be the benefits, etc.?

Focusing on the client

During any assessments and meetings with the client, it is important to make him or her the most important person in the room and demonstrate this by:

- facing forwards and looking at him or her;
- removing any barriers such as desks;
- being interested and attentive to what s/he is saying;

Table 14.2	Change and sustain
Change talk	**Sustain talk**
I know that if I start exercising more I will feel better	I just feel too tired to exercise
I know that if I stop drinking my health will improve	I just can't imagine what my life would be like without alcohol

- being sensitive to your own facial expressions and body language;
- minimising distractions (for consultations) by using a private room, placing a 'do not disturb' sign on the door and ensuring mobile phones are switched off;
- leaning forwards slightly – but not so far that you appear aggressive;
- keeping an open body and upright posture that is comfortable but not too stiff;
- maintaining eye contact without staring;
- reflecting warmth by demonstrating the core conditions (empathy, unconditional positive regard, congruence);
- smiling naturally and being present for the client;
- avoiding fidgeting.

COMMUNICATION SKILLS
Questioning

Questioning is a method of inquiry that can help the exercise professional to gain a fuller picture of the person's subjective experience and gather information. However, asking too many questions may block some clients from speaking, as they may feel they are under interrogation. Asking too many questions may also prevent active listening to what the client is saying, because the exercise professional may be focused more on asking the questions than really listening and hearing the client's responses. There are different types of questions that can be used.

Open questions These are most effective for gathering information in greater depth. They are questions that begin with the words: What? Who? How? Where? Why? When? These types of question, when asked in the presence of the core conditions, will generally enable the client to relax and speak openly. Examples of such questions are: 'How did you feel when you heard about your diagnosis?', 'How did you feel when you broke from your diet?'

Further information can be gathered from open questioning by using probing questions to encourage the client to expand on his or her initial response; or by using focusing questions to inquire more closely about a specific response that may help to define the problem more clearly.

Probing questions For example: 'Could you explain that?', 'Tell me more about that,' 'Have you ever experienced that sensation before?'

Focusing questions 'Tell me more about the pain in your joint', 'Where exactly are you feeling the discomfort?', 'What does that sensation feel like?'

Active listening

Listening and hearing what the client is saying is a real skill and requires practice and much empathy on behalf of the trainer. It also requires the presence of the core conditions described previously. Active listening can be demonstrated in the following ways:

- Making some acknowledgement as the client speaks, for example, nodding the head, making eye contact, or saying 'yes' or another sound (ummm, uh huh, etc.) that emphasises that they are being heard.
- Summarising what the client has said using your own language, and using a questioning style so that they are able to correct anything misheard. For example: 'Am I hearing you say that you feel anxious when this happens?'
- Reflecting back what the client says by reading between the lines. For example: Client: *I had to travel to hospital with a load of other patients, some had tubes in their throat and everything, and the doctors are just so insensitive.'* Helper: *'Seeing other patients with cancer as you travelled with them made you feel scared?'* Client: *'Yes.'*
- Asking questions if you do not understand or if you need further information from what the client is saying, for example: 'Would you tell me more about that so I can get a better picture?'

ENDING CLIENT WORK AND MAINTAINING RECORDS

Attention should also be given to how the work with the client is ended. The exercise professional should review the client's progress (with them) and identify how s/he intends to move forward into self-management. Any additional support that is available should be pointed out (re-referral, exit routes and follow-up etc.). Time should be spent identifying the coping strategies that the client has established to manage change (internal and external support systems etc.). All records of information that relate to the work with the client should be stored securely (in compliance with confidentiality and data protection legislation) and maintained for future reference as it will be needed for scheme monitoring and evaluation.

BEHAVIOUR CHANGE

15

THE TRANS-THEORETICAL MODEL OF CHANGE

There are many models and theories that offer ideas for what helps people change and what does not and there are a host of textbooks devoted to exploring this (some are listed in the references). One of the most popular models is the trans-theoretical model, which offers a number of *stages* that relate to where an individual may be positioned in relation to the change process; and a number of *processes* (behavioural and cognitive) that may support them. Identifying the position of an individual in the cycle of change can help to identify appropriate strategies to assist with helping the individual to make positive changes. Figure 15.1 provides a diagram of the trans-theoretical model of change.

STAGES OF CHANGE
Pre-contemplation

At this stage the individual is not aware s/he has a problem and is not thinking about making any changes. There may be resistance to the change process (which may be due to underlying feelings of powerlessness or helplessness or possibly because of a fear of failure, which may be masked by denial). At this stage the exercise professional can

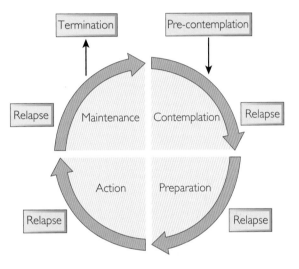

Figure 15.1 Trans-theoretical model of change

provide information that may assist the person to move closer towards contemplating making a change. They can give information in the form of handouts and leaflets that can help raise the client's awareness to the risks associated with continuing their existing behaviour. They can also use sensitive motivational interviewing techniques in a supportive and non-judgmental environment, which can encourage the client to explore any resistance and fears s/he may hold in relation to making a change in behaviour. Validating the client's feelings is

231

important at this stage. Whatever a person feels is real for him or her, these feelings will continually be a barrier to making changes unless they are acknowledged, accepted and managed.

The client's body language and non-verbal language (see Figure 14.1, page 227) can often provide an indication to defences and barriers that they are experiencing. The exercise professional can use open questioning techniques to inquire about the signs that the client is providing, if it seems appropriate for them to do so.

Contemplation

At this stage the individual is aware that a problem exists and is seriously considering making changes. S/he may experience internal conflicts regarding the advantages and disadvantages of making changes and may become stuck at this stage and move no further unless specific interventions are applied.

The exercise professional can help the client to explore the advantages and disadvantages of both changing and not changing, and also explore the risk and harm caused by the existing behaviour. This can be done using the decisional balance sheet outlined in table 15.1. The exercise professional can also help the client to identify their own change and sustain talk (discussed earlier) and encourage the client to speak more from their change position to build motivation.

Preparation

At this stage the individual is getting ready and may have already made some small changes. They may have started using a diary to record their behaviours. They may have enrolled for a yoga class to help release stress, or reduced their coffee intake during the day.

Table 15.1	Decisional balance sheet	
	Advantages	**Disadvantages**
Change	the advantages of making a change are...	the disadvantages of making a change are...
No change	the advantages of not making a change are...	the disadvantages of not making a change are...

The exercise professional can help at this stage by encouraging the steps that have been made and strengthening his or her commitment and building confidence. They can help the client to set small process-focused goals using the SMART method (see page 238) and establish an action plan for achieving these goals.

Action

At this stage the individual is making changes and has committed some time and energy to doing so. S/he may have made the changes for just one day or up to six months.

The exercise professional can help by focusing on the client's successes and positively affirming progress. This positive reinforcement helps to maintain motivation and can build self-efficacy and help the client to stay committed. They can also guide the client towards using positive affirmations that will help the client maintain motivation and self-belief.

Lapse and relapse are always a risk, so the exercise professional can also explore external stimuli that might trigger the old behaviour and look at ways of avoiding or managing these stimuli (stimulus control). For example, a smoker may wish to avoid going to the bar after work where s/he will be tempted to have a cigarette. An alternative behaviour could be proposed, such as attending an exercise session or any other activity that will distract from the stimulus.

The exercise professional could suggest that the client has a massage or another personal reward for maintaining a change of behaviour. S/he can also explore the client's feelings about the change and encourage the client to look at the positive impact of her or his new behaviour. For example, a client who is new to exercise could be encouraged to consider how s/he feels better after the exercise session, even though s/he feels tired before s/he attends. This exploration of both the positive and negative aspects of the change can provide reinforcement that helps to maintain and manage the change of behaviour.

It can also be useful to explore a range of alternative behaviours and other coping strategies. For example, a client who drinks a cup of coffee when s/he is stressed could explore the option of drinking another beverage that will not trigger an additional stress response (see food stressors in chapter 7). S/he could also look at taking five minutes at intervals throughout the day to complete some desk exercises that can help reduce muscle tension. These alternatives provide new and different responses to the stimulus or trigger (counter-conditioning), a strategy that can help one to manage stress more positively. It is also useful to have a contingency plan to help the client maintain motivation when tempted to relapse.

Maintenance

At this stage the individual is sustaining the changes and preventing relapse. The new habit may be established and some coping strategies will already be in place for managing problem situations and avoiding temptation.

The role of the exercise professional is to provide a helpful and supportive relationship and reinforce the positive behaviour by giving plenty of praise and encouragement, which acts as a reward and can help to increase the client's self-efficacy. The client will also need reminding of all her or his successes to help maintain motivation. S/he will also need to be made aware of possible cues that may indicate the likelihood of a relapse and have strategies in place to manage a relapse.

It may be worthwhile educating the client in how his or her thought processes might respond in times of relapse. Some clients will *over-generalise* and see the slip as meaning a complete failure. Others may experience *selective abstraction*, where they focus only on the failure and not on any of the successes. Other clients will take excessive responsibility for the slip and see it as their own personal weakness. Others will *catastrophise*, go totally overboard, and exaggerate how bad the slip was. Some clients use a mixture or even all of these thought processes to throw themselves out of the change cycle.

It is useful if the exercise professional can work with the client to help him or her recognise where potential slips may be attributed. For example, a client who sees a slip as a personal lack of willpower will experience a reduction in self-efficacy and personal power if they relapse, whereas a client who believes a slip is just a temporary lack of coping will maintain self-efficacy and is more likely to get back into the cycle (see locus of control in chapter 14, page 225). It is therefore useful if the exercise professional works with the client and explains that slips are often a natural occurrence until a new habit or change of behaviour is imprinted. It is worth recognising that even changing the way we think is a challenge for most people. For example, if one has spent 30–40 years thinking self-critical or negative thoughts then it will be a big challenge to break that behaviour pattern. A client who has smoked for 20 years will have an equal challenge to break a number of behaviour patterns that include buying cigarettes, lighting them, the hand-to-mouth action, the inhaling, etc. There are many behaviours that would have to change and each step the client makes is a success! It is essential to highlight all of these.

Relapse

At this stage of the cycle of change the client would have returned to his or her old behaviour. For example, s/he may have stopped exercising, returned to old eating or lifestyle patterns, started smoking again, etc. Relapse is a very uncomfortable experience for people who are trying to make changes, as it increases feelings of failure and hopelessness, which discourages them and makes them lose confidence and belief in their ability to make these changes: their self-efficacy.

The exercise professional can give support and encouragement and explore possible causes for the relapse. S/he can then review the client's action plan and work with the client to help him or her to re-enter the change cycle.

Termination

The new behaviour would be permanent at this stage and the client would have achieved his or her goal.

It usually takes clients a few attempts to move through the change cycle, and they experience a few relapses before reaching this stage. The

change process in reality is not orderly; people get stuck at specific stages a few times before they achieve a permanent change of behaviours and habits.

LEVELS

The model represents the different levels of psychological functioning which interrelate and which require work to help the person make the desired changes. These are:

* presenting problem (symptom, situational);
* negative thought processes (maladaptive cognitions/thinking);
* relationship difficulties (interpersonal conflicts);
* social/systemic difficulties (relationship with systems);
* intrapersonal difficulties (relationship with self).

The exercise professional's role is to help the person make change to a specific behaviour (inactivity), so there are boundaries and limitations to helping with the other areas and in most instances counseling support will be needed. Clients may well cross the boundaries and share information because they feel comfortable and safe to do so; however, some areas of difficulty are out of scope of practice and can be too much for the exercise professional to hold. When working in exercise referral it is important to work with other health professionals, using a multi-discipline approach, as most 'problems' are multi-faceted and need to be addressed at different levels and by different professionals.

PROCESSES

Prochaska and Diclemente named 10 common processes that people involved in a change and growth process move through (Jackson, in Feltham & Horton, 2000:400).

Consciousness-raising and self-monitoring

These are methods for gathering information about oneself and one's problem(s) and monitoring and raising awareness of circumstances that trigger specific lifestyle choices. They include:

- keeping a diary to monitor eating patterns (type of food, time of day, quantity, mood etc.); smoking or alcohol use (when, where, mood, thoughts, etc.); to record daily activity levels (how long, how hard, what type, when, etc.);
- writing a hassle list for all the things that add to stress levels (what, when, where, etc.);
- researching a medical condition;
- researching the effects of prescribed medications;
- researching ways for managing a condition.

Self-liberation

Taking a positive approach and believing in the possibility of change and making the choice to commit to take action. For example:

- finding the inner determination to commit to working with and handle the medical condition;
- using positive self-talk to maintain the self-belief that the condition can be managed.

Social liberation

Raising awareness of the increasing opportunity for alternative behaviours in society. For example:

- diabetes groups;
- exercise referral schemes;
- smoking cessation programmes etc.

Counter-conditioning

Introducing alternative behaviours to replace the specific problem behaviour. For example:

- taking a few deep breaths instead of having a cigarette;
- going for a walk before sitting down in front of the television and having a drink.

Stimulus control

These techniques are used to reduce the stimuli that trigger specific behaviours, for example:

- putting cigarettes out of reach when driving;
- buying only healthy foods to keep at home;
- not visiting environments where the behaviour may be triggered (e.g. the pub).

Self re-evaluation

Evaluate how one thinks and feels about oneself in relation to the problem behaviour or medical condition. For example:

- speaking to a therapist or counsellor regarding depression related to diagnosis of cancer or other life-threatening disease.

Environmental re-evaluation

Recognise how the problem behaviour affects the family, relatives, the wider community and the environment. For example:

- recognising that smoking may affect the health of babies and children;
- recognising how the overuse of alcohol impacts others.

Contingency/reinforcement management

Giving oneself a reward or a creature comfort or being rewarded by others, when a single, small change has been made, for example, being more active. Rewards can include:

- small treats (a bubble bath, watching a favourite video etc.);

- medium treats (buying a new outfit, a body massage etc.);
- larger treats (a holiday or health spa retreat etc.).

Dramatic relief

This involves experiencing and expressing feelings that may be linked with the problem behaviour and identifying possible solutions to manage these. For example:

- working with a counsellor or support worker to discuss feelings, for example, clients diagnosed with a life-threatening illness may feel angry. It is essential that this anger is explored so that it is not focused inward towards the self

(causing depression, addictive behaviours, etc.) or outwards in a way that could be destructive to supportive relationships.

Helping relationships and support systems

Receiving appropriate support and encouragement is a key factor in assisting with the management of behaviour change. It is essential to have a support system of people who care and whom the client is able to trust to speak openly about the problems s/he may be experiencing. Support can come from a variety of sources: friends, family, church, mosque, or other spiritual community or other clients within a referral scheme.

STRATEGIES FOR HELPING CHANGE

16

The way the exercise professional works with a client will be dependent on a number of factors, which include:

- **Case conceptualisation** How the trainer conceptualises and understands what the client presents (physical/medical conditions, mental/emotional state, beliefs, attitudes etc.) and the trainer's attunement and empathy to the client's experience.
- **The working contract negotiated** – which is usually short term (10–16 weeks) in commissioned and funded projects.
- **The working alliance** The level of relationship developed and work undertaken. For example, a client who has been working for a longer time and who has made some successful changes will require a different approach from a client who has just been referred and has yet to start making the necessary changes.
- **The client's readiness to change** Where the client is in relation to different stages and processes.

TECHNIQUES FOR ASSISTING THE CHANGE PROCESS

There are a host of different techniques for supporting and helping people to make changes; several methods are introduced in this chapter. The key for the exercise professional is to offer techniques and let the client choose and continue developing their skills and knowledge through CPD to identify other techniques and ways of working.

MODIFYING BEHAVIOUR

These are techniques used for making conscious changes to habitual behaviour, and include:

- eating more slowly and more consciously;
- having short breaks while eating a meal;
- drinking single shots of alcohol rather than double shots;
- using mixers to dilute alcoholic drinks;
- taking a few deep breaths or going for a short walk before having a cigarette.

GOAL-SETTING

Goal-setting techniques can be a positive way of making changes and establishing appropriate time-frames for getting things done. It is more helpful if goals focus on the process of making changes, rather than specific outcomes. For example: I will practise five minutes of relaxation every morning this week (process), rather than I will feel more relaxed (outcome). The SMART method can help to make goals workable:

- Specific
- Measurable
- Achievable
- Reward yourself
- Time-framed

Example: I will walk (specific) for 15 minutes (achievable) on 3 days this week (measurable and time-framed).

ASSERTIVENESS

Learning to become more assertive can help people raise their confidence levels and manage themselves and their lives more effectively (Lawrence, 2005). Methods for developing assertiveness include:

- taking an assertiveness training course;
- reading an assertiveness book;
- personal counselling;
- learning more about and respecting own personal boundaries;
- learning to say 'no' sometimes;
- learning how to keep self safe (emotionally and mentally).

POSITIVE SELF-TALK AND THINKING STRATEGIES

These techniques promote awareness of how the mind works and are a key to making someone their own best friend (Lawrence, 2005). For example:

- becoming aware of the inner dialogue and whether one's thoughts and beliefs are positive or negative;

- sitting for a short while to monitor one's thoughts;
- noticing the negative thoughts and words one uses to describe oneself, for example: 'I am so stupid… useless… no willpower…' etc.;
- replacing negative thoughts with positive self-affirmations that validate the self, for example: 'I can handle this… I am worthwhile… I am valued...' etc.;
- listening to positive affirmation tapes;
- writing down several positive things about oneself on a daily basis.

VISUALISATION

Clients can use visualisation techniques to create picture images of their goals. Clients can be asked to:

- focus on their specific goals (e.g. move around without becoming breathless, performing a series of exercises or an exercise class with ease, seeing themselves eat healthier foods, lose weight, etc.);
- focus on themselves when they have achieved their goals (how they will move, look, feel, speak, walk, etc.);
- make the picture image brighter and bigger and add colour to make the picture more visual and alive in their minds;
- explore the thoughts and feelings they hold in relation to seeing themselves achieve this goal, which can be used to assist their motivation;
- connect these memories with a physical gesture (for example, touching the forefinger to the thumb). This connection can be used as a prompt for a daily meditation to remind them of their goals and to maintain focus. It can also be used as a prompt for when times are tough and they feel like giving up.

Visualisation techniques (focusing on how they would like to see themselves) can also be used to increase motivation for change and decrease the vividness of any less pleasant pictures clients might create about themselves. Unpleasant images and pictures can be made smaller, darker and taken further away in their mind's eye by using visualization techniques. Pleasant images can be made brighter, larger and brought closer.

RELAXATION TECHNIQUES

Relaxation techniques are ways of managing the physical symptoms of anxiety, stress and depression that may present in clients with specific medical conditions. Learning to relax can also help with pain management. Some examples are provided in chapter 17.

PROMOTING SELF-MANAGEMENT FOR BEHAVIOUR CHANGE

Encouraging a person to make the decision to change certain aspects of their lifestyle is a positive step, although it can also seem an unmanageable task for many. Sometimes the specific changes can feel very uncomfortable and unnatural and may provide the person with increased stress. Some keys to people making any successful change are:

- to empower them to make their own choices (whether you agree with them or not, they know what is right and works for them);
- to provide education and support them in their decisions (facilitating learning and exploring without dictating);
- encouraging them to take one step at a time and to reflect and learn from their experiences (offering support and encouragement and not

an 'I told you so', self-righteous attitude);
- engaging with and encouraging them to commit to a decision and process (listening to them and reading between the lines, checking their self-belief and readiness to make particular changes);
- encouraging them to keep going and never give up (developing their determination, self-belief and a positive mental attitude).

The following 10 steps can be used as a list of strategies to assist clients with managing their own change processes (e.g. increasing activity, changing lifestyle habits and eating patterns, etc.).

1. Get the client to make lists of all the things they would like to change (thoughtstorm).

2. Let them decide what changes are the most important for them (work on one thing at a time).

3. Raise their awareness of the advantages and disadvantages of changing each behaviour by discussing this with them.

4. Work out specific and realistic goals that can be measured to create the changes they desire (use SMART, see page 238).

5. Encourage them to develop their own self awareness and get to know more about their behaviour (triggers etc.) by keeping a diary.

6. Identify what alternative strategies and behaviours they could use when the desire to relapse into old behaviour is triggered.

7. Prepare to make the changes (identify the resources and support they may need and put some coping strategies in place).

8. Set the date when they will start making changes.

9. Be ready to cope with setbacks (normalise).

10. Encourage them to stay motivated and keep getting support and ask for help when needed!

EXERCISE AND ACTIVITY APPROACHES

17

This chapter offers some ideas for adapted exercise plans which may be appropriate for some referred client groups. The exercise plans included are NOT ready-made sessions; they offer a framework for the exercise professional to adapt and plan their own session. Exercise professionals should conduct a thorough client assessment and should then review and evaluate the appropriateness of the activities for their specific client(s) before programming and delivering. They should also have attended appropriate additional training and CPD to ensure they are qualified to deliver specific types of activity sessions.

This chapter also introduces some alternative approaches to activity, which may be valuable variations to traditional approaches to activity when working with referred clients. Instructors wishing to deliver any of the alternative approaches described would need to be qualified as an exercise referral instructor and would need to attend additional training to specialise in the alternative area. Any alternative approaches would need to be recognised by the Register of Exercise Professionals (REPs) and may need to be appropriately adapted to suit specific conditions.

Contents of this section include:

- **Functional circuit 1 (general) – pages 241–244**
  - Warm-up
  - Functional circuit 1 (courtesy of Keith Smith)
  - Cool-down

- **Functional circuit 2 (chair-based) – pages 245–247**
  - Warm-up
  - Functional circuit 2 (chair-based)
  - Cool-down

- **Functional circuit 3 (low back pain) (courtesy of Lisa Young) – pages 248–251**
  - Warm-up
  - Functional circuit 3 (low back pain)
  - Cool-down

- **Breathing and relaxation – pages 252–256**
  - Breathing activity
  - Benson method of relaxation
  - Active muscular relaxation
  - Passive muscular relaxation
  - Relaxation scripts

- **Pelvic floor exercises – page 257**
  - Back passage isolation
  - Middle passage isolation

- Front passage isolation
- Back to front – the wave
- The flower
- The light switch

- **Alternative activity approaches – page 258**
  - Nia (by Fiona Winter)
  - Seated and Adapted Training
  - The ChiBall® Method (by Sandie Keane)

EXERCISE AND ACTIVITY APPROACHES

FUNCTIONAL CIRCUIT 1 (GENERAL)

Focus: Improve general activity, mobility and functional patterns and improve CV and MSE fitness (low level).

General warm-up for a functional circuit (general)			
Total time: 18 minutes			
Timing	**Purpose**	**Exercise/activity**	**Considerations**
1 minute	Pulse raise and warming	Walk around the area	Walking speed and stride length appropriate for individual
1 minute	Shoulder girdle mobility	March in place with shoulder lift and lower Shoulder rolls	Land lightly while marching Option to keep legs still Controlled range of motion to ability of individual
30 seconds	Pulse raise and warming Knee mobility	Knee bends/shallow squats	Knees unlocked Bending to a comfortable range of motion
30 seconds	Pulse raise and warming	Walk in circle	Option to increase stride length if comfortable
30 seconds	Knee mobility	Face centre leg curls	Comfortable range of motion
30 seconds	Hip mobility	Face centre knee raises	Knee raises to comfortable range, not exceeding hip height
4 minutes	Pulse raise and warming and mobility	Repeat all above	Option to increase stride length and range of motion
30 seconds	Spine mobility	In place trunk rotations/twists	Ensure hips and lower body remain still Isolate trunk Comfortable and controlled range of motion
30 seconds	Spine mobility	In place side bends	Ensure hips and lower body remain still Isolate trunk Comfortable and controlled range of motion

Timing	Purpose	Exercise/activity	Considerations
1 minute	Pulse raise and warming	Brisk walk in circle with direction changes	Option to increase stride length and range of motion Direction changes optional and with control
30 seconds	Pulse raise and warming	Elbow and knee mobility	Knee bend/shallow squat in place with bicep curl arm action Knees unlocked Bending to a comfortable range of motion
30 seconds	Pulse raise and warming	Brisk walk around area	Option to increase stride length and range of motion Mobility and pulse raising for functional circuit 1 (general)
2 minutes	Stay warm and lengthen upper body muscles	Walk in circle and stretch pectorals, triceps and latissimus dorsi	Elbow unlocked during upper body stretches Option to perform stretches standing still or seated Adapt range of movement for comfort
2 minutes	Stay warm and lengthen calf muscles	March in place and face centre	Rear lunges into calf stretch right and left Adapt range of movement for comfort
1 minute	Stay warm and lengthen hamstrings	Heel digs into back of thigh stretch right and left	Adapt range of movement for comfort Can be performed seated in a chair
1 minute	Stay warm and stretch inner thigh	Squat in place into double inner thigh stretch	Adapt range of movement for comfort Can be performed seated in chair
30 seconds	Stay warm and lengthen calf muscles	Quad stretch using wall for balance	Option to decrease range of motion by performing hip/pelvic tilt (and not raising heel to buttocks) or using a towel around ankle
30 seconds	Pulse raise and warming	Brisk walk around area	Option to increase stride length and range of motion Warming and muscle lengthening

Total time: 18 minutes

Functional circuit 1 (general) (courtesy of Keith Smith)

Total time: From 5–15 minutes (variable dependent on number of stations and number of circuits etc.)

Stations	6–10
Exercise type	Encourage movements and exercises that resemble daily lifestyle activities. Maintain activity levels and functional movement. Improvements to fitness will be comparatively less for older populations.
Work time per station	20–40 seconds
Rest ratio after work station	10–20 seconds Active march or walk to next station
Number of circuits	One or two
Music	Can be used as background for socialisation purposes

Purpose	Exercise	Alternative
CV Functional	Walk through crowds (use chairs around room to simulate people)	Shuttle walks
Deltoids, triceps – functional reaching and pushing action	Shoulder press	Lateral raise or chest press
CV – functional lifting action Lower body strengthening	Dead lift (use lightly weighted shopping bags)	Half squat
Anterior deltoid, upper trapezius and biceps Functional pulling	Standing upright row	Single arm upright row
Lower body strengthening	Standing calf raise and toe taps	Perform seated
CV Functional stepping	Crossing the road	Step up with wall support
Wrist strengthening	Towel wring/wrist curl	Seated or standing
CV Functional	Shuttle walks (fartlek style – varying pace/speed)	Shuttle walk even pace

Optional MSE stations

Purpose	Exercise	Alternative
Erector spinae	Lying back raises/extensions	Seated back extension
Pectorals, triceps and anterior deltoid	Box press-ups	Wall press-ups OR Seated chest press using exercise band
Transversus abdominus	Abdominal hollowing – all fours	Abdominal hollowing seated
Pelvic floor	Pelvic floor standing	Pelvic floor seated

Note: Floor-based exercises are only recommended for those persons who can comfortably get up and down from the floor.

General cool-down and stretch for functional circuit I (general)

Total time: 11 minutes

Timing	Purpose	Exercise/activity	Considerations
1 minute 30 seconds	Maintain intensity of circuit prior to lowering	Walk around the area	Walking speed and stride length appropriate for individual
1 minute 30 seconds	Pulse lowering	Gentle side squats right march in place and repeat left	
1 minute	Pulse lowering	Gentle walk around room	
1 minute	Lengthen gastrocnemius and soleus	Calf stretch	Use wall for support and balance
1 minute	Pulse lowering	Walk to another position on wall	
30 seconds	Lengthen quadriceps	Quad stretch	Use wall for support and balance
1 minute	Pulse lowering and upper body stretches	Walk anywhere, slower pace Stretch triceps and pectorals and latissimus dorsi	
1 minute	Pulse lowering	Steady walk	
1 minute 30 seconds	Lengthen hamstrings and adductors Optional relaxation and breathing	Floor seated Hamstring stretch Inner thigh stretch Optional relaxation and breathing exercises	Chair seated and adapt ROM Optional seated relaxation and breathing
1 minute	Gentle wake up	Back to standing, gentle march or walk with shoulder rolls	March in place with gentle mobility

FUNCTIONAL CIRCUIT 2 (CHAIR-BASED)

Focus: Improve general activity, mobility and functional patterns and improve circulation and MSE fitness (low level).

General warm-up for functional circuit 2 (chair-based)

Total time: Approx. 9–18 minutes

Timing	Purpose	Exercise/activity	Considerations
30–60 seconds	Circulation boost	Left and right toe taps	Light movement and maintain control
30–60 seconds	Circulation boost	Seated marching	Gentle movement to start
30–60 seconds	Shoulder girdle mobility	Shoulder lifts Shoulder rolls	Controlled range of motion
30–60 seconds	Circulation boost	Thigh claps	Light clapping
30–60 seconds	Spine mobility	Trunk rotations	Keep lower body still
30–60 seconds	Ankle mobility	Ankle point and flex right and left	Can hold chair for support
30–60 seconds	Circulation boost	Alternate arm sways forward and backwards	Controlled movements Raising arms to comfortable height
30–60 seconds	Spine mobility	Side bends	Reaching gently to the side Care not to lean forwards or backwards
30–60 seconds	Circulation boost	Seated marching	Progressively larger march and can add arm swings or claps
30–60 seconds	Finger mobility	Fingers to thumb mobility, right hand then left hand	Controlled pace
30–60 seconds	Circulation boost	Seated marching	
30–60 seconds	Stretch	Triceps stretch	Work within comfortable ROM
30–60 seconds	Circulation boost	Seated marching	
30–60 seconds	Stretch	Seated hamstring stretch right and left	Body weight supported on bent knee
30–60 seconds	Circulation boost	Seated marching	
30–60 seconds	Stretch	Seated calf stretch, right and left	Raise toe towards shin – active lengthening
30–60 seconds	Stretch	Pectoral stretch	Hands on side of chair or holding rear of chair Draw shoulder blades back and down
I minute	Circulation boost	Seated marching	Progressively larger march and can add arm swings or claps

NB: Time can be reduced

Functional circuit 2 (chair-based)

Total time: From 5 to 15 minutes (variable dependent on number of stations and number of circuits etc.)

Stations	6–8 with an emphasis on functional movements e.g. combing hair
Aims and goals	Encourage movements and exercises that resemble daily lifestyle activities Maintain activity levels, promote mobility and functional movement
Type of circuit and teaching position	Command – everyone performs same exercise at the same time, arrange chairs in a semi-circle with tutor at front for demonstrations (visible to all), tutor should move to observe and support individuals during activity
Pace	Movements to be performed in a slow and controlled manner and focusing on correct technique
Seated exercise position	Sit the client on front third of chair, with feet firmly on the floor in a chair of an appropriate height (at least 90 degree angle at knees with hips positioned slightly higher than knees when seated)
Work time per station	20–30 seconds
Rest ratio after work station	10–15 seconds, can be a static back rest position, shuffling back to a relaxed seated position with back supported by back of chair Rest time can be used by tutor to explain the next movement
Number of circuits	1
Music	Optional – can be used as background for socialisation purposes

Purpose	Exercise	Alternative
Circulation	Seated march	
Calf strengthening to assist walking	Seated calf raises	Both together or alternate
Strengthen upper arm to assist with pushing movements, e.g. assisted movement out of bath etc.	Seated triceps extension	With or without exercise band or small dumbbell
Strengthen upper arm to assist with lifting and carrying	Seated biceps curl	With or without exercise band or small dumbbell
Strengthen front thigh to assist with walking	Seated leg extension	Lift and short hold at top Adapt ROM according to individual
Promote mobility	Seated comb hair action	Wipe brow action to adapt ROM
Strengthen wrist and forearm	Wrist squeeze and pull	Using band to squeeze and pull OR opening and closing hands
Strengthen lower body Assist with standing	Sit to stand	Seated marching as alternative Tutor or helper can assist individual Increase repetitions for more able

General cool-down for functional circuit 2 (chair-based)

Total time: Approx. 5–10 minutes

Timing	Purpose	Exercise/activity	Considerations
30–60 seconds	Circulation	Seated marching	Gentle movement
30–60 seconds	Circulation	Alternate arm sways forward and backwards	Gentle sway action
30–60 seconds	Circulation	Seated marching	Progressively larger march and can add arm swings or claps
30–60 seconds	Shoulder girdle mobility	Shoulder rolls and comb hair	Work to comfortable ROM and a controlled pace
30–60 seconds	Finger mobility	Fingers to thumb mobility right hand then left hand	Both hands together or single hand movements Adapt pace
30–60 seconds	Stretch	Triceps stretch Pectoral stretch	Triceps – start with hand on same shoulder and gently use other arm to ease into stretch position
30–60 seconds	Stretch	Seated hamstring stretch right and left	Lengthen up and forward to increase ROM
30–60 seconds	Stretch	Seated calf stretch right and left	Flex foot further to increase ROM Use towel around ball of foot to assist stretch
30–60 seconds	Strengthen pelvic floor	Pelvic floor	Slow and fast time
30–60 seconds	Relaxation and breathing	Breathing activity Relaxation activity	Abdominal or lateral breathing to assist mobility of rib cage Lengthen and release method of relaxation or Benson method (see page 252)

FUNCTIONAL CIRCUIT 3 (LOW BACK PAIN)

Focus: Improve functional patterns to spare the spine and improve CV and MSE fitness (low level)

Warm-up for functional circuit 3 (low back pain) (courtesy of Lisa Young)			
Total time: 15 minutes, 30 seconds			
Timing	**Purpose**	**Exercise/activity**	**Considerations**
1 minute	Pulse raise warming, evaluate posture and gait	Walk around the area	Clients to walk naturally at own pace
1 minute	Posture and gait improvements, engagement of core	Posture adjustment	Work within client's ability to modify posture
1 minute	Pulse raise warming, evaluate posture and gait	Walk around the area	Clients to walk with improved gait
30 seconds	Shoulder joint	Shoulder rolls, small to larger	To keep torso still to enable movement from the joint and not the whole torso
30 seconds	Thoracic joint mobilisation	Twists	Hips and torso motionless
30 seconds	Pulse raise	March on spot/knee lifts with support	Keep torso still; use wall as required
30 seconds	Shoulder joint	Shoulder rolls, larger	To keep torso still to enable movement from the joint and not the whole torso
30 seconds	Spine mobility	Side bends	Ensure hips and lower body remain still and level Isolate trunk. Ensure there is a comfortable and controlled ROM
1 minute	Pulse raise and warming	Brisk walk with direction changes	Option to increase stride length and range of motion but still with good posture and gait. Direction changes are optional and with control
1 minute	Hips and knees mobility Set up for safe pick-up techniques	Squats to lunges	Keep spine neutral and within pain-free ROM. Use support for lunges

Timing	Purpose	Exercise/activity	Considerations
2 minutes	Practise smaller versions of moves for circuit	Side steps Rotational moves	Ensure good posture throughout
2 minutes	Stay warm and lengthen upper body muscles	Walk in circle and stretch pectorals, triceps and latissimus dorsi	Elbow unlocked during upper body stretches. Option to perform stretches standing still or seated Adapt range of movement for comfort
2 minutes	Stay warm and lengthen calf muscles	March in place and face centre. Rear lunges into calf stretch right and left	Adapt range of movement for comfort
1 minute	Stay warm and lengthen hamstrings	Heel digs into back of thigh stretch right and left	Adapt range of movement for comfort Can be performed seated in a chair
30 seconds	Stay warm and lengthen calf muscles	Quad stretch using wall for balance	Option to decrease ROM by performing hip/pelvic tilt (and not raising heel to buttocks) or using a towel around ankle
30 seconds	Pulse raise and warming	Brisk walk around area	Option to increase stride length and range of motion

Functional circuit 3 (low back pain) (courtesy of Lisa Young)

Total time: 10–20 minutes	
Stations	10
Exercise type	A mixture of CV and MSE exercises that will assist in strengthening muscles required to protect the spine and enhance good posture.
Work time per station	50 seconds
Rest ratio after work station	10 seconds, active march or walk to next station
Number of circuits	1–2
Music	Background
Total time	10–20 minutes

Purpose	Exercise	Alternative
CV Functional	Power walks with a dead-lift of shopping bag	Shuttle walks
Deltoids, triceps, pectorals Functional reaching and pushing action	Shoulder press with a weight or ball to mimic putting items on a shelf	Lateral raise or chest press
Lower limb strength Practise safe lifts	Mini-lunge lift bag	Mini-lunges, no weight or squats
CV Side step awareness and encourage movement control through hips	Side steps over a step or floor-based	Half jacks
Middle trapezius and rhomboids (strengthen weakened muscles)	Standing or seated row	Single arm row
Improve balance and core strength	One leg stance	Use wall for support OR calf raises and hold
CV Functional walking over different levels	Up and over different height steps	Low single height step OR shuttle walk
MSE deltoids, triceps and obliques to mimic placing items on side shelf or pushing heavy door	Side reaches with weighted ball	Side reaches no weight
Balance work (notoriously poor in those with bad backs)	Semi-tandem stance	With support
Lower limb MSE	Plies squats (mimic sit to stand) with support	

Additional core stations post-pulse lower for functional circuit 3 (low back pain)
Total time: 10 minutes

TVA, rectus abdominus, obliques	Single leg slide	TVA, pelvic floor engagement on back
Obliques	Supine torsion resistance	Engagement of core side laying
Erector spinae	Pilates swim	Cat paws or merely engagement on all fours

Note:
Floor-based exercises are recommended for all persons, but the client must be taught to get up and down off the floor first.

General cool-down and stretch for functional circuit 3 (low back pain) (courtesy of Lisa Young)

Total time: 11 minutes

Timing	Purpose	Exercise/activity	Considerations
4 minutes	Pulse lower	Walk around the area, slowly decreasing pace – include some exercises used in the main section but reduced ROM	Adapt according to individual ability
1 minute	Lengthen gastrocnemius and soleus	Calf stretch	Use wall for support and balance
1 minute	Pulse lowering	Walk around – swap places across the room	
2 minutes	Lengthen quadriceps and adductors standing and hip flexors	Quad stretch Adductor lunge stretch Hip flexor front lunge stretch	Use wall for support and balance
1 minute	Pulse lowering and upper body stretches	Walk anywhere, slower pace Stretch triceps and pectorals and latissimus dorsi	
1 minute	Pulse lowering	Steady walk	
1 minute	Lengthen hamstrings	Laying band Hamstring stretch	Chair seated or standing

Note:
Introduce core exercises here then relaxation as required

BREATHING AND RELAXATION

BREATHING ACTIVITY

Breathing exercises can be performed in a lying, standing, seated or kneeling position. The main consideration is that the position feels comfortable and allows the individual to maintain an open posture (see chapter 8 for seated and standing postural instructions).

Lateral/diaphragmatic breathing

Instructions:

- Sit/stand in a comfortable position with open posture.
- Place the hands at the sides of the lower ribcage.
- Breathe in and feel the rib cage expand.
- Breathe out and feel the rib cage release.
- Aim to isolate the lower rib cage and minimise activity of the upper rib cage.
- Focus on deeper, slower breathing.
- Aim to practise for 5 minutes.

Abdominal breathing

Instructions:

- Sit/stand in a comfortable position with open posture.
- Place the hands on the tummy with middle fingers touching at the tummy button.
- Breathe in and the tummy will rise and the fingers move away from the tummy button.
- Breathe out and the tummy lowers and the fingers move back together.
- Focus on deeper, slower breathing.
- Aim to practise for 5 minutes.

RELAXATION METHODS

Learning to relax is helpful in the management of many medical conditions. Stress, anxiety and depression are often co-morbid with other health conditions, and relaxation techniques offer a way for the body and mind to have time to rest and re-focus.

Relaxation exercises can be performed in any position where the body feels relaxed and comfortable, which may include seated, lying (supine or prone) or foetal position.

The environment needs to be prepared in advance and should ideally be warm and comfortable and free of any outside distractions. Individuals will need to be guided to start in a comfortable position and focus on their breathing. A script can be used to deliver active or passive techniques (see scripts 1 and 2 in boxes below). Instructors can speak clients through the script instructions to help them relax. A slow, soft and gentle voice should be used. (NB: the script instructions can be adapted). At the end of the relaxation, individuals should be given time to return their focus back to being in the room and allowed to steadily wake up from any longer relaxation. Encouraging individuals to move at their own pace and in their own time and gently move different body parts can help them to awaken from a relaxation.

BENSON METHOD OF RELAXATION

Herbert Benson originally developed this technique for people with high blood pressure. He suggested that individuals sit still and quiet and focus on saying the word 'one' out loud as they breathed out. He recommended 5 minutes to practise the method.

The technique can be adapted in the following ways:

- The word 'one' can be replaced by other words that an individual may find more natural, such

as: 'calm', 'peace', 'love', 'still', 'silent', 'relax' etc.
- The word can be spoken silently within, rather than out loud.
- The technique can be used in everyday activities, for example, when queuing at a supermarket, on the train, while out walking, at an office desk etc.

ACTIVE MUSCULAR RELAXATION (SEE SCRIPT 1 BELOW)

Active muscular relaxation involves moving specific parts of the body sequentially and can involve lengthening or tensing and releasing; a script is usually followed to ensure all parts of the body have been covered.

Script 1: Active muscular relaxation

- Sit or lie in a comfortable position and allow your body to relax and lengthen.
- Allow the muscles to soften.
- Focus your awareness on your breathing. Notice the depth and pace of your breathing.
- Allow your breath to become slower, softer and deeper.
- Take your mind's awareness to your body, starting with the feet.
- Spread and separate your toes, feeling the tension in the feet.
- Flex your toes towards your knees, feeling the tension in the lower leg.
- Stay aware of the tension, breathe steadily in and out.
- Then let the toes and feet relax, let go of any tension in the lower legs.
- Be still and breathe softly and deeply.
- Take your mind's awareness to the thigh muscles.
- Allow the muscles at the front of the thigh to tighten without locking the knee.
- Tighten the muscles at the back of the thigh.
- Squeeze the buttocks tight.
- Stay aware of the tension in the thighs and buttocks – breathe steadily in and out.
- Then let the thigh and buttock muscles relax.
- Feel the hip joint open and soften.
- Feel the whole of the legs relax and soften.
- Be still and breathe softly and deeply.
- Focus your mind's awareness on the abdomen.
- Draw the abdominal muscles in tightly towards your backbone.
- Feel the sides of the abdomen draw in tight.
- Feel the muscles of the lower back tighten.
- Stay aware of the tension, experience the feeling of a corset tightening around the centre of the body, breathe steadily in and out.
- Then release the tension in these muscles, feeling the centre of the body relax, and let go.
- Be still and breathe softly and deeply.
- Focus your awareness on the shoulders and upper back.
- Squeeze the shoulders towards the ears.

Script 1: Active muscular relaxation continued

- Feel the tension increase in the muscles of the upper back and the back of the neck; breathe steadily in and out.
- Then allow the muscles to let go and release.
- Lengthen the ears away from the shoulder.
- Feel the chin tucking towards the body.
- Feel the muscles in between the shoulder blades drawing downwards and tightening.
- Stay aware of the tension; breathe steadily in and out.
- Then release the tension in these muscles – allow the body to let go.
- Be still and breathe softly and deeply.
- Focus your awareness on the muscles of the arms.
- Extend the arms and tense all the muscles in the upper and lower arms; breathe steadily in and out.
- Clench the fist to increase the tension.
- Stay aware of the tension, breathing steadily in and out.
- Then allow the muscles to release and let go.
- Spread the fingers and open up the hands.
- Extend the fingers as far away from the shoulders as you can.
- Stay aware of the tension in the muscles of the hands and arms; breathe steadily in and out.
- Then release and let go and allow the arms to soften and relax.
- Allow the body to be still; breathe slowly and deeply.
- Focus your mind's awareness on the face and head.
- Open your mouth wide and feel the tension around the mouth and jaw.
- Stay aware of the tension; breathe steadily in and out.
- Then release and let go – allow the jaw to relax, wiggle the jaw a little.
- Stick out your tongue, then allow it to relax back into your mouth.
- Feel the tongue soften and the mouth and jaw relax; breathe steadily in and out.
- Wiggle your nose and then release.
- Feel the eye sockets opening and then release.
- Move the muscles in the forehead, then allow them to soften and relax.
- Let the body sink deeper and relax further.
- Any tension just easing away.
- Tighten the whole body one last time, extending your head and toes and fingers as far away from each other as you can.
- Release and let go; allow yourself to sigh.
- Take your mind's awareness back to your breathing.
- Focus on slower, deeper breathing.
- Allow your body to be still and silent.
- With every breath, allow the body to relax further.
- Allow a feeling of relaxation and calm to spread through your whole body.

PASSIVE MUSCULAR RELAXATION (SEE SCRIPT 2 BELOW)

Passive muscular relaxation involves using the mind to focus on different body areas and using this awareness to relax each specific body part. There is no specific movement of any body part.

Individuals who are able to focus and concentrate all their attention on their body will find this method very relaxing and calming. It is great for providing stillness to people who are very active. It is also a very effective method for people who have injuries or physical disabilities that make it uncomfortable or impossible to move specific body parts.

This method may be frustrating for people who are very active and find it difficult to be still and relax their mind.

Script 2: Passive muscular relaxation

- Sit or lie in a comfortable position.
- Allow your body to relax and lengthen.
- Allow the muscles to soften.
- Focus your awareness on your breathing.
- Notice the depth and pace of your breathing.
- Allow your breath to become slower, softer and deeper.
- Take your mind's awareness to your body, starting with the feet.
- Allow the feet to soften and relax; let go of any tension.
- Allow the ankle joint to open and relax.
- Feel the calf muscles and muscles at the front of the shin soften.
- Take a deeper breath and on the outward breath allow the lower leg to relax and soften even further.
- Take your mind's awareness to the knee joint.
- Allow the knee joint to open and relax.
- Feel the muscles at the front of the thigh soften.
- Feel the muscles at the back of the thigh lengthen and relax.
- Take a deeper breath and on the outward breath allow the whole of the legs to relax and let go.
- Focus your mind's awareness on the hip joint.
- Allow the hip joint to open up and relax.
- Feel the buttock muscles relax and soften.
- Feel the muscles around the hip release and open.
- Focus your mind's awareness on the spine.
- Start at the base of the spine and be mindful of each vertebrae up to the skull.
- Feel each vertebrae open up.
- Allow the muscles around the vertebrae (spine) to relax and lengthen.

Script 2: Passive muscular relaxation continued

- Allow all the tension to ease away.
- Allow the shoulder blades to separate and open up.
- Take a deep breath and allow the whole spine to lengthen and relax.
- Focus on the abdominal muscles.
- Allow them to release.
- Notice how the breath fills the abdominal area.
- Observe the abdomen rising and falling with each breath.
- Notice the rib cage and the breast bone.
- Feel the muscles around the ribs relax.
- Allow the breath to become slower and deeper.
- Allow the ribs and the breastbone to soften.
- Focus your awareness on the shoulder joint.
- Allow the shoulder joint to open up and relax.
- Feel the muscles of the upper arm lengthen and relax.
- Notice the elbow joint.
- Feel the elbow joint relaxing and opening.
- Feel the muscles of the forearm relax and soften.
- Notice the wrists and the hands.
- Allow the tension to ease away.
- Allow the fingers to curl open and the tension to float away.
- Focus your mind's awareness on the head.
- Allow each of the facial muscles to soften and relax.
- Feel the jaw relax.
- Feel the tongue soften.
- Feel the lips gently touching and forming a soft smile.
- Allow the cheek bones to relax.
- Notice the eye sockets relaxing.
- Allow the forehead to relax.
- Any tension just easing away.
- Feel your body soften.
- Allow your body to feel light and relaxed.
- Take your mind's awareness back to your breathing.
- Focus on slower, deeper breathing.
- With every breath allow the body to relax further.
- Allow a feeling of peace and calm to spread through your whole body.

PELVIC FLOOR EXERCISES

Most individuals will benefit from performing pelvic floor exercises. They are especially beneficial for older adults, persons with respiratory conditions (who may experience incontinence from coughing) and for individuals who may have weaker pelvic floor muscles (inactive, obese, low pain back etc.).

The pelvic floor consists of a number of muscles that run underneath the pelvis like a hammock on both right and left sides to surround the lower orifices: the urethra, the vagina (females) and penis and testes (male) and the anus. A number of factors can cause the pelvic floor to become weakened. Weakness is generally more common in females then males (Palastanga et al, 1990). These include:

- pregnancy and childbirth;
- prolonged inactivity;
- urinary diseases and infections;
- constipation and other bowel conditions (irritable bowel);
- obesity;
- excessive coughing (some respiratory conditions);
- excessive and sustained jumping and impact;
- hormonal changes (pregnancy and menopause);
- prostatectomy (males);
- constant heavy lifting as required by some occupations, causing constant pressure on these muscles.

PELVIC FLOOR EXERCISE POSITIONS

Pelvic floor exercises can be performed in the following positions:

- supine crook lying (lying on the back with knees bent);
- prone lying (lying on tummy with face down towards the floor);
- seated (floor or chair);
- standing (when waiting in a queue, walking).

A large percentage (approximately 70 per cent) of the pelvic floor muscles are slow twitch fibres (slow to contract and slow to tire – endurance) and a smaller percentage (approximately 30 per cent) are fast twitch (fast to contract and fast to tire – strength). It is therefore offered as a guideline to include a combination of slower exercises for the pelvic floor and faster exercises to recruit both types of fibre.

Back passage isolation
Inhale to prepare and exhale to isolate and draw up the muscles of the pelvic floor surrounding the anus, without gripping the buttocks or other muscles. Inhale to release.

Middle passage isolation
Inhale to prepare and exhale to isolate and draw up the muscles of the pelvic floor surrounding the vagina, without gripping the buttocks or other muscles. Inhale to release.

Front passage isolation
Inhale to prepare and exhale to isolate and draw up the muscles of the pelvic floor surrounding the urethra, without gripping the buttocks or other muscles. Inhale to release.

Back to front – the wave
Inhale to prepare and exhale to draw up the muscles of the pelvic floor surrounding the anus, vagina and urethra sequentially, without gripping the buttocks. Inhale to release.

The flower

Visualise the whole of the pelvic floor area between the legs as an 'open flower'. Inhale to prepare and exhale to draw the muscles upwards to close the petals of the flower – feeling also the connection with the deeper abdominals.

The light switch

Inhale to prepare, exhale to draw up the pelvic floor muscle (in isolation, sequential or altogether) – visualising the light switching on. Inhale to release – visualising the light switching off.

ALTERNATIVE ACTIVITY APPROACHES
NIA
(Contributed by Fiona Winter)

Nia is a sensory-based movement practice created in the early 1980s by Debbie Rosas and Carlos AyaRosas.

Nia draws from disciplines of the martial arts, dance arts and healing arts. Each class offers a unique combination of 52 moves that correspond with the main areas of the body:

- The base
- The core
- The upper extremities

Nia invites participants to focus inside the body rather than outside, to connect the body, mind, emotions and spirit. Throughout the session, participants are encouraged to recognise how their body responds to the five sensations of:

1. Flexibility
2. Agility
3. Mobility
4. Stability
5. Strength

They are then asked to use their personal knowledge of that response, modifying the moves to suit their own body and to create conditioning and relaxation as required. This 'mindful' approach to movement also encourages recognition of stress and tension within the body and mind and the class provides various opportunities and ways to release this.

The benefits of Nia and its contribution to physical and total fitness include the following:

- Strengthens muscles, improves muscle tone, and increases muscle definition.
- Increases flexibility.
- Improves organ function, particularly that of the heart and lungs.
- Improves circulation of blood and lymphatic drainage.
- Improves posture and even increases height.
- Enhances sensory awareness.
- Increases endorphins, helping to alleviate depression, anxiety and stress.
- Balances the autonomic nervous system.
- Strengthens immunity.
- Improves concentration and cognitive function.
- Facilitates weight loss and proper weight maintenance.
- Calms the mind and relieves stress.

Nia is suitable for people of all fitness levels (lower to higher), ages, shapes and sizes as every movement can be adapted to meet individual needs and abilities. Nia can be adapted so that individuals can personalise their intensity levels. It is great for those new to exercise and older adults, and can be modified for clients who have chronic health conditions, including overweight and obesity, diabetes, arthritis, osteoporosis, back care, hip and knee replacement, asthma,

COPD, hypertension, high blood cholesterol, stroke, depression, anxiety and stress, Parkinson's, multiple sclerosis, and combinations of the above. The method has also been used with clients with fibromyalgia, cancer survivors, substance misuse, mental health and intellectual disabilities.

Specific considerations

The Nia technique creates standard 'routines' for teachers to share in class. In an exercise referral setting a teacher would need to give appropriate consideration to the pace, complexity, intensity and stability of the standard movements for some individuals and target groups, and offer seated and/or adapted options where appropriate.

Training and qualifications

Nia training is delivered worldwide. Information is available from www.nianow.com

Nia training (like traditional martial arts training) includes several progressive belt levels – white, blue, green, brown and black – and each belt addresses five core-competency areas (movement, music, anatomy, science and philosophy) while exploring 13 unique Nia principles. The exception is the green belt, which focuses on teaching, and the five stages training, which offers a healing focus. Each belt includes 50+ hours of training, which includes movement, discussion and reflection. The recommended and required reflection period between each training belt is 12 months to ensure graduates fully embody the potential of each level before moving on to the next.

Please note: to work in an exercise referral setting, a Nia teacher would need to have completed the Level 3 Diploma in Exercise Referral in addition to Nia training (white and blue belt training minimum). (In the UK, seated and adapted movement training is offered to Nia teachers through www.energymoves.co.uk).

SEATED AND ADAPTED TRAINING

Seated energy moves is a seated or adapted alternative to a traditional 'exercise' class developed by Fiona Winter. It is designed to provide a holistic movement experience and focuses on engaging the body, mind, emotions and unique spirit of the participant, providing an opportunity for every individual to move in their own way, with the pleasure and joy of movement. The session guides the participant through de-stressing and re-energising movements, using imagery, visualisation, sound and breath to connect with the sensations of the moves.

The programme offers an excellent starting point for those who are less mobile or unused to activity, and has been used to work with individuals with neurological conditions, overweight and obesity, diabetes, intellectual disabilities, arthritis, osteoporosis, fibromyalgia, cancer survivors, mental health, low back pain, hip and knee replacement, asthma, COPD, hypertension, high blood cholesterol, stroke, depression, anxiety and stress, Parkinson's, multiple sclerosis and combinations of the above.

The session structure

The session follows a traditional structure and builds in opportunities to develop skills in coordination, stability, balance, agility, sensory awareness and memory.

- **Warm-up** This provides opportunities for joint mobilisation, increasing circulation, breathing and heart rate. The de-stressing moves provide a gateway into mindful movements, changing the focus from 'external' to 'internal' and from 'doing' to 'sensing and feeling'.

- **Get moving** During the get moving section bigger movements create an increase in the demand on the cardiovascular system while working muscles to improve tone and strength.
- **Cool-down** During the cool-down the body is prepared for resting, relaxing and focusing on steady breathing and releasing tension.

Training on the principles of simplifying and adapting movement and seated movement is available from: www.energymoves. There is also a DVD to accompany the programme.

THE CHIBALL® METHOD
(contributed by Sandie Keane)

The ChiBall® Method was created in Australia in 1997. It was designed to provide an exercise programme that promotes balance, health and well-being. The method draws on the philosophy and principles within Traditional Chinese Medicine (TCM) and the exercise disciplines that are introduced and integrated in the Method are Tai Chi, Qi Gong, yoga, Pilates, Feldenkrais, relaxation and meditation.

The method works alongside the laws of nature and aims to bring attention to areas that are in need of nurturing and out of balance. The basic principles work towards re-aligning and re-balancing the whole structure to bring health and well-being back into the body by balancing the ebb and flow of energy, which may become blocked or imbalanced by life struggles.

According to TCM there is only one cause of illness – a disharmony of yin and yang. When our energy systems are functioning optimally, yin and yang are harmonised just like the ebb and flow of the tides. The principles of yin and yang are evident through our everyday lives. There are days when our energy is up (yang), and others when our energy is down (yin). Without one we cannot have the other and to have too much of one will cause an imbalance. e.g. Causes of imbalance may include: the amount of time spent voluntarily sitting at computers or watching television, being indoors, the foods we eat, etc. Exercise has been proven to help reduce the symptoms that are associated with the 'low ebb, no flow' condition.

Low ebb, no flow condition

The first Chinese medical book, *The Yellow Emperor's Classic of Medicine* (Huang Ti) was written over 2000 years ago and is still in publication today. Practitioners in Traditional Chinese Medicine (TCM) use it as their bible. Within its philosophy, mental, physical or emotional problems are attributed to an imbalance or blockage in one or more of the internal organs and the energy pathways (meridians) that are associated with them; and where disease and dysfunction can manifest. The teachings state that there is no such single, simple diagnostic term, characterising illnesses according to common collections of symptoms, bodily and/ or emotional signs, which differs to the modern conventional medical approach of naming each symptom individually.

In recent years, TCM practice has seen a dynamic revival in China and elements of this time-honoured therapy, including acupuncture and the harmony of mind, body, spirit exercise have been embraced in the West (by those who have had no success or who want an alternative to conventional medication. Some western medical practitioners are also open to alternative approaches).

Benefits of the ChiBall® Method and session structure

The ChiBall® Method follows the cycles of the seasons and in the ChiBall year there are five seasons:

1. Spring
2. Summer
3. Late summer
4. Autumn
5. Winter

The five seasons all have an element attributed to them, with a physical and emotional association, each of which carries energy. Appreciating and understanding this energy leads towards better health.

A ChiBall® class is structured to work alongside the energy of each season. Every class starts with the energy of spring represented by Tai Chi-Qigong. This will be followed by a dance section, yoga section, Pilates and Feldenkrais section.

Tai Chi-Qigong

(pronounced Tie Chee-CheeGung)
Tai Chi is often described as 'meditation in motion', but it might well be called 'medication in motion'. Due to its precision and slowness, it can often be hard for new students to slow down, especially if they are living life in the fast lane. At the other end of the scale, those who

have ended up 'on the hard shoulder' often have to deal with their own demons and instead of fighting the outside enemy, they end up fighting the enemy within. Slowing down, like speeding up, is a muscle that develops with training and with Tai Chi it's our mind we need to train to slow down.

Qigong is a powerful system of healing. It is the art and science of combining breathing techniques, gentle movement and moving meditation to cleanse, strengthen, and circulate your energy (qi). Both Tai Chi and Qigong help to mobilise the joints, stimulate the immune system, produce the proper enzymes for digestion, repair damaged cells, flush away bodily toxins and balance the emotions.

Dance section:

All cultures around the world have their own distinctive music and rhythms and it is through dance that we can unleash suppressed emotions, tension and, most importantly, liberate the mind. Dance lifts our heart energy and brings warmth to the body giving us a sense of well-being.

Yoga section:

Yoga integrates and balances all of the body's systems, especially the nervous system. The postures are performed with an 'energised calm' so that on completion of the practice the mind and body are relaxed. The sequence is a progression from one stage to another as reflected in nature. A plant grows up out of the earth while its roots sink further into the earth in perfect symbiosis with time, weather and seasons. Yoga postures similarly develop with time and help us to move with the ebb and flow of life rather than resist it.

Pilates section:

Pilates is one of two modern Western approaches to exercise used within the ChiBall® Method. The principle philosophy of Pilates is to bring the whole structure of the body back towards a better alignment (improved posture); improving the way the muscles perform and increasing flexibility, core strength and mobility, which are useful components to include within an activity programme for many referred groups (see exercise recommendations for specific conditions). Joseph Pilates himself studied and understood the benefits of Tai Chi and yoga and saw beyond the condition of his clients. He would modify and adjust his exercises to accommodate his client's needs so that results were achieved by all.

Feldenkrais section:

The Feldenkrais Method is the second Western exercise discipline used. Moshe Feldenkrais studied human movement and qualified in acupuncture, kinesiology, physiology, neurology, anatomy and psychology.

Feldenkrais developed a unique understanding of sensory-motor function and its relationship to thought, emotion and action. His Awareness Through Movement and Functional Integration uses the body's central nervous system to bring about a more effective, comfortable and healthier way of moving. The Feldenkrais Method is used towards the end of a class, releasing and relaxing the body before entering relaxation and meditation.

Breath work

Improving breathing habits and increasing the daily intake of oxygen has been proven to have a significant effect on the immune system. All ancient physical disciplines emphasise the importance of the breath and its link to a healthy mind and body. Our breath acts as a signpost, clearly indicating either the degree of resistance and suppression or the receptiveness and expression of our emotions. Fullness of breath demonstrates our ease and equanimity with the natural flow of life. It is estimated that the average person breathes about 14–26 breaths per minute. For Yoga, Tai Chi and Qigong Masters the breath is slow and deep at a rate of 3–6 breaths per minute, which is why they are able to sustain mental alertness and tranquility in every situation. Therefore, if we have better control of our breath we can have better control of our life. The emphasis on breathing is of paramount importance. It is seen as the thread that connects the mind to the body. Breath work is valuable for working with all referred client groups and is particularly beneficial for helping with respiratory conditions as well as anxiety and depression (which accompanies many physical health conditions). Some simple breathing exercises were introduced earlier in this chapter.

When we begin to change our movement patterns and focus on our breath we will potentially move parts of the body that may have been immobile for many years and when reaching deep down we may stir up old memories. Emotional experiences and memories can be stored by the body. The five senses – sight, hearing, taste, smell and touch, are the external connections to our past memories and emotions, and the breath is the internal connection. This can be unnerving if unprepared. Holistic activity approaches offer a way of preparing and managing this.

The following exercise is simple and easy to follow. It is recommended that the intention for better health is included as the mindful focus of the practice, which is a moving meditation.

For more information on the ChiBall® Method visit sandie@therapiauk.com

Balance your ebb and flow

- Feet are close together, toes are pointing forward, lips are slightly apart and hands are relaxed by your sides.
- Posture is upright but relaxed. Chest is soft and open and nose is pointing forward.
- Palms face down towards the ground, fingers pointing towards one another, with some space between them.
- Arms are as straight as comfortably possible.
- Chin tilts down, as if looking at the hands, while the body remains upright and shoulders remain relaxed.

- The arms move out in front and up above the head.
- Breathe in gently through the nose.
- The nose follows the movement of the hands.
- The head ends tilting back comfortably.
- At the top, you lift up gently from your heels to your hands, while the arms remain comfortably straight.
- The arms drop smoothly down, like birds wings. The wrists are no longer bent.
- Breathe out gently through the mouth as your arms are descending.
- The neck gradually returns to normal with the nose pointing forward.

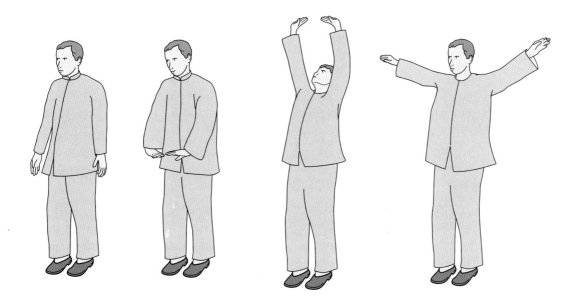

Figure 17.1 Balance your ebb and flow

REFERENCES

NB: All websites were correct at the time of writing

Ainsworth et al. (2000) Update of 'Compendium of Physical Activities: Classification of Energy Costs of Human Physical Activities'. *Medicine and Science in Sports and Exercise* 32: S498–S504.

Ambrosino, N. and Scano, G. (2004) 'Dyspnoea and Its Measurement', *Breathe*, 1/2, available from: www.ersnet.org.

American College of Sports Medicine (ACSM) (2000) 6th edn. *Guidelines for Exercise Testing and Prescription* (Philadelphia: Lippincott, Williams & Wilkins).

— (2001) *Clinical Certification Review* (Philadelphia: Lippincott, Williams & Wilkins).

— (2005a) 7th edn. *Guidelines for Exercise Testing and Prescription* (Philadelphia: Lippincott, Williams & Wilkins).

— (2005b) 5th edn. *Resource manual for Guidelines for Exercise Testing and Prescription* (Philadelphia: Lippincott, Williams & Wilkins).

— (2010) 8th edn. *Guidelines for Exercise Testing and Prescription* (Philadelphia: Lippincott, Williams & Wilkins).

American Diabetes Association (ADA) (2003) *Physical Activity/Exercise and Diabetes Mellitus*. Diabetes Care 26:S73–S77. Available from http://care.diabetesjournals.org/.

— (2004) *Physical Activity/Exercise and Type 2 Diabetes*. Diabetes Care 27:2518–2539. Available from http://care.diabetesjournals.org/.

— (2005) *Recommendation for Management of Diabetes During Ramadan*. Diabetes Care 28:2305–2311. Available from http://care.diabetesjournals.org/.

American Psychological Association (APA) (2000) *The Diagnostic and Statistical Manual of Mental Disorders (DSM)* (USA: American Psychiatric Association).

American Thoracic Society (ATS) (1999) 'Pulmonary Rehabilitation', *American Journal of Respiratory and Critical Care Medicine* 159:1666–82, available from: www.thoracic.org.

— and European Respiratory Society (2005) COPD Guidelines, available from www.ersnet.org.

Asthma UK (2004) *Asthma and Exercise*, Fact Sheet 36, available from www.asthma.org.uk.

— (2005) *Take Control of your Asthma*, available from www.asthma.org.uk.

— (2012) *Asthma: Journalist Key Facts and Statistics*, available from http://www.asthma.org.uk/news_media/media_resources/for_journalists_key.html.

Australian Lung Foundation and Australian Physiotherapy Association (2012) *Draft Toolkit for Pulmonary Rehabilitation*, available from http://www.pulmonaryrehab.com.au/index.asp?page=62.

Benson, H., MD (1975) *The Relaxation Response* (New York: Avon Books).

Berry, M. J., Woodward, C. M. (2003), in J. K. Ehrman, P. M. Gordon, P. S. Visich, and S.J. Keteyian, *Clinical Exercise Physiology* (Champaign, Ill.: Human Kinetics).

Betts L. (2005). *Exercise for People with MS*. Multiple Sclerosis Trust. Available from: www.mstrust.org.uk.

Biddle, S., Fox, K., and Boutcher, S. (eds.) (2000) *Physical Activity and Psychological Well-Being* (London and New York: Routledge).

Biddle, S.J.H., Mutrie, N. (2008, revised) *Psychology of Physical Activity* (USA: Routledge).

Bloomfield, S., and Smith, S. (2003) 'Osteoporosis', in J. Larry Durstine and G. E. Moore 2nd edn. *ACSM's Exercise Management for Persons with Chronic Diseases and Disabilities* (Champaign, Ill.: Human Kinetics). First published 1991.

Borg, G. (1998) *Perceived Exertion and Pain Scales* (Champaign, Ill.: Human Kinetics).

Boud, D., Keogh, R., and Walker, D. (1985) *Reflection: Turning Experience into Learning* (London: Kogan Page).

British Association of Cardiac Rehabilitation (BACR) (2000) (Revised edition) *Phase IV Exercise Instructor Training Module* (UK: BACR).

— (2005) *Exercise Protocols for Management of CHD Patients*, BACR Cardiac Rehabilitation Phase IV Training Course Handout.

British Heart Foundation (BHF) (2003a) *Active for Later Life* (London: British Heart Foundation National Centre for Physical Activity and Health).

— (2003b). *Take Note of your Heart: A Review of Women and Heart Disease in the UK* (London: BHF).

— (2004a) Cardiac Care and Education Research Group Patient Questionnaires, available from www.cardiacrehabilitation.org.uk/dataset.

— (2004b) *Updated Guidelines on Cardiovascular Disease Risk Assessment*, Factfile 08/2004, available from www.bhf.org.

— (2005a). *Blood Pressure.* Heart Information Series 4, available from: www.bhf.org.uk.

— (2005b) *Any Questions: What is Angina?* Medical Information Department, available from www.bhf.org.uk.

— (2005c) *Statistics*, available from www.heartstats.org.uk.

— (2005d) *Risk Groups* (online), available from www.bhf.org.uk/smoking/sn_risk_groups.asp.

— and Sport England (2005e) Summary brief on *Physical Activity and Health*, available from www.bhf.org.uk.

BHF (2008) *Modelling the UK Burden of Cardiovascular Disease to 2020*, available from http://www.bhf.org.uk/plugins/PublicationsSearchResults/DownloadFile.aspx?docid=ad18e5a0-7da6-4c7c-8142-f68f27cde451&version=-1&title=Modelling+the+Burden+of+Cardiovascular+Disease+to+2020&resource=Z154.

British Hypertension Society (n.d.a) *Measuring Blood Pressure Using a Digital Monitor*, available from www.bhsoc.org.

— (n.d.b). *Measuring Blood Pressure Using a Mercury Blood Pressure Device*, available from www.bhsoc.org.

— (2004) *Guidelines for Hypertension Management* (BHS-1V): Summary. BMJ 2004 Mar. 13; 328 (7440):634–40, available from www.bhsoc.org.uk.

British National Formulary (BNF) (2005) *Joint National Formulary Committee. British National Formulary* (50th edn.) (London: British Medical Association and Royal Pharmaceutical Society of Great Britain), available from www.bnf.org. uk.

British Nutrition Foundation (2005) *Balance of Good Health* (online), available from www.nutrition.org.uk.

British Thoracic Society (BTS) (1997) *The British Guidelines on Asthma Management: 1995 Review and Position Statement*, Thorax 5 (suppl. 1), S1–S20.

— (2005) COPD Consortium: *Spirometry in Practice: A Practical Guide to Using Spirometry in Primary Care* (2nd edn.).

British Medical Association (BMA) (2011) *New Guide to Medicines and Drugs* (London, UK: Dorling Kindersley).

Brownlee M. Durward B. (2005) *Exercise in Treatment of Stroke and other Neurological Conditions.* In: Gromley J. Hussey J. eds (2005). *Exercise Therapy: Prevention and treatment of disease.* (Blackwell Publishing: UK).

Buckley, J. et al. (1999) *Exercise on Prescription:*

Cardiovascular Activity for Health (Champaign Ill.: Human Kinetics).

Buckley J. and Jones, J. (2005) Assessing Functional Capacity and Monitoring Intensity in Cardiac Patients, training course.

BUPA (n.d.a) *Osteoarthritis*, available from http://hcd2.bupa.co.uk/fact_sheets/html/osteoarthritis.html.

— (n.d.b) *Rheumatoid Arthritis*, available from http://hcd2.bupa.co.uk/fact_sheets/html/osteoarthritis.html.

BUPA (2005). *Stroke. Health fact sheet.* Available from: www.bupa.co.uk.

Burningham S. (2002). *After your stroke: a first guide.* The Stroke Association. London. Available from: www.stroke.org.uk.

Canadian Society for Exercise Physiology (2002) *Screening Forms. Physical Activity Readiness Questionnaire and Physical Activity Readiness Medical Examination*, available from www.csep.ca/.

Cantopher, T. Dr (2003) *Depressive Illness. The Curse of the Strong*, (6) (London, UK: Sheldon Press).

Carlin, B. W. and Seigneur, D. (2003) 'Asthma', in J. K. Ehrman, P. M. Gordon, P. S. Visich and S. J. Keteyian, *Clinical Exercise Physiology* (Champaign, Ill.: Human Kinetics).

Cooper, C. B. (2003) 'Chronic Obstructive Pulmonary Disease', in J. Larry Durstine and G. E. Moore, *ACSM's Exercise Management for Persons with Chronic Disease and Disabilities*, 2nd edn. (Champaign, Ill.: Human Kinetics).

Cooper, C. (2009) 'Chronic Obstructive Pulmonary Disease', in J. Larry Durstine et al, *ACSM's Exercise Management for Persons with Chronic Disease and Disabilities*, 3rd edn. (Champaign, Ill.: Human Kinetics).

Daines, B., Gask, L. and Usherwood, T. (1997) *Medical and Psychiatric Issues for Counsellors* (London: Sage Publications).

Davies, T. and Craig, T. eds (2009) *ABC of Mental Health*, 2nd edn. (UK: BMJ Books, Wiley-Blackwell Publishing).

Davison, G. and Neale, J. (2001) *Abnormal Psychology*, 8th edn. (California: John Wiley & Sons).

Department of Health (1996) *Strategy Statement on Physical Activity* (London: Department of Health).

— (1999a) *Saving Lives: Our Healthier Nation*, available from www.dh.gov.uk.

— (1999b) *National Service Framework for Mental Health*, available from www.dh.gov.uk.

— (2000a) *National Service Framework for Coronary Heart Disease: Main Report* (London: Department of Health).

— (2000b) NHS Plan, available from www.dh.gov.uk.

— (2001*a*) *Exercise Referral Systems: A National Quality Assurance Framework* (London: Department of Health).

— (2001*b*) *Good Practice in Consent. Implementation Guide: Consent to Examination or Treatment*, available from www.doh.org.uk.

— (2001*c*) *National Service Framework for Diabetes*, available from www.dh.gov.uk.

— (2001*d*) *National Service Framework for Older People*, available from www.dh.gov.uk.

— (2003*a*) *On the State of Public Health*, Report from the Chief Medical Officer (London: Department of Health).

— (2003*b*) *Tackling Health Inequalities: A Programme for Action*, available from www.dh.gov.uk.

— (2004*a*) *At Least Five a Week. Evidence on the Impact of Physical Activity and Its Relationship to Health*, Report from the Chief Medical Officer (London: Department of Health).

— (2004*b*) *Choosing Health: Making Healthier Choices Easier* (London: Department of Health).

— (2005*a*) *Choosing Activity: A Physical Activity Action Plan* (London: Department of Health).

— (2005*b*) *Self Care – A Real Choice. Self Care Support – A Practical Option* (London: Department of Health).

— (2005*c*) *The National Service Framework for Long-term Conditions: Information Leaflet*, available from www.dh.gov.uk.

Diabetes UK (2000) *Impaired Glucose Tolerance*, available from www.diabetes.org.uk.

— (2001) *Care Recommendation. New Diagnostic Criteria for Diabetes*, available from www.diabetes.org.uk.

— (2003*a*) *Information: Hyperglycaemia, ketoacidosis and HONK*, available from www.diabetes.org.uk.

— (2003*b*) *Physical Activity and Carbohydrate Intake*, available from www.diabetes.org.uk.

— (2004*a*) *Physical Activity and Diabetes: Information Sheet*, available from www.diabetes.org.uk.

— (2004*b*) *Weight Management – Managing Diabetes in Primary Care*, available from www.diabetes.org.uk.

— (2005) *Tablets available in the UK*, available from www.diabetes.org.uk.

Department of Health (2009) *Be Active, Be Healthy*, available from http://www.dh.gov.uk/prod_consum_dh/groups/dh_digitalassets/documents/digitalasset/dh_094359.pdf.

Department of Health (2011) *Start Active, Stay Active*, available from http://www.bhfactive.org.uk/userfiles/Documents/startactivestayactive.pdf.

Directgov (2005) *Disabled People*, available from www.direct.gov.uk/DisabledPeople/.

Durstine, L. J. and Moore, G. E. (2003) *ACSM's Exercise Management for Persons with Chronic Diseases and Disabilities*, 2nd edn. (Champaign, Ill.: Human Kinetics).

Durstine, L. J. et al (2009) *ACSM's Exercise Management for Persons with Chronic Diseases and Disabilities*, 3rd edn. (Champaign, Ill.: Human Kinetics).

Ehrman, J. K., Gordon, P. M., Visich, P. S. and Keteyian, S. J. (2003) *Clinical Exercise Physiology* (Champaign Ill.: Human Kinetics).

Eleverton, P. (2004) *Taming the Black Dog* (Oxford, UK: How To Books).

Feltham, C. and Horton, I. (eds.) (2000) *Handbook of Counselling and Psychotherapy* (London: Sage Publications).

Fernando, S. (1988) *Race and Culture in Psychiatry* (London: Croom Helm).

Gitkin, A., Canulette M. and Friedman, D. (2003) 'Angina and Silent Ischemia', in J. L. Durstine and G. E. Moore, ACSM's Exercise Management for Persons with Chronic Disease and Disabilities (Champaign, Ill: Human Kinetics).

Durstine and G. E. Moore, *ACSM's Exercise Management for Persons with Chronic Disease and Disabilities* (Champaign, Ill.: Human Kinetics).

Gross, R., and McIlveen, R. (1998) *Psychology: A New Introduction* (London: Hodder & Stoughton).

Gross, R. (1996) *Psychology: The Science of Mind and Behaviour* (London, UK: Hodder & Stoughton).

Halliwell, E. (2005) *Up and Running? Exercise Therapy and the Treatment of Mild or Moderate Depression in Primary Care*, available from http://www.mentalhealth.org.uk.

Health and Safety Executive (2003) *Five Steps to Risk Assessment*, available from www.hse.gov.uk.

— (2005) *Stress-Related and Psychological Disorders*, available from http://www.hse.gov.uk/statistics/causdis/stress.htm.

HSE (2012) Management Standards and Stress-Related Work Outcomes, in Occupational Medicine (59:574–579), available from http://www.hse.gov.uk/stress/management-standards.pdf.

Health Development Agency (2001) *Coronary Heart Disease: Guidance for Implementing the Preventive Aspects of the NSF*, available from www.publichealth.nice.org.uk.

— (2005*a*) *The Effectiveness of Public Health Interventions for Increasing Physical Activity Among Adults: A Review of Reviews*, available from http://www.had.nhs.uk.

— (2005*b*) *Getting Evidence into Practice in Public Health*, available from http://www.had.nhs.uk.

— (2005*c*) *Choosing Health? Choosing Activity: Comments on the Consultation Document from the Health Development*

Agency, available from http://www.had.nhs.uk.

Health Education Authority (2000) *Black and Minority Ethnic Groups in England: The Second Health and Lifestyles Survey*, Executive Summary (London: HEA), available from www.had-online.org.uk.

Health and Social Care Information Centre (2010) *Statistics on Obesity, Physical Activity and Diet*, available from http://www.ic.nhs.uk/webfiles/publications/opad10/ Statistics_on_Obesity_Physical_Activity_and_Diet_ England_2010.pdf.

Hornsby, G. and Albright, A. (2009) in Durstine et al (eds) *ACSM's Exercise Management for Persons with Chronic Diseases and Disabilities (Diabetes)*, 3rd edn. (182) (Champaign, Ill.: Human Kinetics).

Hughes, J. and Martin, S. (2002), in C. Waine, *Obesity and Weight Management in Primary Care* (Oxford: Blackwell Science).

IPAQ (2002) *International Physical Activity Questionnaires*, available from https://sites.google.com/site/theipaq/ questionnaire_links and http://www.ipaq.ki.se/scoring.pdf.

Jackson, K. and Mulcare, J. (2009) *Multiple Sclerosis* in J. Larry Durstine et al. *ACSM's Exercise Management for Person's with Chronic Diseases*, 3rd edn. (Champaign, III: Human Kinetics).

Joint British Societies (JBS) (2005) *Guidelines on Prevention of Cardiovascular Disease in Clinical Practice* (Heart 2005;91v1–v52;doi:10.1136/ hrt.2005.079988), available from www.diabetes.org.uk.

Joint Health Surveys Unit (1999) *Health Survey for England: Health of Minority Ethnic Groups 1999*. (London: Stationery Office).

— (2003) *Health Survey for England 2003* (London: Stationery Office).

— (2006) *Health Survey for England 2006* (London: Stationery Office).

Karpatkin H. I. (2005). Multiple Sclerosis and Exercise. A Review of the Evidence. International Journal of MS Care. 2005;7:36-41. Available from: www.mscare.org.

Lago, C. and Thompson, J. (2003) *Race, Culture and Counselling* (Buckingham: Open University Press).

Lawrence, D. (2004a) *The Complete Guide to Exercise in Water*, 2nd edn. (London, UK: A & C Black).

— (2004b) *The Complete Guide to Exercise to Music*, 2nd edn. (London, UK: A & C Black).

— (2005) *The Complete Guide to Exercising Away Stress* (London, UK: A & C Black).

— and Hope, B. (2005) *The Complete Guide to Circuit Training* (London, UK: A & C Black).

— and Sheppard, M. (2011a) *Exercise Your Way to Health: Osteoporosis* (London, UK: A & C Black).

— and Burns, J. (2011b) *Exercise Your Way to Health: Depression* (London, UK: A & C Black).

— and Bolitho, S. (2011c) *The Complete Guide to Physical Activity for Mental Health* (London, UK: A & C Black).

Leith, Larry M. *Foundations of Exercise and Mental Health* (1994) (21) (Morgantown, USA: Fitness Information Technology).

McArdle, W., Katch, F. and Katch, V. (1991) *Exercise Physiology. Energy, Nutrition and Human Performance* (Philadelphia: Lea & Febiger).

McLaughlin, C. (2000). *Communication problems after stroke*. The Stroke Association. London. Available from: www. stroke.org.uk.

Mental Health Foundation (2000) *Fact sheet*, available at www.mentalhealth.org.uk.

Mental Health Foundation (2010) *Mindfulness Report*. (UK: Mental Health Foundation).

Mindell, A. (1995) *Sitting in the Fire: Large Group Transformation Using Conflict and Diversity* (Portland, Ore.: Lao Tse Press).

Minor, M. and Kay, D. (2003) 'Arthritis', in J. Larry Durstine and G. E. Moore, *ACSM's Exercise Management for Persons with Chronic Diseases and Disabilities*, 2nd edn. (Champaign, Ill.: Human Kinetics).

Moore, S. (2001). *Cognitive Problems after Stroke*. Stoke Association. Available from: www.stroke.org.uk.

Multiple Sclerosis Trust (2005). *Information for Health and Social Care Professionals*. UK. Available from: www.mstrust.org.uk.

Multiple Sclerosis Trust (2004). *Multiple Sclerosis Explained*. UK. Available from: www.mstrust.org.uk.

NHS Choices (2012a) *The Eatwell Plate*, available from http://www.nhs.uk/Livewell/Goodfood/Pages/eatwell-plate.aspx.

NHS Choices (2012b) *8 Tips for Healthy Eating*, available from http://www.nhs.uk/Livewell/Goodfood/Pages/ eight-tips-healthy-eating.aspx.

NHS Choices (2012c) *Arthritis*, available from, http://www. nhs.uk/Conditions/Arthritis/Pages/Introduction.aspx.

NHS Choices (2012d) *Osteoarthritis*, available from http://www.nhs.uk/conditions/Osteoarthritis/Pages/ Introduction.aspx.

NHS Choices (2012e) *Rheumatoid arthritis*, available from http://www.nhs.uk/Conditions/Rheumatoid-arthritis/ Pages/Introduction.aspx.

NHS Choices (2012f) *Obesity*, available from http://www.

nhs.uk/Conditions/Obesity/Pages/Introduction.aspx.

NHS Choices (2012*g*) *Diabetes*, available from http://www. nhs.uk/Conditions/Diabetes/Pages/Diabetes.aspx.

NHS Choices (2009*h*) *Low Back Pain*, available from http:// www.nhs.uk/Conditions/Back-pain/Pages/Prevention.

NHS Choices (2010) *Hypertension*, available from http:// www.nhs.uk/Conditions/Blood-pressure-(high)/Pages/ Introduction.aspx.

National Institute of Health & Clinical Excellence (NICE) (2002) *A Guide for Adults with Type 2 Diabetes and Carers*, available from www.nice.org.uk.

— (2003). *Multiple Sclerosis – Management of multiple sclerosis in primary and secondary care*. NICE clinical Guideline 8. London: NICE.

— (2004*a*) *Quick Reference Guide: Chronic Obstructive Pulmonary Disease, Management of Chronic Pulmonary Disease in Adults in Primary and Secondary Care*, Clinical Guideline 12 (London, UK: NICE).

— (2004*b*) *Type 1 Diabetes in Adults: Understanding NICE guidance, Information for Adults with Type 1 Diabetes, their Families and Carers, and the Public*, Clinical Guideline 15, available from www.nice.org.uk.

— (2004*c*) *Hypertension – Management of Hypertension in Adults in Primary Care, Information for Adults with Hypertension, their Families and Carers, and the Public*, Clinical Guideline 18 (London, UK: NICE).

— (2005) *Review of Hypertension Guidelines*, available on www.nice.org.uk.

— (2006*a*) *A Rapid Review of Exercise Referral Schemes to Promote Activity in Adults*, available from http://www. nice.org.uk/nicemedia/live/11373/43926/43926.pdf.

— (2006*b*) *Quick reference guide 1: Obesity. Guidance on the Prevention, Identification, Assessment and Management of Overweight and Obesity in Adults and Children*, available from http://www.nice.org.uk/nicemedia/ live/11000/30363/30363.pdf.

— (2009) *Depression Guidelines 90-91: Quick Reference Guide* (UK: NICE).

— (2009) *Anxiety: Management of Anxiety in Adults in Primary, Secondary and Community Care*, Clinical Guideline 22 amended (London, UK: NICE).

— (2009) *Low Back Pain*, available from http://guidance. nice.org.uk/CG88/PublicInfo/pdf/English.

— (2010*a*) *Quick Reference Guide: Chronic Obstructive Pulmonary Disease: Management of Chronic Pulmonary Disease in Adults in Primary and Secondary Car*e (London, UK: NICE).

— (2010*b*) *Chronic Pulmonary Disease in Adults in Primary and Secondary Care*, available from http://www.nice.org. uk/nicemedia/live/13029/49425/49425.pdf.

— (2010*c*) *Quick Reference Guide: Cardiovascular Disease*, www.nice.org.uk.

— (2011) *Hypertension: Clinical Management of Hypertension in Adults* (London, UK: NICE).

National Institute of Mental Health (NIMH) (1999) *Schizophrenia Research at the National Institute of Mental Health*, available from http://www.nimh.nih.gov/publicat/ schizresfact.cfm.

NOO (2009) *Measures of Central Adiposity as an Indicator for Obesity* (UK: National Obesity Observatory).

National Osteoporosis Society (2011a) *All About Osteoporosis* (UK: National Osteoporosis Society (NOS)), available at www.nos.org.uk.

National Osteoporosis Society (2011b) *Complementary and Alternative Therapies and Osteoporosis* (UK: National Osteoporosis Society (NOS)), available at www.nos.org.uk.

— (2004) *The Complete Guide to Stretching*, 2nd edn. (London, UK: A & C Black).

Palmer-McLean, K., Harbst, K. B. (2009). 3rd edn. *Stroke and brain injury*. In Durstine L., Moore G. E., eds. *ACSM's Exercise Management for Persons With Chronic Diseases and Disabilities*. 2nd ed. (Champaign, Ill.: Human Kinetics).

Parkinson's Disease Society (2003) *Falls and Parkinson's Disease*, Society Information Sheet 39. Available from www.parkinsons.org.uk.

Parkinson's Society (2004) *Foot Care in Parkinson's*. Society Information Sheet 51. Available from www.parkinsons. org.uk.

Parkinson's Disease Society (2004) *Motor Fluctuations in Parkinson's*. Society Information. Sheet 73. Available from www.parkinsons.org.uk.

Parkinson's Disease Society (2004) *Keeping Moving. Exercise and Parkinson's disease*. Available from www.parkinsons. org.uk.

Parkinson's Disease Society (2005) *Complementary Therapies and Parkinson's disease*. Available from www.parkinsons. org.uk.

Parkinson's Disease Society (2005) *The Drug Treatment of Parkinson's Disease*. Available from www.parkinsons.org.uk.

Parkinson's Disease Society (2003). *Communication*. Information Sheet 6. Available from www.parkinsons. org.uk

Patient UK (2004) *Primary Prevention of Cardiovascular Disease (CVD)*, available from www. patient.co.uk.

— (2005) 'Stroke Rehabilitation', *Patient Plus*, available

from www.patient.co.uk.

Patient UK (2011) *Asthma*, available from http://www.patient.co.uk/health/Asthma.htm.

Patient UK (2012) *Alcohol and Sensible Drinking*, available from http://www.patient.co.uk/health/Alcohol-and-Sensible-Drinking.htm.

Patient UK (2012a) *Non-Specific Low Back Pain*, available from http://www.patient.co.uk/health/Back-Pain.htm.

Patient UK (2012b) *COPD*, available from http://www.patient.co.uk/health/Chronic-Obstructive-Pulmonary-Disease.htm.

Patient UK (2012c) *Hypertension*, available from http://www.patient.co.uk.

PRODIGY (2003a) *Angina*, available from www.prodigy.nhs.uk.

— (2003b) *Coronary Heart Disease Risk Identification and Management*, available from www.prodigy.nhs.uk.

— (2003c) *Diabetes Type 2 – Blood Glucose Management*, available on www.prodigy.nhs.uk.

— (2004) *Chronic Obstructive Pulmonary Disease*, available from www.prodigy.nhs.uk.

— (2005a/2011) *Asthma*, available from http://prodigy.clarity.co.uk/patient_information_leaflet/asthma.

— (2005b) *Depression*, available from http://www.prodigy.nhs.uk.

— (2005c) *Low Back Pain*, available from http://www.prodigy.nhs.uk.

— (2005d) *Osteoarthritis*, available from http://www.prodigy.nhs.uk.

— (2005e) *Osteoporosis*, available from http://www.prodigy.nhs.uk.

— (2005f) *Overweight and Obesity*, available from http://www.prodigy.nhs.uk.

— (2005h) *Rheumatoid Arthritis*, available from http://www.prodigy.nhs.uk.

— (2005i) *Parkinson's disease*. Available from: www.prodigy.nhs.uk.

Protas, E. J. and Stanley, R. K. (2003), in J. L. Durstine and G. E. Moore, (eds.) *ACSM's Exercise Management for Persons with Chronic Diseases and Disabilities*, 2nd edn. (Champaign, Ill.: Human Kinetics).

Rack, P. (1982) *Race, Culture and Mental Disorder* (London: Tavistock).

Ram, F. S. F., Robinson, S. M., Black, P. N. and Picot, J. (2005) *Physical Training for Asthma*, Cochrane Library, available from www.cochrane.org/cochrane/revabstr/ab001116.htm.

Ramaswany, B., Webber, R. 2003. *The Keep Moving Parkinson's Exercise Programme: A rationale for physiotherapists and other health and social care professionals*. Parkinson's Society Information Sheet 79. Available from: www.parkinsons.org.uk.

Rogers, C. and Stevens, B. (1967) *Person to Person: The Problem of Being Human* (Moab, Ut.: Real People Press).

Royal College of Physicians (2004). *Primary Care Concise Guidelines for Stroke*, London. Available from: www.rclondon.ac.uk.

Scottish Intercollegiate Guidelines Network (SIGN) (2001a) *Diabetes*, Publication 55 (Edinburgh: SIGN), available from www.sign.ac.uk.

— (2001b) *The Management of Stable Angina* (Edinburgh SIGN), available from www.sign.ac.uk.

— (2002) *Cardiac Rehabilitation* (Edinburgh: SIGN), available from www.sign.ac.uk.

— and British Thoracic Society (2005) *Update to the British Guidelines on the Management of Asthma*, Report 63 (Edinburgh: SIGN and BTS), available from www.sign.ac.uk.

— and British Thoracic Society (2011) *British Guidelines on the Management of Asthma*, (Edinburgh: SIGN and BTS), available from www.sign.ac.uk.

Sietsema, K. (2001) 'Cardiovascular Limitations in Chronic Pulmonary Disease', in *Medicine and Science in Sports and Exercise*, 33/7 Suppl. S656–S661, July 2001.

Simmonds, M. and Derghazarian in Durstine, L. J. and Moore, G. E. (2009) *ACSM's Exercise Management for Persons with Chronic Diseases and Disabilities (Lower Back Pain Syndrome)*, 3rd edn. (Champaign, Ill.: Human Kinetics).

Smith, T., Wang, C and Bloomfield in Durstine, L. J. and Moore, G. E. (2009) *ACSM's Exercise Management for Persons with Chronic Diseases and Disabilities (Osteoporosis)*, 3rd edn. (Champaign, Ill.: Human Kinetics).

Smith, S. C., Jackson, R., Pearson, T. et al. (2004) *Principles for National and Regional Guidelines on Cardiovascular Disease Prevention: A Scientific Statement from the World Heart and Stroke Forum*, 109: 3112–21, available from www.heart.bmjjournals.com/.

Stewart, I. and Joines, V. (1987) *TA Today. A New Introduction to Transactional Analysis* (Nottingham, UK: Lifespace Publishing).

Strock, M. (2000) *Depression*, available from http://www.nimh.nih.gov/publicat/depression.cfm.

Stroke Association (2005). *Facts and figures about stroke*. Available from www.stroke.org.uk.

Stroke Association (2005). *Act Fast. Article in Stroke News.* Volume 23.3. Available from www.stroke.org.uk.

Stroke Association (2005). *Fact Sheet. Subarachnoid Haemorrhage.* Available from www.stroke.org.uk.

Stroke Association (2006). *Preventing a stroke.* Available from www.stroke.org.uk.

Stroke Association (2005). *Stroke is a Medical Emergency.* Available from www.stroke.org.uk.

Waine, C. (2002) *Obesity and Weight Management in Primary Care* (Oxford: Blackwell).

Walker, R. and Rogers, J. (2004) in association with Diabetes UK, *Diabetes: A Practical Guide to Managing Health* (London: Dorling Kindersley).

Wallace, J. (2003), in J. Larry Durstine and G. E. Moore, *ACSM's Exercise Management for Persons with Chronic Diseases and Disabilities*, 2nd edn. (Champaign, Ill.: Human Kinetics).

Wallace, J. and Ray, S. in Durstine et al (eds) (2009) *ACSM's Exercise Management for Persons with Chronic Diseases and Disabilities (Obesity)*, 3rd edn. (Champaign, Ill.: Human Kinetics).

World Health Organization (1999) *Definition, Diagnosis and Classification of Diabetes and its Complications* (Geneva: WHO), available from www.diabetes.org.uk.

World Health Organization (2003) *World Health Report 2002* (Geneva: WHO).

World Health Organization (2011) *Obesity Factsheet no. 311.*, available from http://www.nhs.uk/Conditions/Obesity/Pages/Introduction.aspx.

USEFUL WEBSITES

American Diabetes Association (ADA) www.diabetes.org

Arthritis Research UK http://www.arthritisresearchuk.org

Asthma UK http://www.asthma.org.uk/

Blood Pressure Association http://www.bpassoc.org.uk

British Lung Foundation (BLF) www.lunguk.org

British Association of Sports and Exercise Science (BASES) http://www.bases.org.uk/

British Heart Foundation (BHF) http://www.bhf.org.uk

British Hypertension Society (BHS) http://www.bhsoc.org

British National Formulary http://bnf.org/bnf/extra/current/450002.htm

The Cochrane Library http://www.thecochranelibrary.com

Department of Health (DoH) www.dh.gov.uk

Diabetes Education and Self Management for Ongoing and Newly Diagnosed (DESMOND) www.desmond-project.org.uk

Diabetes UK www.diabetes.org.uk

Dose Adjustment for Normal Eating (DAFNE) www.dafne.uk.com/

Inclusive Fitness Initiative (IFI) www.inclusivefitness.org

Map of Medicine http://www.mapofmedicine.com/

Medinfo http://www.medinfo.co.uk

Mental Health Foundation (MHF) www.mentalhealth.org.uk

MIMS http://www.mims.co.uk/drugs/a/

MIND www.mind.org.uk

National Institute of Arthritis and Musculoskeletal and Skin (NIAMS) http://www.niams.nih.gov

National Institute for Health and Clinical Excellence (NICE) www.nice.org.uk

National Institute of Mental Health (NIMH) http://www.nimh.nih.gov

National Obesity Forum http://www.nationalobesityforum.org.uk/

The National Osteoporosis Society www.nos.org.uk

National Rheumatoid Arthritis Society (NRAS) http://www.nras.org.uk/

NHS Choices www.nhs.uk

NHS National Library for Health www.evidence.nhs.uk

Patient UK www.patient.co.uk

Scottish Intercollegiate Guidelines Network (SIGN) http://www.sign.ac.uk/

The Society of Chiropodist and Podiatrists (foot care for diabetes) www.feetforlife.org

World Health Organization (WHO) http://www.who.int

USEFUL JOURNALS

British Journal of Sports Medicine

British Medical Journal (BMJ)

Journal of Public Health

Medicine and Science in Sports and Exercise

Psychology of Sport and Exercise

Research Quarterly for Exercise and Sport

INDEX